Clinical Guide for
Overseas Dental Examination
(UK, Europe & Australia)

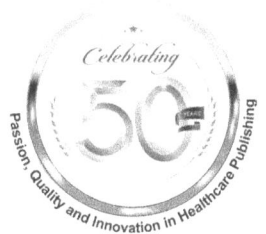

Clinical Guide for
Overseas Dental Examiation
(UK, Europe & Australia)

Pooja Verma Ahmad
BDS (Lon) MBA (Glas) MFDS RCS (Edin) MFGDP RCS (Eng)
General Dental Practitioner
Essex, United Kingdom

Co-author
Priya Verma Gupta
BDS MDS (Pedo) PhD (Pedo) FPFA
Professor and Head
Department of Pedodontics and Preventive Dentistry
KD Dental College and Hospital
Mathura, Uttar Pradesh, India

Foreword
Manesh Lahori

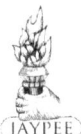

JAYPEE BROTHERS MEDICAL PUBLISHERS
The Health Sciences Publisher
New Delhi | London | Panama

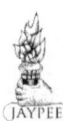 **Jaypee Brothers Medical Publishers (P) Ltd**

Headquarters

Jaypee Brothers Medical Publishers (P) Ltd
4838/24, Ansari Road, Daryaganj
New Delhi 110 002, India
Phone: +91-11-43574357
Fax: +91-11-43574314
Email: jaypee@jaypeebrothers.com

Overseas Offices

J.P. Medical Ltd
83 Victoria Street, London
SW1H 0HW (UK)
Phone: +44 20 3170 8910
Fax: +44 (0)20 3008 6180
Email: info@jpmedpub.com

Jaypee-Highlights Medical Publishers Inc
City of Knowledge, Bld. 235, 2nd Floor, Clayton
Panama City, Panama
Phone: +1 507-301-0496
Fax: +1 507-301-0499
Email: cservice@jphmedical.com

Jaypee Brothers Medical Publishers (P) Ltd
Bhotahity, Kathmandu, Nepal
Phone: +977-9741283608
Email: kathmandu@jaypeebrothers.com

Website: www.jaypeebrothers.com
Website: www.jaypeedigital.com

© 2019, Jaypee Brothers Medical Publishers

The views and opinions expressed in this book are solely those of the original contributor(s)/author(s) and do not necessarily represent those of editor(s) of the book.

All rights reserved. No part of this publication may be reproduced, stored or transmitted in any form or by any means, electronic, mechanical, photocopying, recording or otherwise, without the prior permission in writing of the publishers.

All brand names and product names used in this book are trade names, service marks, trademarks or registered trademarks of their respective owners. The publisher is not associated with any product or vendor mentioned in this book.

Medical knowledge and practice change constantly. This book is designed to provide accurate, authoritative information about the subject matter in question. However, readers are advised to check the most current information available on procedures included and check information from the manufacturer of each product to be administered, to verify the recommended dose, formula, method and duration of administration, adverse effects and contraindications. It is the responsibility of the practitioner to take all appropriate safety precautions. Neither the publisher nor the author(s)/editor(s) assume any liability for any injury and/or damage to persons or property arising from or related to use of material in this book.

This book is sold on the understanding that the publisher is not engaged in providing professional medical services. If such advice or services are required, the services of a competent medical professional should be sought.

Every effort has been made where necessary to contact holders of copyright to obtain permission to reproduce copyright material. If any have been inadvertently overlooked, the publisher will be pleased to make the necessary arrangements at the first opportunity. The **CD/DVD-ROM** (if any) provided in the sealed envelope with this book is complimentary and free of cost. **Not meant for sale.**

Inquiries for bulk sales may be solicited at: jaypee@jaypeebrothers.com

Clinical Guide for Overseas Dental Examination (UK, Europe & Australia)

First Edition: **2019**

ISBN: 978-93-5270-021-9

Dedicated to

Mom and Dad

Foreword

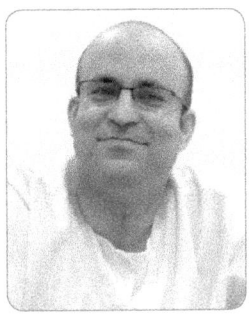

I am extremely happy to pen down a few words about this conscientiously written book. Books play a major role in any education process where they are envisioned to facilitate self-learning beyond classroom exercises.

This book, *Clinical Guide for Overseas Dental Examination (UK, Europe & Australia)* authored by Dr Pooja Verma Ahmad and co-authored by Dr Priya Verma Gupta is presented with such a systematic approach that it demonstrates their skill in preparing students for examinations, it is good to see that they have shared their vast experience in academics with the students through this book.

The authors have made sincere attempt to present all the topics in the form of multiple choice questions (MCQs) thus fulfilling the long-term need for such a clinical guide for overseas dental examinations.

Designing such a book is a challenging task especially if it is to be concise and comprehensive in scope. This outstanding resource is perfect for those studying or preparing for overseas examination and I am confident that this book is undeniably appropriate for overseas exam-going students, who are craving for thorough review of subjects in a short period.

Manesh Lahori
BDS MDS FICOI FISOI FAOI DAOI FICD
Vice-President, Indian Prosthodontic Society
Director, Principal and Dean
KD Dental College and Hospital
Mathura, Uttar Pradesh, India

Preface

The book aims to provide students with various approaches on tackling multiple choice questions (MCQs). The MCQs are arranged in combinations of single best answer (SBAs), extended matching questions (EMQs) or conventional True and False statements. SBAs have more than one answer correct, but there will be one answer to the question that will be superior than others and is best suited answer for the question. EMQs test the applied knowledge to test diagnostic reasoning.

This revision text offers essential MCQ examination practice for both dental undergraduates and postgraduates to build confidence for examination success. The book features over 750 questions and answers to ensure thorough examination preparation. This revision text is best suited for students preparing for Member of the Faculty of Dental Surgery (MFDS), Membership of the Joint Dental Faculties (MJDF), Overseas Registration Examination (ORE), Licence in Dental Surgery (LDS) and dental school final examinations.

The book comprises chapters on history and examination, paediatric dentistry, orthodontics, periodontics, conservative dentistry, endodontics, prosthodontics, oral medicine and pathology, oral radiology, oral surgery, human disease and medical emergencies, drugs and therapeutics, dental materials, law and ethics, and general dental council. Each chapter has a number of MCQs of the conventional true/false variety, single best answer, extended matching questions, coloured clinical pictures and related case studies to consolidate students' theoretical knowledge and clinical experience. The answers to each question are at the end of each chapter with some short notes which attempt to provide a brief explanation for false statements to allow candidates to focus on their revision.

The book intends to provide the perfect practice to build confidence for examination success.

Pooja Verma Ahmad
Priya Verma Gupta

Contents

1. History and Examination 1
2. Paediatric Dentistry 25
3. Orthodontics 46
4. Periodontics 67
5. Conservative Dentistry 83
6. Endodontics 102
7. Prosthodontics 120
8. Oral Medicine and Pathology 139
9. Oral Radiology 178
10. Oral Surgery 202
11. Human Disease and Medical Emergencies 228
12. Drugs and Therapeutics 248
13. Dental Materials 266
14. Law and Ethics and General Dental Council 292

Annexures 311
    Standards for Dental Team 311
    Eligibility Criteria for Registration 312
    Eligibility to Apply for Individual Assessment of
    Knowledge and Skill 312
    Overseas Registration Exam 312
    Contact Information 314
    Application form for Registering as a Dentist with the
    General Dental Council (Overseas Qualified) 315
    Application Process 328
    Processing Times 330
    Registration for Overseas Qualified Practitioners in Australia 331
    Application for Practical Examination–Dentist 335
    Application for Written Examination 342

Contents

1. History and Examination 1
2. Paediatric Dentistry 23
3. Orthodontics 40
4. Periodontics 67
5. Conservative Dentistry 83

Chapter 1
History and Examination

Identify the following Statements as True (T) or False (F)

1. **With regards to assessing dental patients:**
   a. History may not include social factors
   b. Visual appearance may not be of importance
   c. A systemic approach with consistent series of questions should be followed
   d. Closed questions should be used
   e. Patient's response can be paraphrased
   f. Occupation does not have any relevance to clinical conditions.

2. **Extra-oral examination:**
   a. Lymph node examination should start from parotid region and run downwards towards retromandibular to submandibular to submental region
   b. If node is enlarged, record the size of the node
   c. Questions about nail biting is not relevant
   d. Cartilage hard nodes can be seen in Hodgkin's disease
   e. Rubbery hard nodes are found in pleomorphic adenomas
   f. Neoplasm are painless
   g. Pulsation in a swelling can indicate presence of fluid
   h. Patient with disturbed sensation in upper lip has a lesion affecting mandibular division of trigeminal nerve
   i. Paralysis of the lower face indicates lower motor neuron lesion
   j. Paralysis of facial muscles indicates upper motor neuron lesion
   k. A misplaced inferior dental block can affect facial expression.

3. **Intra-oral examination:**
   a. Teeth are first tissues to be examined when conducting intra-oral examination
   b. Most oral swellings are inflammatory
   c. Site of ulcers are not of importance in diagnosis
   d. Base of ulcer is important during assessment of ulceration
   e. Glossopharyngeal nerve supplies anterior 2/3 of the tongue
   f. Sensory disturbance in the tongue is usually due of damage of the function of hypoglossal nerve
   g. There is a problem with speech as lingual sounds such as l, t, d gets affected due to vagus nerve lesions

Clinical Guide for Overseas Dental Examination

    h. If single cusp is tender to percussion, it may be indicative of cracked tooth syndrome
    i. Examination of dentition should only involve assessment of mobility, periodontal probing and pressure test.

4. **Laboratory investigations:**
   a. It is important to have differential clinical diagnosis while advising investigations
   b. Human immunodeficiency virus (HIV) infection tests should be undertaken only by the specialist in the field
   c. Suspected oral cancer should be referred directly to the specialist for biopsy
   d. Specimen can be collected in any container
   e. Tests have sensitivities and specificity.

5. **Microbiology:**
   a. Viral swab may be required for diagnosis of herpes simplex
   b. Glandular fever can be detected by rising titres of antibodies in patient's serum
   c. Denture related stomatitis requires direct smears for diagnosis
   d. Infected mucosa can be stained by periodic acid Schiff method
   e. Bacterial infections of oral cavity, jaws and salivary glands can be identified by sending specimen of pus to laboratory for culture and antibody sensitivity
   f. Swabs or oral rinses cannot be used to discriminate various Candida species.

6. **Biopsy:**
   a. Aspirational biopsy requires special needle and syringe to collect fluid from suspected cyst
   b. Odontogenic keratocysts contain brown shimmering fluid due to presence of cholesterol crystals
   c. Pale greasy fluid of odontogenic cyst contains keratotic squames
   d. Mucosal biopsy specimen is fixed in volume of 1% neutral buffered formalin
   e. Incisional biopsy is suitable of mucoceles
   f. Excisional biopsy is suitable for diagnosis of lichen planus
   g. Specimen of non-healing ulcer should include margins of ulcer with some normal tissue
   h. Immuno-fluorescence requires fresh tissue.

7. **Haematology:**
   a. Patients with haematological disease should be treated by specialist
   b. Full blood count and assays of hematinics are important for patient presenting with lingual papillary atrophy
   c. Patients on anticoagulant therapy should have their International Normalised Ratio (INR) checked before any examination

History and Examination

    d. Sickledex test may be used to prior general anaesthesia (GA)
    e. Coagulation studies and platelet counts are required for recurrent oral ulceration.

8. **Biochemical and immunological investigations:**
   a. Biochemical investigations are required when patients have systemic manifestation of oral disease
   b. Alkaline phosphate in Paget's disease of bone will be assessed by biochemical investigation
   c. Serum calcium of giant cell granuloma is present will require immunological investigations
   d. Detection of Sjorgen's syndrome A (SSA) and Sjorgen's syndrome B (SSB) antibodies for diagnosis of Sjorgen's syndrome requires immunological investigations
   e. HIV testing can be undertaken by dental practice.

9. **Imaging:**
   a. X-ray examination should be based on specific selection criteria
   b. Radio-opaque contrast imaging is commonly used for sialography
   c. Computed tomography (CT) scan does not use Hounsfield scale
   d. In CT scan, soft tissue are dark gray and fat is black
   e. Cone beam computed tomography (CBCT) have higher radiations dose than conventional CT
   f. Voxel size CBCT are bigger than CT, therefore, provides a better image resolution
   g. Ultrasound can be used for soft tissue lumps in the neck and salivary glands
   h. Technetium-99 m labelled methylene diphosphonate is used in radioisotope imaging in Paget's disease and arthritis
   i. Magnetic resonance imaging (MRI) is safe in patients with intra-cranial vascular clips and cardiac pacemakers
   j. Salivary scanning uses sodium pertechnetate-99 m in radioisotope imaging for diagnosis of Sjogren's syndrome.

10. **Referral letter:**
    a. Referral letter does not require detailed history of patient
    b. It should not include results of dental examination/dentist finding
    c. It should not include provisional diagnosis
    d. It should include history of complaint and medical history
    e. It can include special factors or consideration
    f. Patient does not have access to their referral letter
    g. Primary care dentist can also directly contact the department concerned for advice for urgent referral
    h. The National Institute of Health and Care Excellence (NICE) produces referral guidelines.

Give the Single Best Answer for the following Questions

11. **The responsibilities of a dental professional are:**
    a. Putting patient's interest first and protecting them
    b. Not protecting patients confidentiality
    c. Non-maintenance of professional knowledge and competence
    d. Being untrustworthy.

12. **The importance of case history is:**
    a. To extract patient's information for nonprofessional purpose
    b. To decline the treatment on the basis of patient selection
    c. To gather information regarding etiology in order to establish the differential diagnosis
    d. None of the above.

13. **According to the site, type of lesion suspected in anterior neck region can be:**
    a. Thyroglossal cyst
    b. Ludwig angina
    c. Fibroma
    d. Sialolithiasis.

14. **All options are the factors that affect body temperature, *except*:**
    a. Time of the day
    b. Exercise
    c. Smoking
    d. Hormones
    e. Infection
    f. Hypothyroidism.

15. **All options are the factors that affect body pulse rate and respiration, *except*:**
    a. Age
    b. Medication
    c. Hot and cold liquids
    d. Stress
    e. Fever.

16. **All these options are the six phases of comprehensive treatment plan, *except*:**
    a. Acute phase
    b. Promotive phase
    c. Control phase
    d. Rehabilitation phase
    e. Surgical phase.

17. **The procedure undertaken in preventive phase is:**
    a. Oral hygiene instructions
    b. Diet advice/counselling

c. Endodontic therapy
d. Topical fluoride application
e. Crowns and bridges.

18. All are the procedures undertaken in the rehabilitation, *except*:
    a. Crown and bridges
    b. Reconstruction prosthesis
    c. Composite restorations
    d. Complete partial dentures
    e. Removable partial dentures.

19. Ethical consideration of treatment planning includes the following, *except*:
    a. Placing the patient's interest and well-being as the most important criteria
    b. Patients should not feel pressurised to accept treatment plan
    c. To be truthful to the patient
    d. No harm will be done to the patient.

20. The biomechanical loading force causes loss of hard tooth substance. This type of loss causes flexure and chemical fatigue, degradation of enamel and/or dentin away from actual site where force was applied. This type of tooth surface loss is known as:
    a. Abfraction
    b. Attrition
    c. Erosion
    d. Abrasion.

21. The wearing away of a substance or structure particularly enamel due to some unusual or abnormal mechanical process other than mastication is:
    a. Abfraction
    b. Erosion
    c. Abrasion
    d. Attrition.

22. What is localized collection of purulent exudates formed due to disintegration of tissues in oral cavity is known as?
    a. Abscess
    b. Granuloma
    c. Inflammation
    d. Cyst.

23. In a fixed or removable prosthesis, which is used to anchor or support tooth, root and an implant?
    a. Edge
    b. Crown
    c. Appliance
    d. Abutment.

24. A patient has history of pain with rapid onset, spontaneous in nature. It is tender to percussion and during occlusal loading. Presence of inflammatory exudate and swelling of associated tissue is observed. What will be the diagnosis of such an inflammatory reaction?
    a. Acute apical abscess
    b. Periapical cyst
    c. Periapical granuloma
    d. Apical periodontitis.

25. A patient has history of pain which is of abrupt onset and is of short duration. The swelling is characterized by the exudation of fluid, serum proteins, inflammatory mediators and cells mainly polymorphonuclear leukocytes. If injurious agent persists, what will this condition be known as:
    a. Chronic inflammation
    b. Acute inflammation
    c. Cellulitis
    d. Purulis.

26. What is the relief of pain without loss of consciousness called as:
    a. Syncope
    b. General anaesthesia
    c. Analgesia
    d. Local anaesthesia.

27. An immediate allergic reaction that is mediated via histamine lasting for seconds to minutes after exposure to an antigen is:
    a. Anaphylactic shock
    b. Vasoactive shock
    c. Iatrogenic shock
    d. Septic shock.

28. The term used to describe any deviation from normal anatomy, development or function is called:
    a. Incongruity
    b. Deviation
    c. Aberration
    d. Anomaly.

29. The substance or agent that inhibits or prevents the blood from bleeding is:
    a. Plasma
    b. Anticoagulant
    c. Antihemorrhagic
    d. Serum.

30. A method used to induce a calcified barrier in a root with an open apex or the continued apical development of an incompletely formed root in teeth with necrotic pulp is:
    a. Pulpotomy
    b. Apexification
    c. Apexogenesis
    d. Apicoectomy.

31. Inflammation and destruction of apical periodontium without any clinical symptoms which appears as an apical radiolucent area radiographically is:
    a. Cyst
    b. Abscess
    c. Asymptomatic apical periodontitis
    d. Granuloma.

32. A diminution in the size of a cell, tissue or organ is known as:
    a. Hypertrophy
    b. Dystrophy
    c. Atrophy
    d. Hyperplasia.

33. The physiological wearing away of a substance or structure of the tooth during the course of normal use is known as:
    a. Abrasion
    b. Avulsion
    c. Erosion
    d. Attrition.

34. This syndrome is characterized by continuous aching or throbbing pain of long duration without any established neural pathways. On clinical examination, it does not reveal an apparent cause. What can be the probable diagnosis?
    a. Muscle pain
    b. Neuritis
    c. Atypical facial pain
    d. Abscess.

35. The removal of tissue for histologic examination and diagnosis is called as:
    a. Biopsy
    b. Incisional biopsy
    c. Excisional biopsy
    d. All the above.

36. The use of a chemical agent to treat tooth discolorations is called as:
    a. Apexification
    b. Apexogenesis
    c. Bleaching
    d. Staining.

37. An oral habit of rhythmic or spasmodic nonfunctional clenching of teeth is called as:
    a. Bruxism
    b. Night grinding
    c. All of above
    d. None of above.

38. The process of conversion from liquid to solid, especially of blood is known as:
    a. Coagulation
    b. Clotting
    c. Bleeding
    d. Both A and B.

39. An organic, polymerizable resin mix which contains inorganic particles treated with a bonding or coupling agent and polymerized by chemical mechanisms is:
    a. Amalgam
    b. Compomer
    c. Glass ionomer cement
    d. Composite.

40. A traumatic tooth injury characterized by tenderness to percussion and no mobility or displacement is:
    a. Concussion
    b. Avulsion
    c. Fracture
    d. Apposition.

41. Diffuse radiopaque lesion representing a localized bony reaction to a low-grade inflammatory stimulus, usually seen at apex of tooth is:
    a. Condensing osteitis
    b. Osteomyelitis
    c. Garre's osteomyelitis
    d. Fibrous dysplasia.

42. This phenomenon involves fractures, usually, of the marginal ridges, occurring primarily in minimally restored mandibular first and second molars. There is presence of pain during chewing and the tooth becomes sensitive to heat. The likely diagnosis is:
    a. Cracked root
    b. Green stick fracture
    c. Ellis fracture I
    d. Cracked tooth.

43. The tooth contact relation that occurs when few upper teeth are inside the lower teeth during mastication is termed as:
    a. Cross bite
    b. Anterior bite

c. Deep bite
d. Lateral occlusion.

44. The misalignment and abnormal contact relationships due to teeth discrepancy between tooth sizes and arch length and/or tooth positioning is known as:
    a. Diastema
    b. Supernumerary teeth
    c. Spacing
    d. Crowding.

45. The exaggerated painful response, short in duration initiated when exposed dentine is subjected to certain thermal, mechanical, and/or chemical stimuli:
    a. Dentinal hypersensitivity
    b. Chronic hyperplastic pulpitis
    c. Irreversible pulpitis
    d. Reversible pulpitis.

46. A space between two adjacent teeth in a permanent dental arch is called as:
    a. Diastema
    b. Physiological space
    c. Leeway space
    d. Nance space.

47. What is an accumulation of fluid in a tissue?
    a. Oedema
    b. Purulis
    c. Transudate
    d. Exudate.

48. A pathological accumulation of gas or air in tissue spaces. It may be caused by an air-driven dental handpiece, syringe, coughing, or blowing the nose:
    a. Emphysema
    b. Embolism
    c. Abscess
    d. Granuloma.

49. What is redness of the skin or mucous membranes is also known as?
    a. Plaque
    b. Macule
    c. Erythema
    d. Rash.

50. The physiological loss of primary dentition is known as:
    a. Exfoliation
    b. Eruption

c. Sublimation
d. Degradation.

51. A bony prominence projecting outward from the surface of a bone towards periphery is called as:
   a. Papilloma
   b. Exostosis
   c. Acanthoma
   d. Neavus.

52. The movement of a tooth that occurs in an incisal or occlusal direction can be either physiologic or traumatic:
   a. Rotation
   b. Avulsion
   c. Intrusion
   d. Extrusion.

53. The lateral view of face outline:
   a. Facial profile
   b. Lateral profile
   c. Oblique view
   d. Vertical view.

Select the most appropriate answer to the following extending matching questions

54. Regarding the types of head:
   a. Average shape of the head with normal dental arches
   b. Cephalic index value is less than 75.9
   c. Cephalic index value is 81.0-85.4
   d. Long and narrow head with narrow dental arches
   e. Extremely wide head
   f. Cephalic index value is more than 85.5
   g. Broad and short head with broad dental arches
   h. Cephalic index value is 76.0–80.9

| 1. Mesocephalic | 3. Hyperbrachycephalic |
| 2. Brachycephalic | 4. Dolichocephalic |

55. Regarding the types of facial forms:
   a. Average or normal face form with normal U-shaped arches
   b. Facial index value is 79.0–83
   c. Short face with low facial index
   d. Long and narrow face form
   e. Facial index area is 88.0–92.9
   f. Extremely long face form
   g. Facial index value is greater than 93.0
   h. Facial index value is 84.0–87.9
   i. Face is broad and short
   j. Facial index value is less than 78.9

1. Leptoprosopic	4. Hyperleptoprosopic
2. Mesoprosopic	5. Hypereuroprosopic
3. Europrosopic	

56. **Which aetiologic agent is responsible for following occupational diseases?**
    a. Carpenters
    b. Bakers
    c. Explosives
    d. Cobblers
    e. Pavers
    f. Cement workers
    g. Musicians
    h. Chemical workers
    i. Smokeless powder and shoe factory workers
    j. Bismuth handlers
    k. Miners stone cutters
    l. Candy makers
    m. Distillery
    n. Metal refiners
    o. Asphalt and coal tar workers

1. Instruments used	7. Coal
2. Tar	8. Arsenic
3. Copper	9. Bismuth
4. Iron	10. Sugar
5. Nickel	11. Amyl acetate
6. Chromium	

57. **Which of the following is associated with the below mentioned orofacial soft tissue swelling?**
    a. Seborrheic keratosis
    b. Peripheral ossifying fibroma
    c. Squamous cell carcinoma
    d. Sialolithiasis
    e. Mucocele
    f. Salivary neoplasm
    g. Space infection
    h. Fibroma
    i. Sialadenitis
    j. Lymphadenopathy
    k. Melanoma
    l. Thyroglossal cysts
    m. Metastatic carcinoma
    n. Thyroid neoplasm
    o. Pyogenic granuloma
    p. Jaw cysts and tumors
    q. Ranula
    r. Goiter
    s. Abscess

1. Face	7. Gingiva
2. Parotid region	8. Lips and buccal mucosa
3. Submandibular region	9. Dorsolateral tongue
4. Masseteric region	10. Ventral tongue and oral floor
5. Lateral neck	11. Palate
6. Anterior neck	

58. Classify the following orofacial pain according to the below mentioned categories:

 a. Facial arthromyalgia
 b. Pre-trigeminal neuralgia
 c. Nerve compression
 d. Glossopharyngeal neuralgia
 e. Optic neuritis
 f. Cluster headache
 g. Cranial arteritis
 h. Ramsay Hunt syndrome
 i. Dentinal pain
 j. Thermal sensitivities
 k. Pulpal pain
 l. Trigeminal neuralgia
 m. Burning mouth syndrome
 n. Pain of periodontal origin
 o. Internal derangements
 p. Cracked tooth syndrome
 q. Temporomandibular joint (TMJ) pain
 r. Atypical facial pain/idiopathic orofacial pain
 s. Postherpetic neuralgia
 t. Myofascial pain

1. Neurological/vascular
2. Dentoalveolar
3. Muscular/ligamentous/soft tissue

59. Which type of swelling among the following is associated with below mentioned palpation characteristics?

 a. Fibroma
 b. Sialocysts
 c. Melanoma
 d. Salivary
 e. Ranula
 f. Developmental cysts
 g. Lipoma
 h. Gingival cysts
 i. Mesenchymal tumors
 j. Space infections and abscesses

k. Granulomas
l. Seborrheic
m. Basal cell carcinoma
n. Adenomas adnexal skin tumors
o. Keratoacanthoma
p. Sarcomas
q. Keratosis
r. Granular cell tumor
s. Mucocele
t. Myofascial pain

1.	Soft, nonfluctuant	4.	Firm, fixed
2.	Soft, fluctuant	5.	Indurated, fixed
3.	Firm, movable		

60. **Match the following oral ulcers based on their characteristics:**
    a. Acute necrotizing ulcerative gingivitis
    b. Herpes simplex virus
    c. Allergies
    d. Chemotherapy
    e. Chancre
    f. Herpes simplex virus
    g. Paraneoplastic pemphigus
    h. Mucous patches
    i. Aphthae
    j. Herpangina
    k. Apthae
    l. Epidermolysis bullosa
    m. Fungi (deep)
    n. Necrotizing sialometaplasia
    o. Mucous membrane pemphigoid
    p. Tuberculosis
    q. Allergies
    r. Herpes zoster virus
    s. Bullous pemphigoid
    t. Lupus erythematosus
    u. Squamous cell carcinoma
    v. Pemphigous vulgaris

1.	Acute	3.	Solitary ulcers
2.	Multiple ulcers	4.	Chronic

CASE DISCUSSION

Case 1: A patient attends your practice with complaint of pain and clicking of temporomandibular joint (TMJ). Please discuss the examination of the patient.

Golden Rule

Before attempting any clinical examination certain points have to be considered as mandatory:
- Self-introduction be polite and courteous
- Obtaining consent before examination
- Confidentiality to be maintained throughout the examination.

Examination

Examination starts visually as soon as the patient walks into the surgery with dental practitioner observing them. However, the formal examination starts after complete history is taken. The general rule of thumb is to start with general examination of the patient and then specific systemic examination.
- Introduce yourself to patient.

Extra-oral examination

- Lip competency to be looked for/or recorded
- Look for any lip incompetence and associate etiology
- Facial symmetry to be recorded
    > Palpate lymph nodes for any tenderness or swelling
    > Palpate left and right TMJs for any pain or tenderness to touch. TMJs should be palpated while patient open their mouth slowly. This is done by placing fingers over the joints or in patient's ear **(Figs 1.1A to C)**
    > Any noise from the joints need to be noticed **(clicking or crepitus)**
    > The path traced by the lip of lower central incisors through the opening and closing cycle should be noted **(Look for tear drop cycle)**
    > TMJs should also be palpated throughout lateral, protrusive excursive and movements
    > Measure the lateral and protrusive, excursive movements (normal is around 10 mm)
    > Measure maximum opening between incisor tips (normal is 45 mm)
    > Palpate muscles of mastication: masseter and temporalis are palpated extra-orally. Lateral pterygoids are evaluated by asking patient to try to open mouth while dentist restricts the movement by placing hand

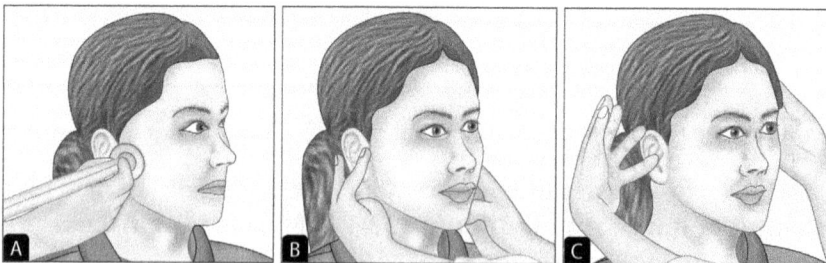

Figs 1.1A to C: Extra-oral examination of temporomandibular joint (TMJ) (A) Ausculation; (B) Lateral palpation; (C) Posterior palpation

under the chin. If pain is elicited from preauricular region, it is from lateral pterygoid muscle. The medial pterygoid muscle can be palpated intra-orally along the medial aspect of the mandible.
- Joint noises:
  › A click implies that there is a displaced disc that reduces back to normal position
  › Crepitus or grating noise implies degenerative changes within the joint.
- Mandibular movement:
  › Obstruction of movement within the joint will cause mandible to deviate on opening and closing.

Intra-oral examination

- Examine the number of teeth present
- Generalised condition of dentition
- Pattern of tooth wear
- Examine intercuspal position (ICP) and retruded contact position (RCP)
- Examine group function and canine guidance in lateral excursions and protusive movements
- Any displacements or premature contacts
- Examine buccal mucosa—grinding (white striae)
- Radiographic examination for TMJ are shown in **Figures 1.2 and 1.3A and B**.

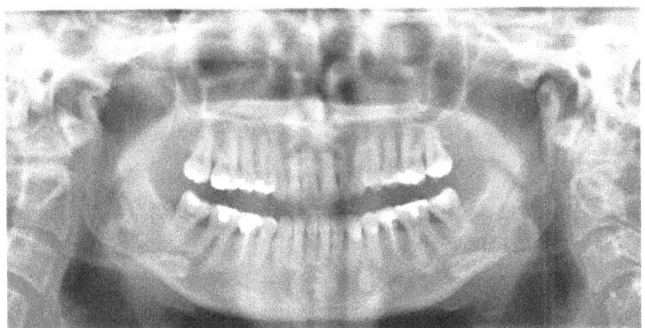

Fig. 1.2: OPG done for overall view of detention of TMJ

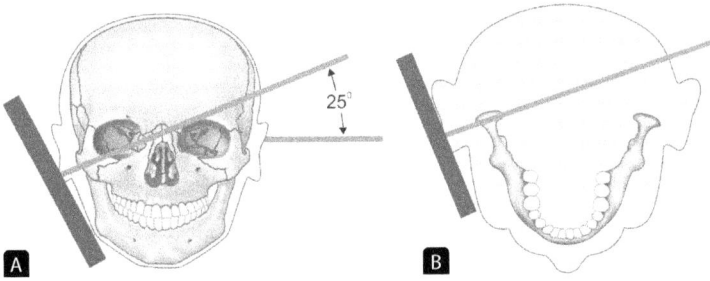

Figs 1.3A and B: Transcranial imaging

Case 2: Examine patient's cranial nerves.

Examination Procedure
- Bring the patient to penectomy and make him comfortable
- Introduce yourself politely to the patient
- Take the general history of pain poor to examination
- Explain the procedure for examination
- Start examinary the 12 cranial nerves (CN) **(Fig. 1.4)**.

Olfactory Nerve CN I—Sense of smell
- Ask patient if they have altered sense of smell
- Test with aromatic substances
- Anosmia is common following head or midface trauma.

Optic Nerve CN II—Sight
- Examine pupil for both direct and consensual reflex
- Assess visual field
- Check visual acuity.

Oculomotor Nerve CN III
- Motor supply to extraocular muscles except lateral rectus and superior oblique
- Supplies ciliary muscles, constriction of pupil and levator palpebrae superioris
- The injury of CN III can cause impairment of upward, downward and inward movement of the eye
- Diplopia, ptosis, absence of consensual reflexes.

Trochlear Nerve CN IV
- Supplies superior oblique muscle

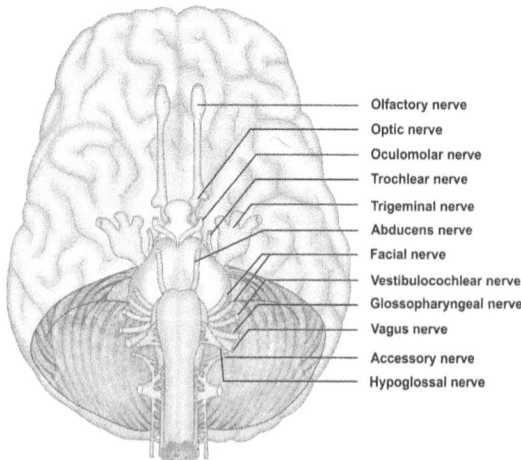

Fig. 1.4: Cranial nerves

- Paralysis can cause diplopia
- Worst on looking downwards and inwards.

Trigeminal Nerve CN V

- Major sensory nerve to face, oral, nasal, conjunctival sinus mucosa and part of tympanic membrane
- Motor supply to muscles of mastication
- Check all three divisions—ophthalmic, maxillary and mandibular
  - Is the sensation of the skin normal over these divisions—use pin-prick and gentle touch
  - Does patient have corneal reflex?
  - Can patient clench jaw muscles?
- Motor weakness is best assessed on jaw opening and excursions.

Abducens Nerve CN VI

- Supplies lateral rectus
- Defect causes paralysis of abduction of eyes.

Facial Nerve CN VII

- Motor to muscles of facial expression
- Provides taste sensation to anterior 2/3 of tongue
- Secretomotor to the lacrimal, sublingual and submandibular gland
- Innervates stapedius muscle of middle ear
- Lower face is innervated by contralateral motor cortex
- Upper face has bilateral innervation
- Assess facial movements and expressions—can patient smile, pout, wrinkle her forehead or raise eyebrows?

Vestibulocochlear Nerve CN VIII

- Is sensory for balance and hearing
- Symptoms such as deafness, vertigo and tinnitus.

Glossopharyngeal Nerve CN IX

- Provides sensation and taste to posterior third of the tongue
- Motor to stylopharyngeus
- Secretomotor to parotid
- Gag reflex is impaired if damaged
  - Ask patient to say 'aah' and look for deviation uvula and movement of soft palate.

Vagus Nerve CN X

- Motor to palatal, pharyngeal and laryngeal muscles
- Impaired gag reflex, hoarseness and deviation of the soft palate to the unaffected side are seen, if damaged
- Vagus has huge parasympathetic output to viscera of the thorax and abdomen
- Ask patient to say 'aah' and look for deviation of uvula.

Accessory Nerve CN XI
- Motor to sternomastoid and trapezius
- Check if patient can shrug their shoulders
- Turning the head away from the affected side.

Hypoglossal Nerve CN XII
- Motor supply to the tongue
- Lesion cause dysarthria (impaired speech)
- Deviation towards affected side on protrusion.

Case 3: Examine the swelling in the front of the neck.
- The neck of seated patient is observed from the front
- Ask the patient to swallow (offer a glass of water to the patient)
- Stand behind the patient and palpate the thyroid gland
- Percuss the manubrium for retrosternal extension
- Auscultate for bruit
- Palpate the triangle of the neck and supraclavicular fossa for lymph nodes
- Lumps in the neck can be divided into—malignant and benign
- They can also be classified based on location of the lump:
  - Is there a single lump or multiple lump
  - Where is the lump?
  - Is lump solid or cystic?
  - Does it move with swallowing?

  Figure 1.5 shows lump of neck.

Malignant Lumps
- Primary:
  - Thyroid cancer.
- Secondary:
  - Metastatic lymph nodes.

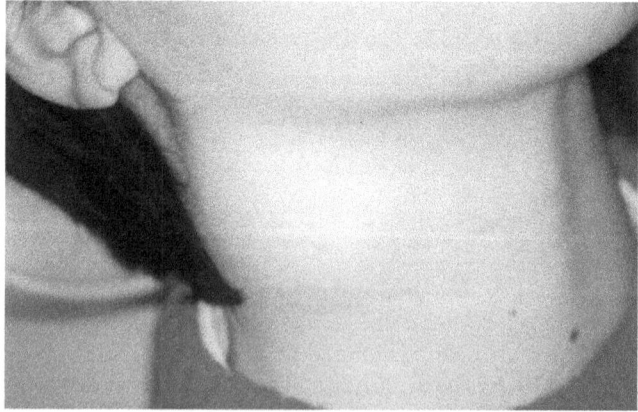

Fig. 1.5: Lump of neck

Benign Lumps

- Congenital
  - Lymphangiomas
  - Dermoidcyst
  - Thyroglossal duct
  - Branchial fistula.
- Acquired
  - Ranulae
  - Laryngoceles
  - Pharyngeal pouches.
- Infective
  - Bacterial
  - Viral.
- Neurogenic tumours
  - Neurofibromas
  - Carotid body tumours
  - Glomus jugulare tumours.

Neck lumps relative to location (Flowcharts 1.1 to 1.3)

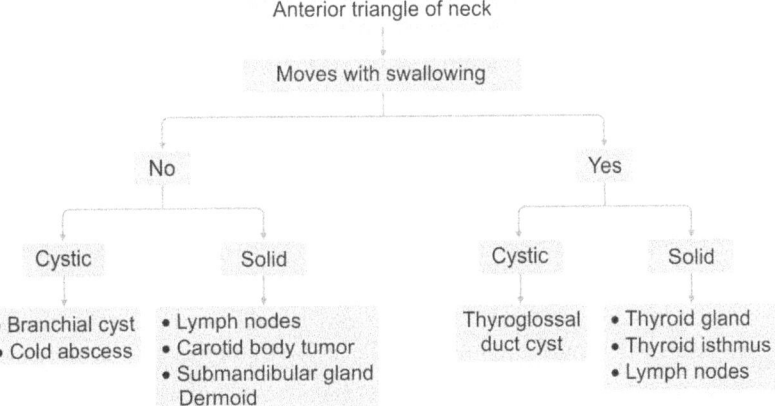

Flowchart 1.1: Anterior triangle of neck

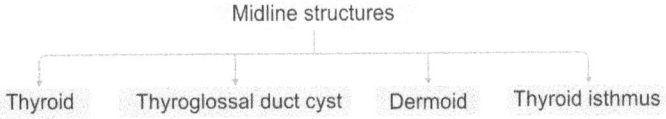

Flowchart 1.2: Midline structures

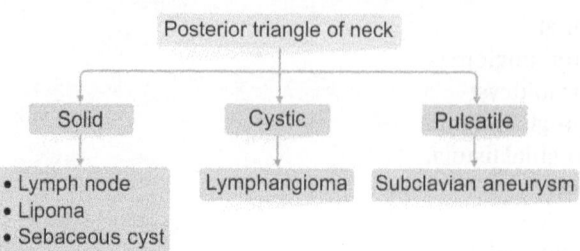

Flowchart 1.3: Posterior triangle of neck

Case 4: Examine patient for suspected mandible fractures.

Examination for all patients follows the standard pattern. It starts with general examination and proceeds to specific problem. Visual examination based on observation of the patient, the history and degree of trauma sustained. Examine whole facial skeleton to discount other injuries.
- Explain the examination procedure after taking complete history.

Extra-oral Examination
- Examine patient directly in front or in same level as patient and note any asymmetry
- Examine for any swelling, bruising and lacerations. Check behind ears for bruising and for evidence of bleeding or cerebrospinal fluid (CSF) leak from the ears
- Check any sensory disturbance of the skin of lower lip—damage of ID nerve
- Palpate mandible gently (will be painful for the patient) from the condyle to the symphysis on both sides. Check for any step deformities in the continuity of bone and also any swelling or discomfort in any particular region
- Assess the patient if he is able to perform mandibular movement to watch the degree of mouth opening and deviation of mandible
- Palpate the condyles while patient is carrying out mandibular movements.

Intra-oral Examination
- Check for bruising or swelling within mouth
- Examine buccal and lingual sulcus, and sublingually
- Check for laceration within the mouth, gingival tears
- Any empty sockets, missing or broken teeth should be accounted for as there is always a possibility that patient has swallowed, avulsed tooth post-traumatic injury
- Check for loose or-fractured teeth or fractured denture

- Look for step deformities in the occlusion. Palpate steps in lingual and buccal sulcus
- Check occlusion—presence of certain malocclusion can give clue regarding the site of fractures in the malocclusion, e.g. anterior open bite is seen with bilateral fractured condyles
- Ask patient to carry out full range of mandibular movements and note the location of discomfort with limited movement
- If possible hold angle of mandible with both hands and check for movement across suspected fractures. This will cause pain to the patient and can turn an undisplaced fracture into a displaced fracture. Only performed, if there is no other way to determine the location of fracture.

X-rays

- Orthopantomogram (OPG) and posterior-anterior mandible are essential
- Right and left lateral oblique, if OPG unavailable
- Rotated PA mandible—for fracture between symphysis and canine
- Periapical radiograph, occlusal radiograph, high OPG or reverse towne view for condylar fractures
- Lower anterior occlusal view for anterior mandibular fracture
- CT scan showing a three dimensional (3D) image of panfacial fracture involving mandibular fracture is shown in **Figure 1.6.**

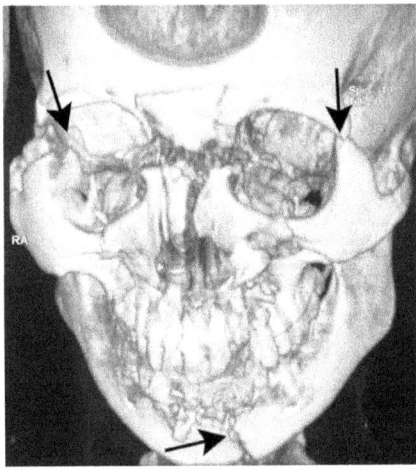

Fig. 1.6: CT scan showing panfacial fracture involving mandibular fracture by 3D image construction

Answers

1.	a. F	b. F	c. T	d. F	e. F
	f. F				
2.	a. F	b. F	c. F	d. F	e. F
	f. T	g. F	h. F	i. F	j. F
	k. T				
3.	a. F	b. T	c. F	d. T	e. F
	f. F	g. F	h. T	i. F	
4.	a. T	b. T	c. T	d. F	e. T
5.	a. F	b. T	c. F	d. T	e. T
	f. F				
6.	a. F	b. F	c. T	d. F	e. F
	f. F	g. T	h. T		
7.	a. F	b. T	c. F	d. T	e. F
8.	a. F	b. T	c. F	d. T	e. F
9.	a. T	b. T	c. F	d. F	e. F
	f. F	g. T	h. T	i. F	j. T
10.	a. F	b. F	c. F	d. T	e. T
	f. F	g. T	h. T		

11. a	12. c	13. a	14. d	15. c
16. e	17. d	18. c	19. b	20. a
21. c	22. a	23. d	24. a	25. b
26. c	27. a	28. d	29. b	30. b
27. a	28. d	29. b	30. b	31. c
32. c	33. d	34. c	35. d	36. c
37. c	38. d	39. d	40. a	41. b
42. d	43. a	44. d	45. a	46. a
47. a	48. a	49. c	50. a	51. b

52. d   53. a
54. a. 1   b. 4   c. 2   d. 4   e. 3
    f. 3   g. 2   h. 1
55. a. 2   b. 3   c. 5   d. 1   e. 1
    f. 4   g. 4   h. 2   i. 3   j. 5
56. a. 1   b. 10   c. 11 d. 1   e. 2
    f. 3,4,5,6,7   g. 1   h. 8   i. 11 j. 9
    k. 3,4,5,6,7   l. 10 m. 11 n. 8   o. 2
57. a. 1   b. 7   c. 1   d. 2   e. 10
    f. 3   g. 4   h. 9   i. 2   j. 5
    k. 1   l. 6   m. 5   n. 6   o. 7
    p. 4   q. 10   7   s. 6   t. 11
58. a. 3   b. 1   c. 1   d. 1   e. 3
    f. 1   g. 1   h. 1   i. 2   j. 2
    k. 2   l. 1   m. 3   n. 2   o. 3
    p. 2   q. 3   r. 3   s. 1   t. 3
59. a. 1   b. 2   c. 5   d. 3   e. 2
    f. 2   g. 1   h. 2   i. 3   j. 2
    k. 3   l. 4   m. 5   n. 3   o. 4
    p. 5   q. 4   r. 4   s. 1   t. 5
60. a. 1   b. 2   c. 1   d. 1   e. 3
    f. 1   g. 4   h. 1   i. 2   j. 1
    k. 3   l. 4   m. 3   n. 3   o. 4
    p. 3   q. 4   r. 1   s. 4   t. 4
    u. 3   v. 4

CORRECT ANSWER FOR FALSE STATEMENTS

1. b. Swelling and Nerve dysfunction.
   a. Open questions.
   b. Should not be paraphrased.
   c. Physical and psychological stress.
2. a. Start submental → submandibular → jugulo-diagastric node → parotid → retromandibular → cervical chain of nodes.
   a. Record texture; hard node (metastasizing malignancy, soft node (inflammatory process).
   b. Shows personality type (anxiety and stress), temporomandibular pain and dysfunction syndrome (TMPDS)—Grinding.
   c. Pleomorphic adenomas.
   d. Hodgkin's disease.
   a. Vascular lesion.
   b. V2.
   c. Upper motor neurone.
   d. Lower motor neurone.
3. a. Last.
   a. Posterior one-third.
   b. Motor disturbance.
   c. Hypoglossal nerve.
4. d. Right specimen container and fluid is required.
5. c. History and appearance of mucosa.
6. a. Standard gauge needle and syringe.
   b. Radicular cyst.
   d. 10%.
   a. Excisional biopsy—Benign polyps, papillomas epulides and reactive lesions.
   b. Incisional biopsy.
7. a. Should be referred for specialist opinion.
   c. Surgical procedure.
   e. Excessive bleeding.
8. a. Oral manifestation of systemic disease.
   c. Biochemical to exclude hyperparathyroidism.
   a. By specialist, requires informed consent and counselling. However, general dental practitioner (GDP) should be able to recognise oral manifestation of immunodeficiency and arrange proper referral.
9. d. Dense bone (white), soft tissue (mid-grey), flat (dark grey), air (black).
   b. Similar.
   i. Contraindicated and also cannot be used on patient with fixed orthodontic appliance.

Chapter 2

Paediatric Dentistry

Identify the following Statements as True (T) or False (F)

1. **In the development of caries:**
   a. Non-milk extrinsic sugars are not broken down by oral flora
   b. Acid formation lowers pH below critical pH
   c. The pH within plaque will rise through inward diffusion of acids and their metabolism and neutralisation, therefore remineralisation
   d. *Streptococcus mutans* predominates
   e. Sucrose has ability to facilitate production of extracellular polysaccharide in plaque
   f. The concentration of calcium in plaque is most important in remineralisation process.

2. **Diagnosis of caries can be made by:**
   a. Visual examination
   b. Visual and tactile
   c. Dental panoramic tomographs are usually suffice
   d. Bitewing radiographs
   e. Fibre-optic transillumination
   f. Electrical resistance method
   g. Diagnodent
   h. Caries detector dyes.

3. **Fluoride in reducing dental decay:**
   a. It has ability to decrease acid production in plaque
   b. Pre-eruptive effects show more rounded cusps and fissure patterns
   c. Its concentration in tooth moves towards enamel-dentine junction
   d. Its reduced concentration in plaque inhibits the synthesis of extracellular polysaccharide
   e. When pH drops in oral cavity, free ionic fluoride is released.

4. **Safety and toxicity of fluoride:**
   a. Water, salt and milk are examples of systemic delivered fluoride
   b. Fluoride is rapidly absorbed from small intestine
   c. Pre-natal ē is effective as placenta can allow large amounts of ē to cross

d. Fluorosis is caused by increased porosity in the inner third of the enamel
e. Lethal dose is 5 mg ē/kg body weight and requires hospitalization.

5. **Indications of fissure sealant:**
   a. Patients with medical/physical/intellectual disability
   b. Caries in primary dentition
   c. Occlusal surface of permanent molars and cingulum pits of upper incisors
   d. Glass ionomer cement can be used as permanent fissure sealant
   e. Isolation is essential for success.

6. **Aetiology of extrinsic staining:**
   a. Chromogenic bacteria
   b. Iron supplements
   c. Chlorhexidine
   d. Food and beverage
   e. Micro-abrasion is treatment of choice
   f. Bleaching
   g. Fluorosis.

7. **Intrinsic discolouration can occur due to:**
   a. Injury/infection of primary predecessor
   b. Internal resorption
   c. Amelogenesis imperfecta
   d. Haemolytic disease of new born
   e. Smoking
   f. Food and beverages can commonly cause intrinsic stains
   g. Congenital porphyria
   h. Root canal fillings
   i. Drugs.

8. **Regarding restorative materials for restoring primary dentition:**
   a. Compomer is material of choice for restoring minimal approximal cavity with no dovetail occlusally
   b. Approximal cavities with occlusal extension should be restored with amalgam
   c. Glass ionomer cements is material of choice for pits and fissure caries
   d. Stainless steel crowns is used for restoring cusps and endodontically treated teeth
   e. Nursing caries is best treated with glass ionomer cements.

9. **Regarding restoration of permanent dentition:**
   a. Fissure biopsy should not be performed on stained fissures with no radiographic caries
   b. Composite restoration can be used for pit and fissure caries, if occlusal contacts are on enamel

c. Amalgam is the material of choice for approximal cavities
d. A macroscopically intact sealant is not necessary to be microscopically intact
e. Occlusal caries is easy to diagnose clinically.

10. **Regarding endodontics in primary teeth:**
    a. Direct pulpal capping is the treatment of choice over vital pulpotomy
    b. Calcium hydroxide is the material of choice for vital pulpotomy
    c. Mineral trioxide aggregate stimulates cytokine release from pulpal fibroblasts
    d. Treatment is indicated in children with immunosuppression
    e. Treatment is indicated in children with behavioural problems.

11. **In permanent teeth with open apices:**
    a. Direct pulp capping is indicated when there is no history of swelling or spontaneous pain
    b. Ferric sulfate is the material of choice for pulpotomy
    c. Cvek pulpotomy is indicated for permanent vital incisors
    d. Apexogenesis is indicated for non-vital incisors with immature apices
    e. Non-vital teeth with immature apices should be removed unless required for orthodontic reason.

12. **Regarding primary tooth trauma:**
    a. Luxation is the most common type of injury in primary dentition
    b. Mostly occurs at the age of 5–6 years
    c. Avulsed teeth should be re-implanted immediately
    d. Buccal luxation carries highest risk to secondary dentition
    e. Dilaceration is common after traumatic injury to primary dentition.

13. **Regarding injuries to permanent teeth:**
    a. Treatment depends upon size of exposure and root development stage
    b. Treatment is directed towards retaining vitality of fractured or displaced tooth
    c. Open apices have better prognosis compared to closed apices
    d. Root fractures occur frequently in the coronal third of the root
    e. Functional splinting should be done for 4 months minimum, if the fracture is in coronal third of the root.

14. **Regarding splinting:**
    a. Apical and middle third of root fracture requires 3–4 months of functional splinting
    b. Coronal third root fracture requires 4 weeks of rigid splinting
    c. Dento-alveolar fracture requires 4 weeks of functional splinting
    d. Exarticulation injuries requires 2 weeks of splinting
    e. Splinting is done to encourage healing with calcified tissue
    f. Rigid splints have one abutment tooth on each side of injured tooth
    g. Acrylic resin is suitable for all type of splinting
    h. Lone-standing luxated tooth can be supported by sling suture.

15. **Regarding luxation injuries:**
    a. In subluxation, there is rupture of periodontal ligament fibres and pulp
    b. In extrusive luxation, there is rupture of periodontal ligament fibres only
    c. In lateral luxation, there is rupture of periodontal ligament fibres and pulp only
    d. Lateral luxation requires functional splint for 4 weeks
    e. The chances of pulpal survival at 5 years after injury involving periodontal ligament are high in teeth with open apices as compared to closed apices.

16. **In intrusive luxation injuries:**
    a. There is extensive damage to PDL and alveolar plates
    b. Teeth with closed apices periodontal ligament require orthodontic extrusion immediately
    c. Risk of pulpal necrosis is low in teeth with closed apices
    d. Functional splint is required for 2 weeks
    e. Early pulp extirpation for teeth with closed apices within two weeks
    f. Calcium hydroxide in the root canal does preclude orthodontic movement.

17. **With regards to prescription of radiographs in children:**
    a. Bitewings should be taken every 6–12 months for primary dentition in high caries risk
    b. Bitewings should be taken every 6–12 months for mixed dentition in low caries risk
    c. Bitewings should be taken every 6–12 months for permanent dentition in low caries risk
    d. Bitewings should be taken every 6–12 months for mixed dentition with high caries risk
    e. Bitewings should be taken every 12–24 months in mixed dentition with low caries risk.

18. **Regarding avulsion of re-implantation of tooth:**
    a. Re-implanted tooth can act as natural space maintainer
    b. Successful healing after re-implantation depends upon type of extra-alveolar storage medium and time
    c. Immature tooth may undergo pulp re-vascularisation, if extra-alveolar time is less than 45 minutes
    d. Dry storage will result in vital periodontal ligament cells.

19. **In non-accidental injury (NAI):**
    a. The aim of intervention is to diagnose and treat disordered parenting
    b. Usually older children are involved
    c. Usually the story of the injury does not vary from child to parent
    d. Bruises of different vintage may present on examination
    e. More than 50% of abused children have signs on the head and neck

f. Abrasions and laceration are common type of orofacial injuries in non-accidental injury
g. Frenal tears can be caused by forcible feeding
h. Most of these children live in rural community
i. The children act of 1989 states 5 categories of abuse.

20. **In dental anomalies:**
    a. The incidence of hypodontia occurring is greater in primary dentition than permanent dentition
    b. Hypodontia can be also found in Ellis-van Creveld and Roger syndromes
    c. Supernumerary tuberculate or inverted conical forms can be removed non-surgically
    d. True generalized macrodontia occurs in pituitary gigantism
    e. True localized microdontia can also be associated with hypertrichosis.

21. **Regarding dental anomalies:**
    a. Dens invaginatus commonly occurs on maxillary central incisors
    b. Dens invaginatus is more common in females
    c. Dens evaginatus is usually unilateral
    d. Dens evaginatus commonly occurs in mandible
    e. Talon cusp may reach and contact incisal edge
    f. Taurodontism can be associated with Klinefelter's syndrome and hypophosphatasia.

22. **Regarding defects in enamel and dentine:**
    a. Amelogenesis imperfecta results from single gene defects
    b. Incidence of amelogenesis imperfecta is 1:100,000
    c. In hypoplastic amelogenesis imperfecta, enamel is not mineralised
    d. Dentinogenesis imperfecta type II is associated with osteogenesis imperfecta
    e. Dentinogenesis imperfecta is associated with hypophosphataemic rickets but not vitamin D dependent rickets
    f. Dentiogenesis imperfecta type II mainly affects permanent dentition than primary dentition
    g. Dentine dysplasia type II shows short and blunt roots radiographically.

23. **Regarding eruption and exfoliation disorder:**
    a. Premature eruption is not inherited
    b. Natal and neonatal teeth are associated with Ellis-van Creveld and Hallermann-Streiff syndrome
    c. Delayed eruption in primary dentition can be associated with nutritional deficiencies
    d. Premature exfoliation of teeth is not seen in children with neutropenia and histiocytosis-X
    e. Delayed exfoliation can be associated with double primary teeth
    f. Infra-occlusion commonly occurs in males.

24. **In patients with congenital heart disease:**
    a. Patent ductus arteriosus prevails commonly
    b. Antibiotic cover is required for scaling and polishing
    c. Chlorhexidine mouthwash should be offered prophylactically to patient at risk of infective endocarditis
    d. Penicillin is the antibiotic of choice for prophylaxis
    e. Mortality associated with infective endocarditis is around 10%.

25. **In patient with bleeding disorders:**
    a. Defects in primary haemostasis results in deep-seated muscle and joint bleeding
    b. Haemophilia presents with defects in secondary haemostasis
    c. More than 25% of factor VIII levels in haemophillia A presents as severe disease
    d. Platelet count of $90 \times 10^9/L$ is safe for invasive dental procedure in general practice
    e. Von Willebrand's disease is X-linked recessive
    f. In haemophilia C, the missing factors is XI
    g. Desmopressin should be given for mild to moderate haemophilia A instead of factors replacement.

26. **In patients with red and white cells disorders:**
    a. Glucose-6-phosphate dehydrogenase deficiency is an autosomal condition
    b. In sickle cell anemia, there is a substitution of single amino acid in haemoglobin chain
    c. Homozygotes have sickle cell traits
    d. Chediak-Higashi syndrome, lazy leucocyte syndrome and leucocyte adhesion defects are quantitative neutrophil disorders
    e. Recurrent aphthous ulceration and recurrent herpes simplex infection can be due to neutrophil deficiencies and T-cells defects
    f. T-cell deficiencies can lead to recurrent bacterial infections
    g. Acute lymphocytic leukaemia is the common childhood malignancy
    h. Bone marrow transplant is the treatment of choice for acute lymphoblastic leukaemia
    i. Fungal and viral infections are common in immunosuppression
    j. Prophylactic antibiotics can be given, if functional neutrophil count is depressed
    k. Regional block local anaesthesia is not contraindicated.

27. **In patients with respiratory disease:**
    a. Asthma affects 25% of children in UK
    b. Nitrous oxide is contraindicated in asthmatic patient
    c. Cystic fibrosis is autosomal dominant disorder
    d. Cystic fibrosis is not a cause for decreased saliva formation
    e. Use of steroids may cause candidiasis.

28. **In patients with metabolic and endocrine disorders:**
    a. Diabetic patients can present with xerostomia
    b. Steroid supplementation is indicated for routine restorative care in patients with adrenal insufficiency
    c. Hyperthyroidism results in delayed eruption and increased spacing
    d. Hypothyroidism can results in osteoporosis
    e. Oral infections can exaggerate hyperthyroidism
    f. Anti-thyroid drugs can produce agranulocytosis
    g. Hypoparathyroidism does not cause circumoral parasthesia
    h. Osteoporosis with cortical resorption is common bone lesion of hyperparathyroidism.

29. **Neoplastic disease in children:**
    a. Lymphomas are the most common form of cancer in children
    b. Acute lymphoblastic leukaemia has 70%-80% cure rate
    c. Teeth with poor prognosis should be restored
    d. Systemic antifungal antivirals are not prescribed
    e. Acute myloblastic leukaemia is the most common leukaemia of children
    f. Prophylactic antibiotics are contraindicated.

30. **In children with organ transplantation:**
    a. Bone marrow transplant is treatment of choice for acute lymphoblastic leukaemia
    b. Use of chlorhexidine mouthwash or spray is not indicated
    c. Prophylactic anti-viral and anti-fungal is prescribed during immunosuppression therapy
    d. Gingival hyperplasia is associated with treatment with nifedipine and cyclosporine
    e. Prophylactic antibiotics are contraindicated
    f. There could be delayed eruption and exfoliation of primary teeth
    g. Artificial saliva prescribed in case of xerostomia.

31. **In patients with renal and hepatic disease:**
    a. Renal disease can be associated with high caries rate
    b. Paracetamol is not contraindicated in renal disease
    c. Renal patients may develop uraemic stomatitis
    d. Biliary atresia is the most common cause of liver transplantation in children
    e. There are coagulation problems in patients with hepatic disorder
    f. Hepatitis C is infectious disease.

32. **In patients with co-existing disease or developmental disorders:**
    a. Febrile convulsions occur after the age of 3 years
    b. Female convulsions proceed to epilepsy
    c. Epilepsy affects 0.5-1% of the population
    d. Patients with cerebral palsy are mentally impaired

e. Visually impaired patients are not photophobic
f. Deaf patients are sensitive to vibrations
g. Developmental disability is not commonly associated with other multiple medical problems.

Identify the Single Best Answer for the following

33. What would be recommended fluoride supplement for 5-year-old child with high caries risk living in non-fluoridated area?
    a. 0.25 mg F⁻ per day
    b. 0.25 mg F⁻ per week
    c. 0.5 mg F⁻ per day
    d. 0.5 mg F⁻ per week
    e. 0.75 mg F⁻ per day
    f. 0.75 mg F⁻ per week
    g. 1 mg F⁻ per day
    h. 1 mg F⁻ per week.

34. Regarding calcification of upper first molar (D) begins at:
    a. 12-16 weeks in utero
    b. 13-16 weeks in utero
    c. 15-18 weeks in utero
    d. 14-17 weeks in utero
    e. 12-15 weeks in utero
    f. 16-23 weeks in utero.

35. Upper first molar (D) will erupt at:
    a. 6-7 months
    b. 7-8 months
    c. 18-20 months
    d. 12-15 months
    e. 24-36 months
    f. 16-23 months.

Please provide answers to the following Extended Matching Questions

36. Regarding calcification of permanent teeth:
    a. Calcification of lower central incisor.
    b. Calcification of first molar.
    c. Calcification of canine.
    d. Calcification of lower lateral incisor.
    e. Calcification of upper lateral incisor.
    f. Calcification of upper first premolar.
    g. Calcification of lower first premolar.
    h. Calcification of upper second premolar.
    i. Calcification of lower second premolar.

1. 3–4 months	7. 27–30 months
2. 4–5 months	8. 30–36 months
3. 10–12 months	9. 84–108 months
4. 18–21 months	10. 96–120 months
5. 21–24 months	11. At birth
6. 24–27 months	

37. **Regarding eruption of permanent teeth:**
    a. Eruption of upper central incisor
    b. Root calcification of upper central incisor
    c. Eruption of upper canine
    d. Root calcification complete of upper canine
    e. Eruption of lower first premolar
    f. Root calcification complete of lower first premolar
    g. Eruption of upper second premolar
    h. Eruption of second molar
    i. Root calcification complete of upper first molar
    j. Root calcification complete of second molar.

1. 6–7 years	9. 17–21 years
2. 7–8 years	10. 8–10 years
3. 8–9 years	11. 9–11 years
4. 9–10 years	12. 11–13 years
5. 10–11 years	13. 12–14 years
6. 10–12 years	14. 12–15 years
7. 11–12 years	15. 13–16 years
8. 12–13 years	

CASE DISCUSSIONS

Case 1: Management of unerupted central incisors.

A 9½-year-old patient presents to your practice with unerupted upper right central incisor. Discuss the causes of unerupted central incisor and management of this patient.

History

History of complaint to be recorded with special emphasis to any trauma history of primary dentition, e.g. falls, fractures, avulsions, extractions, etc.

Medical history

If patient suffers from any ailments, or head and neck syndromes, please check for hypodontia.

Dental history

If patient have or currently under the care of General Dental Practitioner, attends regularly or not?

Clinical Examination
- Extra-oral examination:
  - Assess patient's skeletal pattern, vertical relationship, soft tissues, lip competency, facial symmetry or any abnormal temporomandibular joint signs or symptoms.
- Intra-oral examination:
  - Examine patient's soft tissues and hard tissues
  - Assess patient's general condition of mouth and dentition with special emphasis to the following:
    Oral hygiene; (calculus and plaque control)
    Dentition present; (mixed dentition)
    Any restorations present (DMFT/dft)
    Occlusal relationship; class I/II/III
    Incisor relationship, (midline deviation)
    Crowding or spacing in quadrants.

Causes of Unerupted Incisors
- Missing:
  - Congenitally missing
  - Avulsed
  - Extracted.
- Unerupted:
  - Dilaceration
  - Ectopically positioned
  - Pathology (cyst/odontomes)
  - Crowding
  - Supernumerary.

Investigations
- Clinical:
  - Palpation of labial and buccal mucosa in upper right area to detect unerupted upper right central incisor.
- Radiographs:
  Dental panoramic tomograms
  - To check the state of developing dentition and to detect presence or absence of unerupted teeth.

  Periapical view:
  - To visualize roots of adjacent teeth and to detect any periapical changes or pathologies.

  Upper standard occlusal:
  - Better view of anterior maxilla and to check presence of any supernumerary teeth or any pathology.

  Using principle of vertical parallax, the orthopantomogram standard occlusal or periapical view can be used to localize the position of unerupted or supernumerary tooth.

Discussion
- Congenitally absence of upper right incisors is very rare and unlikely as upper left central incisor is present
- Avulsion/extraction of upper right incisors is excluded as it was never erupted or had any trauma history
- Ectopic position can be due to pathology or presence of supernumerary
- Scar tissue to be excluded as there is no history of trauma
- Supernumerary is the most likely cause with incidence of 1-3% in premaxilla
- Crowding is unlikely as very severe crowding can prevent eruption of upper central incisors
- Pathology can be present but unlikely as there should be expansion of premaxilla likely due to cyst formation from unerupted upper right incisors, supernumerary or odontome.

Effects of Supernumerary Teeth
- Midline diastema
- Deviations in midline
- Crowding
- Displacements
- Root resorption of adjacent teeth.

Treatment Options
- No treatment: This is not a suitable option as eruption of upper right incisors has already been delayed
- Wait for supernumerary to erupt and then extract: It is unlikely as child is over 9 years with unerupted upper right incisors so supernumerary might not ever erupt.
- Surgical removal of supernumerary and upper right incisors to erupt by itself: Orthodontic treatment may be indicated, if there is not adequate space for upper right incisors to erupt or space maintenance is required to allow upper right incisors to erupt. Removal of supernumerary to be carried out under general anaesthesia as child is 9½-year-old.
- Surgical removal of supernumerary, bonding of the unerupted incisor with bracket and gold chain to pull it into the place. This procedure is to be carried but under general anaesthesia.
- Ask patient's parents if they have any questions or require some more information.

Case 2: Management of fractured permanent incisor root.
A 12-year, old boy attends to your practice after a football tackle and sustains injury to upper left permanent central incisor upper right incisors middle third root fracture. Discuss your management for this patient.

Patient's Complaint
Should be recorded in patient's own word.

History
Establish how injury occurred and circumstances around injury.

Medical history
General medical status of the child and emphasis on the questions below:
- Any loss of consciousness?
- Any pain or discomfort while opening or closing jaw? Rule out the possibility of condylar fracture
- Status of vaccionation aganst tetauns.

Dental history
If the patient have been currently under care of general dental practioner and or not.

Clinical Examination
- Extra-oral examination:
  - Facial swelling, bruising, any double vision due to stepping of infra-orbital margin or altered sensation of the cheek.
- Intra-oral examination:
  - Soft tissues and hard tissues, check displacement of crown and mobile teeth.

Clinical Investigations
- Radiographs:
  - Periapicals or anterior occlusal view to diagnose root fractures. Upper laterals to be checked for any injuries.
- Vitality test for all upper and lower incisors.

Treatment
The treatment depends upon the position of the fracture and prognosis of the injury depends upon the communication of fracture line with the gingival crevice.

Positions of Root Fracture and Treatment
- Apical one-third root fracture:
  - Usually no treatment unless there is increased mobility and displaced coronal fragment
  - Reposition and splint for three to six weeks
  - To be kept under observation for necrosis of two-thirds coronal pulp
  - Root canal therapy (RCT) of coronal pulp, if non-vital as apical one-third usually retain vitality

- ➢ If extraction required, apical one-third can be left in-situ to preserve bone.
- Middle third one-third root fracture:
  - ➢ Coronal fragment is usually loose, requires repositioning and flexible-functional splint for three to six weeks in order to repair of fracture line with hard tissue union
  - ➢ If loss of vitality of coronal part, RCT to fracture line
  - ➢ Calcium hydroxide to be used as interim dressing to limit inflammation and resorption
  - ➢ If extraction is required, leave apical fragment in-situ.
- Coronal one-third root fracture:
  - ➢ This fracture usually communicates with gingival crevice and allows ingress of bacteria into pulp
  - ➢ Extraction of both part or removal of coronal part
  - ➢ Root canal therapy
  - ➢ Placement of dressing to prevent gingival overgrowth
  - ➢ Permanent restoration: Post-retained crown
  - ➢ Orthodontic extrusion or gingivectomy for crown fabrication
  - ➢ Over denture and retained root to maintain alveolar bone height.

Case 3: Management of fracture of immature crown.

A 10-year-old boy presents to your practice after being hit by the football during games session. He sustained enamel, dentine and pulp fracture on his upper central incisors. Discuss the management of this patient.

Patient's Complaint

To be recorded in patient's own words.

History

History of complaint—When, where, how? Any other injuries?

Medical history

History of illness, loss of consciousness, dizziness, vomiting:

Dental history

- Regular attender? Any treatment under LA and how did patient cope.
- Locate the place of fractured tooth, if unable to below chest X-ray may be required to check the status of fragment if it has been aspirated during the loss of consciousness.

Clinical Examination

- Extra-oral examination:
  - ➢ Lip swelling, mucosal laceration to check if tooth fragment retained in the lip.

- Intra-oral examination:
  - Check for enamel, dentine and pulp fracture and note the diameter
  - Mobility to check for root fracture or PDL injury
  - Colour for pulpal haemorrhage into dentinal tubules
  - Percussion for periapical damage and oedema
  - Vertical crown or root fracture
  - Vitality testing
- Loss of vitality to electric pulp testing (EPT); hot and cold stimuli. Readings can serve as baseline and subsequent tests during review examination can be compared.

Clinical Investigations

- Periapical radiographs, to detect:
  - Foreign body
  - Apical status
  - Root fractures
  - Dento-alveolar fracture.
- Vitality testing for all upper and lower incisors.

Treatment

- Treatment depends upon the type of fracture.
- Enamel only:
  - For small enamel fracture, smooth the tooth surface with white stone burr so patient does not feel any sharp surface.
- Enamel and dentine fracture:
  - Protect exposed dentine
  - Use of hard setting calcium hydroxide cement
  - To be restored with acid etched retained composite restoration **(Figs 2.1A and B)**.
- Enamel dentine and pulp fracture:
  - Treatment depends upon size of exposure and state of root development and time since injury. Radiologically, the roots of upper central incisors complete around 10–11 years and histologically, 14–15 years

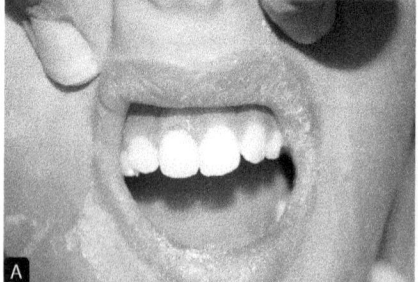 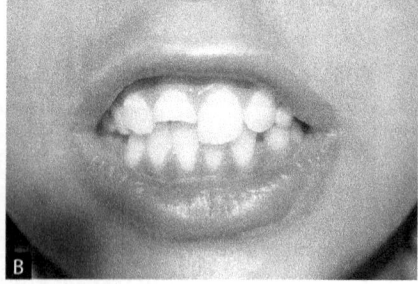

Figs 2.1A and B: (A) Pre-treatment and (B) Post-treatment of fracture of immature crown

- ➢ If open apices, the aim of the treatment is to retain vitality of the pulp to allow root closure to continue (Fig. 2.2B).
- Direct pulp capping:
  - ➢ If there is a tiny exposure
  - ➢ The treatment should be direct pulp capping with calcium hydroxide and coverage with acid etch retained composite restoration
  - ➢ Review at every 1, 3 and 6 months.

Partial Pulpotomy (Cvek)

- Removal of the outer layer of exposed and hyperaemic tissue to maintain vitality of the pulpal tissue which will allow full growth of root
- To be performed under local anaesthesia and rubber dam
- Access site of exposure with high speed, and water coolant and amputate 2-4 mm into healthy pulp tissue
- Arrest bleeding with moist sterile cotton wool
- Place calcium hydroxide to cover amputation site
- Seal with Glass ionomer cement
- Review at 1, 3 and 6 months.

Complete Pulpotomy

- Removal of coronal pulp tissue and placement of dressing at canal orifice. This will arrest dentine formation in pulp chamber and allow completion of root growth
- Local anaesthesia and rubber dam
- Amputate coronal pulp to cervical constriction

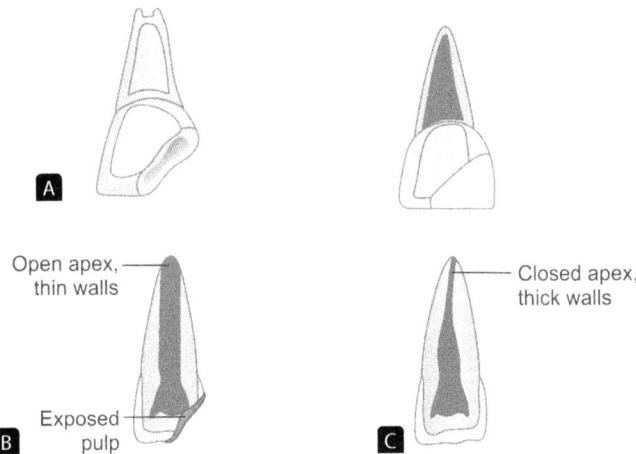

Figs 2.2A and B: (A) Diagrammatic presentation of apexogenesis (B) Diagrammatic presentation of apexification in immature tooth (C) mature tooth

- Wash with sterile water
- Place non-setting calcium hydroxide
- Seal with Glass ionomer cement and acid-etch composite restoration
- Clinical and radiographical review at 1, 3 and 6 months to check vitality and normal growth of the root
- If evidence of non-vitality, then extirpate the pulp and place calcium hydroxide to stimulate root closure prior to obturation with gutta percha.

Case 4: Management of avulsed incisor.

A 9-year-old girl has fallen down while playing with her friends and avulsed one of her upper front teeth. Mother has got the tooth but does not know what to do? Discuss the management of this patient.

Patient's Complaint
In patient's own words.

History
History of complaint—How and when the injury occurred?

Medical history
General medical status of the patient, any head injury. In case of known medical history of heart defects immunosuppression and history of rheumatic fever to not consider reimplantation.

Dental history
If patient attends regularly for dental appointments.

Factors Affecting Prognosis
- Time from tooth loss to re-implantation:
  - PDL cells survive less than 60 minutes (extra-orally). The earlier the tooth is re-implanted within 15 minutes, the better the prognosis and chance of tooth survival.
- Storage medium:
  - Prognosis is better if stored in preferred storage media—milk and normal saline. Dry storage damages periodontal ligament cells.
- Splinting:
  - 7–10 days flexible splinting. Any longer splinting time can promote ankylosis.
- Viability of pulp:
  - Revascularisation is possible in tooth with open apex, if replaced within 30 minutes.

Treatment

- Immediate treatment:
  - Hold by crown and wash gently in saline to remove any debris for 10 seconds. Irrigate socket and place tooth in socket and bite on gauze for 15–20 minutes, compress buccal and lingual alveolar plates
  - Use 0.6 mm stainless steel wire to splint and includes one tooth either side of avulsed tooth
  - Prescribe chlorhexidine mouthwash 0.2% twice daily
  - Amoxycillin 125 mg TDS for 5 days
  - Erythromycin 125 mg QDS for 5 day, if allergic to amoxicillin
  - Review 7–10 days later.
- Intermediate treatment:
  - 7–10 days later
  - Review splinting and mobility (If mobile after 2 week, check for root fracture or loss of vitality)
  - If closed apex—extirpate pulp, clean canal, place initial intra canal dressing calcium hydroxide
  - If open apex—monitor closely, institute RCT if there is a sign of pulpal necrosis
  - If calcium hydroxide is placed in canal, it should be renewed every 3 month until apical barrier is formed and then gutta percha is placed.

Sequelae Following Trauma

Types of resorption:
- **Surface resorption:** Occurs as a result of minor trauma to PDL. It can be seen as blunting of tooth apices after application of excessive orthodontic forces or due to canine tooth impaction on the roots of upper laterals. The teeth are usually vital and require no treatment.
- **Replacement resorption:** Ankylosis is caused by damage to PDL cells during extra-alveolar drying time and prolonged splinting. There is absence of PDL and bone is fused to cementum and dentine. This allows resorption of tooth and replacement by bone. In growing child, it causes infra-occlusion of affected tooth. Usually progressive and eventually results in loss of tooth.
- **External inflammatory resorption:** This is dependent upon presence of damaged PDL and pulpal necrotic products diffusing through dentinal tubules. Occurs rapidly within 1–2 weeks after injury, progressive with poor prognosis if evident on radiographs. Treatment will be pulp extirpation and placement of non-setting calcium hydroxide. If resorption stops, obturate with gutta percha root filling.
- **Internal inflammatory resorption:** This originates from root canal due to inadequate mechanical and chemical debridement of root canal system of non-vital tooth.

Answers

1.	a.	F	b.	T	c.	F	d.	T	e.	T
	f.	F								
2.	a.	T	b.	T	c.	F	d.	T	e.	T
	f.	T	g.	T	h.	T				
3.	a.	T	b.	T	c.	F	d.	F	e.	T
4.	a.	T	b.	F	c.	F	d.	F	e.	T
5.	a.	T	b.	T	c.	T	d.	F	e.	T
6.	a.	T	b.	T	c.	T	d.	T	e.	F
	f.	F	g.	F						
7.	a.	T	b.	T	c.	T	d.	T	e.	F
	f.	F	g.	T	h.	T	i.	T		
8.	a.	T	b.	F	c.	T	d.	T	e.	F
9.	a.	F	b.	T	c.	T	d.	T	e.	F
10.	a.	F	b.	F	c.	T	d.	F	e.	T
11.	a.	T	b.	F	c.	T	d.	F	e.	T
12.	a.	T	b.	F	c.	F	d.	T	e.	F
13.	a.	T	b.	T	c.	T	d.	F	e.	T
14.	a.	F	b.	F	c.	F	d.	T	e.	T
	f.	F	g.	F	h.	T				
15.	a.	F	b.	F	c.	F	d.	T	e.	T
16.	a.	T	b.	T	c.	F	d.	T	e.	T
	f.	F								
17.	a.	T	b.	F	c.	F	d.	T	e.	T
18.	a.	T	b.	T	c.	T	d.	F		
19.	a.	T	b.	F	c.	F	d.	T	e.	T
	f.	F	g.	T	h.	F	i.	F		
20.	a.	F	b.	T	c.	F	d.	T	e.	F
21.	a.	F	b.	F	c.	F	d.	T	e.	T
	f.	T								

22.	a.	T	b.	F	c.	F	d.	F	e.	T
	f.	F	g.	F						
23.	a.	F	b.	T	c.	T	d.	F	e.	T
	f.	F								
24.	a.	F	b.	F	c.	F	d.	F	e.	F
25.	a.	F	b.	T	c.	F	d.	T	e.	F
	f.	T	g.	T						
26.	a.	F	b.	T	c.	F	d.	F	e.	T
	f.	F	g.	T	h.	T	i.	T	j.	T
	k.	F								
27.	a.	F	b.	F	c.	F	d.	F	e.	T
28.	a.	T	b.	F	c.	F	d.	F	e.	T
	f.	T	g.	F	h.	T				
27.	a.	F	b.	F	c.	F	d.	F	e.	T
28.	a.	T	b.	F	c.	F	d.	F	e.	T
	f.	T	g.	F	h.	T				
29.	a.	F	b.	T	c.	F	d.	F	e.	F
	f.	F								
30.	a.	F	b.	F	c.	T	d.	T	e.	F
	f.	T	g.	T						
31.	a.	F	b.	F	c.	T	d.	T	e.	T
	f.	T								
32.	a.	F	b.	F	c.	T	d.	F	e.	F
33.	c	34.	d	35.	d					
36.	a.	1	b.	11	c.	2	d.	1	e.	3
	f.	4	g.	5	h.	6	i.	7	j.	8
37.	a.	2	b.	11	c.	7	d.	15	e.	6
	f.	14	g.	6	h.	8	i.	10	j.	15

CORRECT ANSWER FOR FALSE STATEMENTS

3. c. Towards surface of enamel.
   d. Increased F–.
4. b. Stomach.
   c. Ineffective as placenta allows a small amount of F– to cross.
   d. Outer.
6. f. For intrinsic.
8. e. With strip crown technique.
9. e. It is difficult and requires radiographs.
10. b. Ferric sulfate.
    d. Extraction.
11. b. Calcium hydroxide.
    d. Apexification.
12. b. 2-4 years.
    e. Hypoplasia.
13. d. Middle or apical third.
14. a. 3-4 weeks.
    b. 3-4 months of functional splint.
    c. Four weeks of rigid splinting.
    f. Two abutments on either side.
    g. Except root fractures.
15. a. Only PDL fibres.
    b. Both PDL fibres and pulp.
    c. Also compression injury to alveolar plate.
16. c. High is closed apices.
    f. Does not.
18. d. Non-vital PDL cells.
19. f. Contusions and ecchymosis.
    h. Urban and metropolitan.
    i There are 4 categories; physical, sexual, emotional, neglect.
21. a. Lateral incisors.
    b. males.
    c. Bilateral.
22. b. 1:10,000.
    c. It is mineralised.
    d. Type I is associated.
    f. Affects both dentition.
    g. Type I.
23. a. Inherited.
    d. Seen in children with these conditions.
    f. Equal incidence.

Paediatric Dentistry

24. a. Ventricular septal defects.
    b. Not required.
    c. Should not be offered.
    d. Amoxicillin.
    a. (20-30%).
25. a. Defect in secondary haemostasis.
    c. <1% severe disease, 1-5% moderate disease, >25% mild disease.
    e. Autosomal dominant.
26. a. X-linked.
    c. Heterozygotes.
    k. Contraindicated.
27. a. 10%.
    b. No contraindications.
    c. Autosomal recessive.
    d. It can cause decrease saliva formation.
28. a. Not indicated, only for extensive oral surgery.
    b. Not indicated, only for extensive oral surgery.
    c. Hypothyroidism.
    g. Does cause and also cause spasm of facial muscles.
29. a. Leukaemia 48%.
    c. To be extracted.
    d. Prescribed.
    e. Adults.
    f. Not contraindicated.
30. a. First/second relapse.
31. a. Low Caries Rate.
32. a. Upto 3 years of age.
    b. Are not.
    e. They have photophobia.

Chapter 3

Orthodontics

Identify the following Statements as True (T) or False (F)

1. **Regarding craniofacial growth:**
   a. In maxilla, growth in width ceases before growth in vertical dimension
   b. Growth in length continues until 17–18 years in girls
   c. Bone is primary determinant of its own growth
   d. Nasal septum acts as independent growth centre
   e. Soft tissue matrix does not contribute to forward and downward maxillary translation.

2. **Regarding growth of craniofacial skeleton:**
   a. The cranial base is formed by intramembranous ossification
   b. Intersphenoid synchondrosis have profound impact on antero-posterior skeletal growth
   c. Spheno-occipital synchondrosis affects maxillary and mandibular relationship
   d. A long cranial base is associated with class III skeletal pattern.

3. **The maxilla:**
   a. Is derived from second pharyngeal arch
   b. Ossifies intra-membraneously, starting in the mesial aspect of nasal capsule
   c. Grows partly via surface remodelling
   d. Moves downward and forward in response to growth of alveolar processes
   e. Growth ceases earlier in males than females.

4. **The mandible:**
   a. Is derived from second pharyngeal arch
   b. Develops mesial to Meckel's cartilage
   c. Growth pattern is dependent on maxillary growth
   d. Growth ceases by 19 years in males.

5. **Growth rotations:**
   a. Have marked effects on the maxilla than mandible
   b. Forward rotation is more common than posterior growth rotation
   c. In forward growth rotation, anterior face height is increased
   d. Posterior growth rotation of mandible results in convex lower border

e. Lower labial segment crowding results from both anterior and posterior growth rotations.

6. **Development of dentition:**
   a. Spacing mesial to upper canine and distal to lower canine in primary dentition is called Leeway space
   b. Leeway space is 1 mm in upper arch and 1.5 mm in lower arch
   c. The permanent lower incisors develop buccal to their primary predecessors
   d. The permanent upper anterior teeth are accommodated by increase in intercanine distance.

7. **Regarding maturational changes in the occlusion:**
   a. Decrease in lower labial segment crowding
   b. Increase in interincisal angle
   c. Increased overbite
   d. Increased overjet
   e. Increase in upper labial segment crowding.

8. **Factors implicated in lower labial section crowding:**
   a. Decrease in mandibular prognathism
   b. Transseptal fibre contraction
   c. Mandibular growth rotations
   d. Presence of aproximal attrition
   e. Mesial drift
   f. Increased forward maxillary growth
   g. Greater in females than males.

9. **Regarding classification of malocclusion:**
   a. Angle's classification is based on incisor relationship
   b. The British Standard Institute (BSI) classification is related to first molar relationship in permanent dentition
   c. The mesio-buccal cusp of upper first permanent molar occludes anterior to the buccal groove of lower first permanent molar is class I relationship
   d. The mesio-buccal cusp of upper first permanent molar occludes posterior to buccal groove of lower first permanent molar is mesio-occlusion
   e. In class II division II, the upper central incisors are retroclined with may be increased overjet
   f. In class II division I, the upper central incisors are proclined with increased overjet.

10. **Aetiology of malocclusion:**
    a. Majority of antero-posterior skeletal problems are caused by environmental factors
    b. Mandibular deficiencies are inherited
    c. Mandibular prognathism is strongly related to patient's race
    d. Dental arch dimensions are not influenced by environmental factors

e. Soft tissues postural effects can contribute in developing anterior open bite
f. Early loss of primary teeth is also a cause for crowding.

11. **Regarding cephalometrics:**
    a. It is not obligatory of orthodontic treatment
    b. It allows assessment of growth
    c. It is used for diagnosis
    d. It is measured with maxillary-mandibular plane angle (MMPA) horizontal
    e. It is used to compare the patient with normal population standard for his racial group
    f. Helps to identify hard tissue pathology
    g. Teeth not to be in occlusion during radiograph
    h. Is taken with head tilted up
    i. It is exact record of facial dimension.

12. **Regarding cephalometric interpretation:**
    a. The cant of the S-N line does not affect SNA values
    b. Skeletal pattern can be classified using ANB values
    c. Mandibular prognathism can be assessed using SNA values
    d. Frankfort plane joins porion and nasion
    e. Mandibular plane joins gonion to menton
    f. The Frankfort mandibular plane angle (FMPA) is average 27°
    g. Maxillary-mandibular planes angle is not related with pattern of mandibular growth
    h. Sella is the most anterior point on the cranial base
    i. ANB can be influenced by position of nasion.

13. **Cephalometric values:**
    a. SNA: 85°
    b. SNB: 79°
    c. ANB: 3°
    d. S-N/Maxilla : 8°
    e. Maxillary Incisors inclination to maxilla plane : 116°
    f. Mandibular Incisors inclination to mandibular plane : 100°
    g. Inter-incisal angle: 130°
    h. MMPA: 22°
    i. Facial proportion: 58%.

14. **Hypodontia:**
    a. The most common missing teeth are lower second premolar in 30% cases
    b. Affects upper lateral incisors more than second premolars
    c. Affects more upper lateral incisors than lower lateral incisors
    d. Third molars are commonly missing teeth
    e. More common in males than females
    f. Does not run in family

15. **Regarding supernumerary teeth:**
    a. Commonly occur in pre-maxilla
    b. Often develops distal to first tooth in each dental series
    c. More common in females than males
    d. Occurs commonly in primary dentition than permanent dentition
    e. Can cause spacing
    f. Can occur in lower incisal section.

16. **Regarding management of first permanent molars with poor long-term prognosis:**
    a. Extraction of lower first permanent molars is best when bifurcation of upper permanent third molar are calcifying
    b. Extraction of upper first permanent molars is best delayed in class II division I until upper permanent second molar erupts
    c. Extraction of upper first permanent molars is delayed in severely crowded mouth until upper permanent second molar erupts
    d. Extraction of lower first permanent molars in class III can be deferred until upper permanent third molar erupts
    e. Timing of extraction of upper first permanent molars is less important.

17. **Regarding serial extractions:**
    a. Was developed by Kjellgren in 1945
    b. Works best in children with class II malocclusion
    c. Extraction of primary canines to encourage alignment of permanent incisors around 8–9 years of age
    d. Extraction of first primary molar is done to encourage eruption of second permanent premolar
    e. Extraction of primary canines as first premolars are erupting.

18. **Regarding extraction of primary canines:**
    a. Loss of primary canines should always be compensated
    b. Extraction of canine can prevent cross bite
    c. Is indicated when permanent upper lateral incisors is erupting palatally
    d. Can prevent loss of periodontal support in lower labial section
    e. To promote alignment of displaced mandibular canine
    f. Unilateral loss of upper canine does not result in centre-line shift.

19. **Regarding extraction of first permanent molars:**
    a. Spontaneous alignment after extraction of permanent lower first molar, if angulation between crypt of permanent lower second molar and permanent lower first molar is > 30°
    b. Increased tendency of mesial drift in mandible
    c. If permanent upper first molar is extracted, the lower tooth has to be compensated
    d. When permanent lower first molar is extracted, the opposing tooth permanent upper first molar should be compensated
    e. Extraction of permanent first molar will relieve labial segment crowding

20. **Regarding maxillary canines:**
    a. Incident of ectopic maxillary canine occurs in 20% of population
    b. 15% are palatal to arch while 85% are buccal
    c. Absence of lateral incisors can cause canines to be displaced
    d. Palatal displacement of canine has familial link
    e. Occurs commonly in males than females
    f. Palatal displacement occurs unilaterally
    g. Transposition is common between lateral incisor and canine.

21. **Spacing of dentition:**
    a. Commonly found in UK population
    b. Median diastema prevails in 98% of 11-year-old
    c. Diastema can be caused by proclination of upper labial segment
    d. Treatment of diastema requires removable appliance
    e. Does not require prolong retention
    f. Frenectomy may be indicated
    g. Thumb sucking habit one of the causative factor.

22. **Increased overjet:**
    a. With increased overjet, trauma is more common in females than males
    b. Anterior oral seal does influence incisor position
    c. Overjet reduction can be difficult in patients with low facial height
    d. Can be caused by digit sucking
    e. Is commonly due to mandible being positioned posteriorly on the cranial base.

23. **Digit sucking habit:**
    a. Can retrocline lower incisors
    b. May increase overjet
    c. May increase overbite
    d. Procline upper labial segment
    e. Does not cause buccal segment crossbite.

24. **Bimaxillary proclination:**
    a. Is common in Caucasians
    b. Represents inclination of upper and lower incisors
    c. May exists in association with class I malocclusion
    d. Increased chance of success post-treatment
    e. Can be due to increased lips pressure than tongue pressure.

25. **Regarding treatment of class II division I malocclusions:**
    a. The antero-posterior skeletal pattern class I will produce favourable results
    b. The forward mandibular growth pattern is unfavourable
    c. Digit sucking habit can persist
    d. Presence or absence of an adaptive tongue thrust can aggravate malocclusion
    e. Overjet reduction to precede overbite reduction

Orthodontics

26. **With regards to functional appliance:**
    a. Are effective for individual tooth movements
    b. Works by restraining mandibular growth
    c. Forward movement of the glenoid fossa
    d. To be worn 14–16 hours per day to be effective
    e. Does not require post-treatment retention.

27. **Increased overbite:**
    a. In increased overbite, upper central incisors are proclined and upper laterals are retroclined
    b. Reduced lower facial height
    c. Is associated with posterior mandibular growth rotation
    d. Is associated with high lower lip line
    e. Reduced inter-incisal angle
    f. Can be advantageous in class III malocclusions
    g. Scissor bite can be present.

28. **Regarding management of increased overbite:**
    a. Extraction to be avoided in upper arch
    b. The inter-incisal angle to be reduced for stable result
    c. Overbite reduction precedes overjet reduction
    d. Upper removable appliance can be used to procline upper incisors alternatively
    e. Does not require long-term retention.

29. **Anterior open bite:**
    a. Only occurs in class III malocclusions
    b. Associated with reduced maxillary mandibular plane angle
    c. Tongue thrust can maintain anterior open bite
    d. Can be seen in cleft lip palate
    e. Extraction of molars can close down bite
    f. Extrusion of incisors can produce favourable stable results.

30. **Reverse overjet:**
    a. Usually associated with class I skeletal pattern
    b. Cross bites are common
    c. Dental crowding is greater in lower arch
    d. The incisor relationship is less severe than skeletal relationship
    e. Becomes worse with growth
    f. In severe cases, surgery is indicated
    g. Is associated with long anterior cranial base.

31. **Cross bites:**
    a. Are usually skeletal in origin
    b. Antero-posterior discrepancies can result is lingual cross bite
    c. Occurs only with displacement
    d. Can predispose patient to temporomandibular pain and dysfunction syndrome

e. Unilateral posterior cross bites cannot be treated with upper removable appliance
f. Bilateral buccal cross bites can mainly due to transverse skeletal discrepancy
g. Bilateral buccal cross bites are associated with functional problems.

32. **Regarding removable appliances:**
    a. Are capable of bodily movement
    b. Cannot be used for moving blocks of teeth
    c. Can be both active and passive
    d. Inter-maxillary traction is possible
    e. Efficient for multiple tooth movement
    f. Can allow differential eruption of teeth
    g. Can be used for correcting unilateral posterior cross bites.

33. **Regarding fixed appliances:**
    a. Effective for multiple tooth movement
    b. Can move teeth to compensate for skeletal discrepancy
    c. Cannot be used in conjunction with other appliances
    d. Inter-maxillary traction is used only to increase anchorage
    e. Stainless steel wires are used for initial stages of treatment.

34. **Functional appliances:**
    a. Requires wax bite to be recorded
    b. Force is in the form of inter-maxillary traction
    c. Twin block is the most common type of functional appliance in UK
    d. Twin block can be used for cases with abnormal soft tissue pattern
    e. Frankel appliances can be worn for meals.

35. **Orthognathic surgery:**
    a. Preferably to be performed before cessation of growth
    b. Pre-surgical orthodontic treatment is not indicated
    c. Usually involves decompensation
    d. Inter-maxillary traction is used post-surgically
    e. Relapse can occur both surgically and orthodontically.

36. **Regarding cleft lip palate:**
    a. Cleft lip palate is more common in females than males
    b. Unilateral cleft lip palate is more common in right side
    c. Cleft palate is more in males than females
    d. Sub mucous cleft is noticed fairly early
    e. Increased prevalence of supernumerary teeth
    f. Cleft palate can be a feature of Treacher Collins syndrome

37. **Management of:**
    a. Lip repair is carried around at 1 month of age
    b. Lip repair can be carried out using Delaire technique
    c. Palatal repair is usually carried out at 6-9 months of age
    d. Millard technique is the method of choice for palatal closure
    e. Alveolar bone grafting is performed before child turns 8 years

f. Alveolar bone grafts allow eruption of permanent canine
g. Rhinoplasty may be indicated as late procedure.

Identify the Single Best Answer for the following

38. Appliance of choice used for expansion in patients with cleft lip and palate:
    a. Hass appliance
    b. Cap splint type of expansion appliance
    c. Hyrax appliance
    d. Spring jet.

39. The process of opening bite is:
    a. Extrusion of posterior teeth and intrusion of anterior teeth
    b. Retroclination of incisors
    c. Intrusion of posterior teeth and extrusion of anterior teeth
    d. Extraction of lower anteriors.

40. The purpose of cephalogram is:
    a. Overjet
    b. Assess facial symmetry
    c. Deep bite
    d. Open bite.

41. ANB angle is used to determine:
    a. Vertical jaw discrepancy
    b. Crowding
    c. Soft tissue profile
    d. Sagittal jaw discrepancy.

42. Optimal force for bodily movement is:
    a. 15–25 gm force per tooth
    b. 50–75 gm force per tooth
    c. 75–125 gm force per tooth
    d. 200–300 gm force per tooth.

43. Prognathic profile is a characteristic feature of:
    a. Skeletal class II malocclusion
    b. Pierre-Robinson syndrome
    c. Skeletal class III malocclusion
    d. Mandibular hypoplasia.

44. The process of cortical drift includes:
    a. Apposition of bone
    b. Deposition of bone
    c. Resorption of bone
    d. Resorption and deposition of bone.

45. **The frequently encountered clinical feature along with lip biting, tongue thrusting and thumb sucking is:**
    a. Deep bite
    b. Posterior cross bite
    c. Anterior cross bite
    d. Proclination of anterior teeth.

46. **The function of night guard is:**
    a. Used to break the habit of tongue thrusting
    b. Used to break the habit of lip biting
    c. Used to break the habit of bruxism
    d. None of the above.

47. **In a spring, loops and helices are included so as to:**
    a. Increase the time interval between their re-activation
    b. Increase the flexibility
    c. Increase the time duration of its activation
    d. All of the above.

Identify the answers to Extended Matching Questions

48. **Regarding pre-natal growth and post-natal growth:**
    a. Intersphenoidal synchondrosis fuses at-------
    b. Cranium to face ratio at birth is-------
    c. Mid-saggital suture between the parietal bone completely closes at-----
    d. Total number of skull bones present at birth is-------
    e. Time of development of major part of face is_____

1. 3rd to 8th weeks of intra-uterine life	6. 6 week of intrauterine life
2. Middle of third decade of life	7. Prenatally
3. 8:1	8. 78
4. At the time of birth	9. First decade of life
5. 45	

49. **Regarding oral habits:**
    a. Hypertonic orbicularis oris activity is seen in
    b. Orthodontic appliance to remove the thumb sucking habit is
    c. Proclination of maxillary anteriors in a child can be due to
    d. Classical adenoid facies is associated with

1. Water test and cotton test is used to diagnose	6. Vestibular screen
2. Thumb sucking habit	7. Bluegrass appliance
3. A passive removable appliance with cribs	8. Asthma
4. Tongue thrusting habit	
5. Mouth breathing habit	

CASE DISCUSSIONS

Case 1: Palatal Incisors

A 17-year-old boy presents to your clinic with both upper retained primary canines. Discuss the cause and management of the patient.

History

Ask for patient's concerns and history of complaint
- Any history of trauma to both primary upper canines and loss of primary dentition
- *Medical history*—if Patient is fit and well and underdrawing any medical treatment
- *Dental history*—if patient has been visiting the dental surgery, and what is the treatment rendered.

Examination

- Extra-oral examination:
  - Skeletal class I/II/III
  - Frankfort mandibular plane angle, lower face heights, soft tissue pattern
  - Temporomandibular joint displacement.
- Intra-oral examination:
  - Oral hygiene
  - Any buccal or palatal swelling in primary upper canine area
  - Look for space discrepancies
  - Incisor and molar relationship
  - Any deviations from bites
  - Midline shifts.

Aetiology of Retained Primary Upper Canines

Absence of permanent canines is rare by affecting only 0.3% of Caucasian population. Ectopic position of canine is likely with 2% of Caucasian population. It occurs bilaterally in 17–25% of cases and more commonly found in females than males.
- Genetic: Palatally displaced canine could be due to inherited polygenic trait associated with missing or short rooted permanent upper lateral incisor and anomalies including hypodontia and microdontia
  - Crypt displacement—grossly displaced position of permanent canines
  - Upper canines have longest path of eruption
  - Arch length discrepancies—could be due to palatally placed permanent upper canines displaced in uncrowded or spaced arch
  - Trauma to anterior maxilla at early stage of development could be another season
  - Occurence of lack of guidance due to missing upper lateral incisors, short or peg-shaped upper lateral incisors therefore leads to palatally impacted canines.

Clinical Investigations
- Palpation and palatal and buccal soft tissue
- Inclination of upper lateral incisors
- Examine position of adjacent teeth, malocclusion and spacing
- Colour, mobility and wear of primary upper canines.

Radiographic Investigations
- To assess position of canine
  - Dental panoramic tomography and intraoral view
  - Vertical or horizontal tube shift parallax.

Assessment
- Vertical placement of primary upper canine to incisor roots
- Root morphology of primary upper canines
- Mesiodistal position of primary upper canine to incisor root
- Axial inclination permanent upper canine
- Apex location permanent upper canine
- Any pathology or incisor root resorption.

Vitality Test
- To check status of upper incisors.

Management
- Interceptive treatment:
  - Removal of primary canines at the age of 10-13 years at mixed dentition stage should induce eruption in case permanent upper canine is slightly palatally impacted between permanent upper lateral incisor and permanent upper first premolar
  - Monitor permanent upper canine to erupt for 6 months
  - If no change, active treatment.
- Retain and observe treatment when:
  - If patient is not keen for treatment
  - No pathology, or root resorption is obeserved
  - Primary canine is not mobile and has good prognosis
  - Permanent upper lateral incisor and permanent upper first premolar are in good contact and aesthetic is not compromised
  - Permanent upper canine is severely displaced but with no associated pathology.
- Expose permanent upper canine and align when:
  - Patient is keen on having treatment and highly motivated for prolonged orthodontic therapy
  - Excellent oral hygiene and health
  - Space of permanent upper canine is available or can be created
  - Permanent upper canine should be in favourable position for orthodontic alignment

- ➤ Expose permanent upper canine, allow it to erupt for 3 months, then orthodontic traction is used to move permanent upper canine towards arch.
- Surgically remove permanent upper canine:
  - ➤ If patient not keen on alignment of permanent upper canine
  - ➤ Cyst formation in permanent upper canine
  - ➤ Poor prognosis of permanent upper canine for alignment
  - ➤ Resorption of adjacent teeth
  - ➤ Permanent upper lateral incisor and permanent upper first premolar are in good contact and aesthetically pleasing
  - ➤ Permanent upper canine has good prognosis and aesthetics
- Transplantation of permanent upper canine:
  - ➤ If there is adequate space to fit larger and permanent tooth in space of deciduous tooth and permanent upper canine is 50–75% formed
  - ➤ If intact, removal of permanent upper canine is possible
  - ➤ Risk of ankylosis/resorption of transplanted permanent upper canine.

Case 2: Missing lateral incisors.

A 11-year old girl presents to your practice complaining of spacing in her upper dentition. On examination, upper lateral have not erupted. Discuss the causes of absent upper lateral incisors and management.

History

- Patient's complaint
- History of complaint
- Medical history—any syndromes of head and neck
- Dental history—history of trauma/avulsion/extraction

Examination

- Extra-oral examination:
  - ➤ Skeletal pattern I/II/III
  - ➤ Facial symmetry
  - ➤ Frankfort mandibular plane angle, lower face heights
  - ➤ Soft tissue profile
  - ➤ Temporomandibular joint displacement
- Intra-oral examination:
  - ➤ Dental hygiene, soft tissue health
  - ➤ Incisor relationship
  - ➤ Occlusion class I/II/III
  - ➤ Any midline shifts
  - ➤ Dentition present
  - ➤ Space discrepancies.

Aetiology
- More common in females (congenitally absent).

Missing teeth
- Incidence occurs in 2% of Caucasian population, 3.5–6.5% permanent dentition, 0.1–0.9% primary dentition
  › Hypodontia—Associated with cleft lip palate, Down syndrome, ectodermal dysplasia
  › Trauma/extraction due to caries.

Teeth absent or failure to erupt
- Crowding
- Ectopic position of crypt
- Supernumerary
- Scar tissue
- Dilaceration
- Cyst/odontoma.

Clinical Investigations
- Patient's motivation for orthodontic treatment
- Skeletal relationship
- Colour, size, shape, inclination of adjacent teeth; permanent upper canine and permanent upper central incisor
- Space discrepancies
- Molar relationship
- Vitality test of permanent upper canine and permanent upper central incisor.

Radiographs
Dental panoramic tomography:
- For absence of teeth and general state of dentition
- Supernumerary, cyst, pathology.

Management
The aim of the treatment is to restore aesthetic, provide adequate function and maintain vertical dimension. The management of missing upper lateral will require either opening of space, maintenance of space for prosthetic replacement or orthodontic space closures. This depends on number of factors:
- Open space:
  › In patients with class I or III skeletal relationship
  › Average or low frankfort mandibular plane angle
  › Uncrowded or mild crowding in upper arch

- Replace permanent upper lateral incisor with bridge (fixed or movable) or upper partial fixed or removable denture or space maintenance for implant placement later.
- Close space:
  - In patient with class II skeletal relationship
  - With increased frankfort mandibular plane angle
  - Crowded upper arch, permanent upper canine and permanent upper central incisor to be of similar colour, permanent upper canine has to be a modified crown
  - Fixed appliances along with or without reserve headgear.
- Accept space:
  - If mild spacing
  - Mesio-distal width of permanent upper canine and permanent upper central incisor with composite build-up or veneers to reduce spacing.

Case 3: Increased overjet.

An 11-year-old girl presents to your clinic and is concerned about the appearance of her upper front teeth. Mother is concerned about her daughter's appearance as she is being teased at school. Discuss the causes and management.

History

Patient's mother and patient is concerned about the appearance of her upper front teeth and anxious to know about treatment options available.
- History of complaint: Since when she started noticing the front teeth sticking out. She is being teased at school and does not like going to school anymore. Any history of trauma to upper labial segment?
- Medical history—Is patient's fit and well orally fit, if the patient is fit enough to go through the orthodontic treatment.
- Dental history—Does patient's regularly attends her general dental practitioner apartments to know about the general compliance of the patient.

Examination

- Extra-oral examination:
  - Examine patient's skeletal pattern in all three planes; anterio-posterior, vertical and lateral
  - Soft tissue pattern, competent lip seal, any digit sucking habit
  - Facial profile, frankfort mandibular plane angle and lower face heights, temporomandibular joint displacement or deviation, facial asymmetry.
- Intra-oral examination:
  - Oral hygiene—plaque or calculus deposits
  - Dentition present

- Space discrepancies
- Incisor relationship
- Molar relationship
- Any buccal/lingual cross bites
- Measure overjet or overbite if present
- Cornics relationship.

Aetiology
- Skeletal:
  - Usually class II malocclusion
  - Mandibular retrognathic
  - Increased horizontal maxillary growth
  - Combined maxillary/mandibular problem.
- Soft tissue:
  - Lower lip trap under upper labial segment
  - Hyperactive lower lip
  - Tongue thrust
- Digit sucking habit:
  - If more than 6 hours in a day, it will procline upper incisors, retrocline lower incisors, anterior open bite tendency and buccal segment cross bite
  - Asymmetric overjet due to digit positing while sucking.
- Crowding:
  - Labial displacement of upper incisor
  - Lingual displacement of upper incisor
  - Combination of both.

Investigations
- Dental panoramic tomography:
  - To check development of dentition
  - Developmental stage, presence and position or any crown/root abnormalities, presence of any unerupted teeth.
- Bitewing:
  - If caries present—check bitewing radiographs.
- Postero-anterior/Upper standard occlusal:
  - History of trauma to upper labial segment—upper anterior occlusal or periapical radiograph to check for any periapical pathology
  - Lateral cephalometric—for antero-posterior and vertical skeletal discrepancies. Also, AP movement to incisor is planned, if angle between > 4 degree which is highly likely in this case
  - Findings of lateral cephalometric analysis to be carried out: SNA, SNB, SN to maxillary plane, Maxillary Incisors to maxillary plane, mandibular incisors to mandibular plane, facial percentage and maxillary-mandibular plane angle.
- Index of treatment need score:

Management

Accept:
- If overjet 4–6 mm
- Competent lips
- Arches are aligned

Patient with skeletal pattern II

- Growing patient: Growth modification
  - Functional appliance:
    Pre-pubertal growth
    Mandibular deficiency
    Posture mandible forward and downward
    Class II intermaxillary traction
    Modify forces generated by orofacial muscles
    Align arches
    Extraction and fixed appliances lateral
  - Head gear:
    Protuded maxilla
    Gummy smile.
  - Functional appliances and headgear:
    To be retained until growth is complete.
- Non-growing patient:
  - Camouflage
  - Mild/moderate skeletal class II pattern
  - Good vertical facial proportion lower face height
  - Aligned arches
  - Extract permanent upper first premolars and fixed appliances.
- Orthognathic surgery
  - Marked skeletal class II malocclusion
  - Decreased or increased facial proportions
  - Gummy smile.
- Stable correction:
  - Overjet complete reduction
  - Lower lip to cover 1/3 to 1/2 of labial surface of upper incisors
  - No abnormal tongue thrust
  - Normal inter-incisal angle
  - Good retention.

Answers

1.	a.	T	b.	F	c.	F	d.	T	e.	F
2.	a.	F	b.	F	c.	T	d.	F		
3.	a.	F	b.	F	c.	T	d.	F	e.	F
4.	a.	F	b.	F	c.	F	d.	F		
5.	a.	F	b.	T	c.	F	d.	F	e.	T
6.	a.	F	b.	F	c.	F	d.	T		
7.	a.	F	b.	T	c.	F	d.	F	e.	F
8.	a.	F	b.	T	c.	T	d.	F	e.	T
	f.	F	g.	T						
9.	a.	F	b.	F	c.	F	d.	T	e.	T
	f.	T								
10.	a.	F	b.	T	c.	T	d.	F	e.	T
	f.	T								
11.	a.		b.	T	c.	F	d.	F	e.	T
	f.	T	g.	F	h.	F	i.	F		
12.	a.	F	b.	T	c.	F	d.	F	e.	T
	f.	F	g.	F	h.	F	i.	T		
13.	a.	F	b.	T	c.	T	d.	T	e.	F
	f.	F	g.	T	h.	F	i.	F		
14.	a.	F	b.	F	c.	T	d.	T	e.	F
	f.	F								
15.	a.	T	b.	F	c.	F	d.	F	e.	T
	f.	T								
16.	a.	F	b.	T	c.	T	d.	F	e.	T
17.	a.	F	b.	F	c.	T	d.	F	e.	F
18.	a.	F	b.	T	c.	T	d.	T	e.	F
	f.	F								
19.	a.	F	b.	F	c.	F	d.	T	e.	F

Orthodontics

20.	a.	F	b.	F	c.	T	d.	T	e.	F
	f.	F	g.	F						
21.	a.	F	b.	F	c.	T	d.	F	e.	F
	f.	T	g.	T						
22.	a.	F	b.	T	c.	T	d.	T	e.	T
23.	a.	T	b.	T	c.	F	d.	T	e.	F
24.	a.	F	b.	T	c.	T	d.	F	e.	F
25.	a.	T	b.	F	c.	F	d.	T	e.	F
26.	a.	F	b.	F	c.	T	d.	T	e.	F
27.	a.	F	b.	T	c.	F	d.	T	e.	F
	f.	T	g.	T						
28.	a.	F	b.	T	c.	T	d.	T	e.	F
29.	a.	F	b.	F	c.	T	d.	T	e.	F
	f.	F								
30.	a.	F	b.	T	c.	F	d.	T	e.	T
	f.	T	g.	F						
31.	a.	F	b.	T	c.	F	d.	T	e.	F
	f.	T	g.	F						
32.	a.	F	b.	F	c.	T	d.	T	e.	F
	f.	T	g.							
33.	a.	T	b.		c.	F	d.	F	e.	F
34.	a.	T	b.	T	c.	T	d.	F	e.	F
35.	a.	F	b.	F	c.	T	d.	T	e.	T
36.	a.	F	b.	F	c.	F	d.	F	e.	T
	f.	T								
37.	a.	F	b.	T	c.	F	d.	F	e.	F
	f.	T	g.	T						
38.	b	39.	a	40.	b	41.	d	42.	d	
43.	c	44.	d	45.	d	46.	c	47.	d	
48.	a.	4	b.	3	c.	2	d.	5	e.	1
49.	a.	3	b.	2	c.	3,4	d.	4	e.	4

CORRECT ANSWER FOR FALSE STATEMENTS

1. b. 14-15 years in girls
   d. sutural growth is reactive and inheritantly programmed
2. a. Endochondral ossification
   b. Spheno-occipital skeletal growth
   d. Small cranial base is associated with class 3 skeletal pattern
3. a. First pharyngeal arch, b:starts in lateral aspect of nasal capsule, d: in response to surrounding soft tissues
4. A. First pharyngeal arch, b: develops lateral to meckel's cartilage
   c. Independent of maxillary growth, d: Endochondral Ossification
   e. Can proceed to grow at very reduced rate upto third decade
5. a. Growth Rotations have marked effects on Mandible
   c. Anterior face height is Reduced in forward growth rotation
   d. Posterior growth rotation of mandible results in Concave lower border
6. a. Primate or Anthorpoid space
   b. 2.5 mm in lower arch
   C. Lingual to their primary predecessors
7. a. Increase in lower labial segment crowding, c:reduced overbite, d: increased overbite, f: decrease in upper labial segment crowding
8. a. Increase in mandibular prognathism, d: lack of approximal attrition
   f. Minimal forward maxillary growth
9. a. Angle's classification is based on Molar relationship
   b. BSI classification is related to Incisor relationship
   c. Class II Relationship
10. a. AP skeletal problems are caused by Genetic factors in majority of cases, d: Dental arch dimensions are influenced by environmental factors.
11. c. Cephalometrics are used as Diagnostic aid.
    d. Cephalometrics is taken horizontal Frankfort mandibular plane angle (FMPA), g: teeth should be in occlusion, h: is taken with natural head position, i: The magnification factor is in the range of 8-12%
12. a. The cant of the S-N line does affect SNA values and position of nasion
    c. Mandibular prognathism is assessed using SNB values
    d. Frankfort planes join Porion and orbitale
    f. MMPA is average 27 degrees
    g. MMPA is related to mandibular growth and facial proportions
    h. Nasion is most anterior point on the cranial base Nasion

Orthodontics

13. a. SNA 81 ± 3°please input correct value as per question 109 ± 6°
    f. 135 ± 10°
    h. 27 ± 4°
    i. 58 ± 2%
14. a. Lower second premolars are commonly missing teeth in 3% cases
    b. Does not affect upper lateral incisors more than second premolars, e. hypodontia is more common in females, f: Hypodontia does run in family
15. b Supernumerary tooth often develops distal to last tooth in each dental series, c:more common in males, d: occurs commonly in permanent dentition
16. a. Permanent Upper second molar calcifying
    d. Eruption of upper Permanent second molar
17. a. Serial extractions was developed by Kjellgren in 1948
    b. Serial extractions works best in children with Class I malocclusion
    d. Extraction of first primary molar to encourage eruption of first premolar
    e. Extraction of permanent first premolar as permanent canines are erupting
18. a. Loss of primary canines should always be balanced
    e. To promote alignment of displaced Maxillary canine
    f. Unilateral loss of primary upper canine results in centre-line shift
19. a. Should be <30°
    b. Increased tendency of mesial drift in Maxilla
    e Extractions of first permanent molars will relieve Buccal segment crowding
20. a. Ectopic maxillary canines occurs in 2% of population
    b. 85% are palatal to arch while 15% are buccal
    f. Palatal displacements occurs Bilaterally
    g. Transposition is common between Maxillary canine and premolars
21. a. Crowding is common in UK population
    b. Median diastema prevails in 49% of 11 years old
    d. Treatment of diastema requires Fixed appliance
    e. It requires prolonged retention
24. a. Bimaxillary Proclination is common in Negros, d:decreased chance of success post treatment, e: results due to increased tongue pressure
33. d. Intermaxillary traction is also used for AP correction
    e. Stainless steel wires are used for planned tooth movements
36. a. CLP is more common in Males
    b. Unilateral CLP is more common in Left side, c: cleft palate is more common in females, d:Submucous palate is usually noticed late

37. a. Cleft Lip repair is carried at around 3 months
    c. Cleft Palatal repair is carried out at 9-12 months
    d. Von Langerbeck procedure is used for palatal closure
    e. Alveolar bone grafting is performed between 8-11 years
22. a. In increased overjet trauma is common in males.
23. c. digit sucking habit increases Overjet
    e. does cause buccal segment crossbite
25. b. forward mandibular growth pattern is favourable
    c. digit sucking habit should not persist
    e. overbite reduction to precede overjet reduction
26. a. Functional appliances are effective for multiple teeth movements
    b. Functional Appliance works by restraining maxillary growth
    e. It does require post treatment retention
27. a. In increased overbite upper central incisors are retroclined and upper laterals are proclined
    c. Is associated with Anterior mandibular growth rotation
    e. Increased Inter-incisal angle
28. a. Extractions to be avoided in lower arch
    e. Management of increased overbite requires long term retention
29. b. associated with increased MMPA
    e. Extractions of molars does not close down bite
    e. extrusion of incisors does not produce stable results
30. a. Reverse overjet is associated with class III skeletal pattern
    C. Dental crowding is increased in upper arch
    g. Associated with short anterior cranial base
31. a Crossbites are usually dental in origin
    c. Occurs with or without displacement
    e. Unilateral posterior crossbites can be treated with URA
32. a. Removable appliances are not capable of bodily movement
    d. Intermaxillary traction is not possible
    e. Not efficient of multiple tooth movement

Chapter 4

Periodontics

Identify the following Statements as True (T) or False (F)

1. **Biological width is:**
   a. 2 mm not including sulcus depth
   b. 3 mm including sulcus depth
   c. 4 mm in total
   d. Composed of epithelial and attached gingival fibres.

2. **Periodontal connective tissues are comprised of:**
   a. Alveloar bone
   b. Periodontal ligament
   c. Principal and oxytalan fibres
   d. Nerves, blood vessels and lymphatics
   e. Cementum.

3. **Regarding Ramjford teeth:**
   a. If one tooth missing, then mesial neighboring tooth should be used
   b. If one tooth missing, then distal neighboring tooth should be used
   c. It is used to monitor plaque control in patient but not in clinical trial and epidemiology studies.
   d. $\dfrac{6/14}{41/6}$

4. **Periodontal disease:**
   a. Prevalent in adults only
   b. Gingivitis is not common in children
   c. Young adults and children are at risk of aggressive and early onset disease
   d. Dental patients should be assessed using basic periodontal examination.

5. **Basic periodontal examination:**
   a. Has evolved from Ramfjord teeth
   b. Is quick method of assessing patient's periodontal status
   c. Has evolved from community periodontal index of treatment needs
   d. The coloured band extends from 3–5 mm from tip
   e. Is measured using World Health Organization (WHO) probe
   f. Code 4 indicates full presence of periodontal disease in each quadrant

g. Does record tooth mobility
   h. Does record furcation involvement.
6. **Errors in measuring probing depth:**
   a. Thickness of probe
   b. Contour of the tooth surface
   c. Angulation of probing
   d. Pressure applied
   e. Presence of calculus
   f. Presence of dental plaque
   g. Position of gingival margin
   h. Integrity of tissue at base of pocket.
7. **Bleeding on probing:**
   a. Is from the base of the pocket
   b. Is not a consequence of trauma
   c. Is from epithelial pocket lining and connective tissue
   d. Is not an indicator of active disease
   e. Probing depth of less than 4 mm will still require sub-gingival scaling.
8. **Furcation:**
   a. Is determined by straight explorer
   b. Lesions are present in multi-rooted teeth
   c. Class III includes instrument not passing between the root
   d. Class I includes cul-de-sac involvement
   e. In Class II furcation lesion, instrument do not completely pass through furcation.
9. **Radiographic features of periodontal disease that can be identified as:**
   a. Pattern of bone loss
   b. Furcation involvement
   c. Supra-gingival calculus
   d. Dental plaque
   e. Widening of periodontal ligament
   f. Periapical lesions
   g. Mobility
   h. Overhanging restoration
   i. Decreased alveolar bone height.
10. **Chronic gingivitis is:**
    a. Dental calculus induced
    b. Swollen and spongy in texture
    c. Indicative of presence of true pockets
    d. Increased sulcus depth
    e. Interdental papillae and marginal gingivae are involved after inflammation spread to attached gingivae
    f. Loss of attachment is present.

Periodontics

11. **In chronic periodontitis:**
    a. Junctional epithelium stays coronal to alveolar crest
    b. Junctional epithelium extends apically beyond alveolar crest
    c. Supra-bony defects are present
    d. Loss of attachment and pocket formation
    e. Bleeding on probing only occurs at inflamed sites.

12. **Alveolar bone destruction in periodontal disease:**
    a. Vertical bone defect have better prognosis than horizontal bone defect
    b. One walled vertical defect can be treated successfully
    c. Radiograph shows sites undergoing active bone loss
    d. Fenestration and dehiscence predispose sites to periodontal breakdown.

13. **Porphyromonas gingivalis:**
    a. Is colonizing species found in early plaque
    b. Invades and replicates within gingival epithelial cells
    c. Is generally not encapsulated
    d. Is the cause of localized aggressive periodontitis
    e. Is obligate aerobe.

14. **Polymorphonuclear neutrophils:**
    a. Are found in gingival sulcus
    b. Secrete matrix metalloproteinase 8
    c. Secrete matrix metalloproteinase 1
    d. Destroy periodontal tissues in periodontitis
    e. Are involved in late response to plaque
    f. Form leukocyte-wall
    g. Are not present in the absence of gingivitis.

15. **Guide tissue regeneration (GTR):**
    a. Is treatment of choice of for class I furcation defect
    b. Increased recession following GTR
    c. Resorbable membrane produce better results than non-resorbable membrane
    d. Initiates osseointegration
    e. Membrane is tented to create space for development of blood clot
    f. Polytetrafluoroethylene (PTFE), and expanded Polytetrafluoroethylene (ePTFE) are resorbable membrane
    g. Polylactic acid and collagen are non-resorbable membrane
    h. Healing occurs by secondary intention (TRUE).

16. **Regarding periodontal surgery:**
    a. Is indicated when non-surgical treatment fails due to poor plaque control
    b. Results in formation of long junctional epithelium
    c. Treatment of choice for drug-induced gingival hyperplasia

d. Results in gingival recession
e. Width of keratinized gingivae cannot be maintained.

17. **Alveolar bone destruction:**
    a. Vertical bony defects have better prognosis
    b. Sites with fenestration are at risk for periodontitis
    c. 3-walled defects can be treated successfully than 2-walled defect
    d. Radiograph shows active bone resorption sites
    e. Osteoclasts are stimulated by cytokines.

18. **In gingivectomy:**
    a. Incision should start at base of pocket
    b. Plaque control is less important following gingivectomy
    c. Gingivectomy heals by primary intention
    d. GTR prevents formation of long junctional epithelium
    e. Full Thickness flap should be raised when repositioning apically.

19. **Traumatic occlusal forces can:**
    a. Initiates inflammatory response
    b. Can cause periodontal disease
    c. Can lead to widening of PDL
    d. Causes increased mobility
    e. Can cause loss of attachment.

20. **In periodontal health:**
    a. Width of keratinised gingivae shows variation throughout the mouth
    b. Gingival cervical fluid is not present
    c. No tooth mobility
    d. No periodontal pocket
    e. Alveolar bone crest and cemento-enamel junction are at same level.

21. **Chlorhexidine:**
    a. Is positively charged
    b. Cannot be incorporated into chewing gums
    c. Does not demonstrate substantivity
    d. Available as 1.2% and 0.2% in UK
    e. Broad spectrum antimicrobial.

22. **Drug-induced gingival hyperplasia is caused by:**
    a. Cyclosporin
    b. Nifedipine
    c. Insulin
    d. Metronidazole
    e. Tetracycline.

23. **Acute necrotising ulcerative gingivitis (ANUG):**
    a. Is viral infection
    b. Is associated with pain
    c. Exhibit vesicles formation

Periodontics

   d. First line of treatment is metronidazole
   e. Metronidazole is effective in controlling NUG.
24. **Maxillary molar with Grade I furcation involvement:**
   a. Has horizontal mobility of 1–2 mm
   b. Is usually non-vital
   c. Has horizontal loss of attachment
   d. Can be managed by tunnel preparation
   e. GTR is not indicated.
25. **Acute periodontal lesion:**
   a. Is associated with non-vital tooth
   b. Can be managed by systemic antimicrobials
   c. Results in buccal sinus
   d. Tender to percussion
   e. Locally delivered anti-microbial is first line of treatment.
26. **Random burst model of periodontal disease progression contains:**
   a. Burst of disease activity is not random
   b. Some site remains disease free
   c. Some sites may remain quiescent for long period of time
   d. Multiple sites break down over a period of disease activity
   e. Sites that bleed are the diseased sites.

Identify the Single Best Answer for the following

27. **The most important features of healthy gingivae is:**
   a. Keratinised
   b. Resilient
   c. Scalloped
   d. Colour.
28. **The depth of gingival sulcus is:**
   a. 0.0–1.5 mm
   b. 0.5–2.00 mm
   c. 2 mm–3 mm
   d. 2 mm–4 mm.
29. **The key feature of oral mucosa is:**
   a. Keratinised
   b. Non-keratinised
   c. Appear paler than adjacent gingivae
   d. Firm
   e. Resilient.
30. **The width of attached gingivae:**
   a. Increases with age
   b. Decreases with age
   c. Remain unchanged
   d. Changes with bone level.

31. The attached gingivae:
a. Extends apical from muco-cemento junction to muco-gingival junction
b. Free gingiva to muco-gingival junction
c. Junctional epithelium to muco-gingival junction
d. Sulcular epithelium to muco-gingival junction.

32. The crest of inter-dental alveolar bone lies:
a. Apical to cemento-enamel junction
b. Coronal to muco-gingival junction
c. Apical to sulcular epithelium
d. Apical to junctional epithelium.

33. The crest of interdental alveolar bone is:
a. 0.5–1.5 mm
b. 0.5–2 mm
c. 0.5–3 mm
d. 1.0–3 mm.

34. Gingival connective tissue contains:
a. Blood vessels, lymphatics, ground substance, nerves, fibroblasts, bundles of gingival collagen fibres
b. Blood vessels, lymphatics, ground substance, erythroblast, dento-gingival fibres
c. Transseptal fibres
d. Sulcular fibres
e. Alveolar gingival fibres.

35. Junctional epithelium is attached to tooth surface by:
a. Basal lamina and hemidesmosomes
b. Basal lamina
c. Hemidesmosomes
d. Gingival crevice.

Identify the answers for Extended Matching Questions

36. Regarding periodontal pathogens:
a. These are associated with diseased sites
b. Early colonizing colonies
c. Associated with chronic periodontitis
d. Invades gingival soft tissues and not removed by root surface instrumentation
e. Inhibits phagocytosis of the organism
f. Found in mature sub-gingival plaque

1. Porphyromonas Gingivalis
2. Aggregatibacter actinomycetemcomitans
3. Fusobacterium nucleatum
4. Streptococci
5. Actinomyces species

37. Inflammatory gingivitis:
a. Established lesion is apparent after_____
b. Predominant cells are_____
c. Associated clinically with increased_____
d. Development of gingivitis disease does not show_____

> 1. 2–4 days of plaque growth
> 2. 2–3 weeks of plaque growth
> 3. Plasma cells
> 4. T-cells
> 5. Gingival crevicular fluid
> 6. Histological changes
> 7. Erythema
> 8. Oedema.

Complete the Statements Correctly using the Appropriate Options

38. In Perio-endo lesions:
A. Necrotic pulp drains into (a)_____ and produces periapical abscess known as (b)_____. There is (c)_____ to vitality test. Radiographically, (d)_____(e)_____can be seen and there is no (f)_____of alveolar bone height. Treatment is (g)_____.

B. Untreated or poorly managed endodontic lesion can be persistant source of infection and is classified as (h)_____with (i)_____ involvement._____(j) probing depth, (k)_____or (l)_____on probing is evident clinically. Radiographically, resorption of (m)_____alveolar bone. Treatment is (n)_____, (o)_____, (p)_____, scaling and prophylaxis. (q)_____is inevitable in extensive lesion.

39. Primary periodontal lesion:
A. Periodontal infection that spreads to periapical tissues is (a)_____ lesion. Clinically, it can be (b)_____, (c)_____pain and has (d)_____ response to vitality test.

B. Radiograph shows (e)_____bone resorption, can be (f)_____, (g)_____or (h)_____defects. Treatment includes (i)_____and (j)_____. In extensive lesion, (k)_____is considered.

40. Primary periodontal secondary lesion:
A. When infection spreads from periodontium to pulp causing (a)_____, it is classified as (b)_____with (c)_____involvement. Clinically, tooth gives (d)_____response to vitality test.

B. Radiographically, bone loss is (e)_____. Treatment includes (f)_____, (g)_____and (h)_____. (i)_____can be considered for deeper pockets and anatomical defects.

41. Combined lesions:
a. Periodontal lesions (a)_____with endodontic lesion of pulpal origin is called (b)_____. Periodontal attachment is (c)_____with (d)_____ tooth mobility. Prognosis is usually (e)_____.

1.	Primary periodontal lesion	19.	Gain
2.	Primary endodontal lesion	20.	Excruciating
3.	Secondary periodontal lesion	21.	Vertical
		22.	Horizontal
4.	Secondary endodontal-lesion	23.	Reduced
		24.	Increased
5.	Negative	25.	Bleeding
6.	Positive	26.	Extensive
7.	Radiolucency	27.	Necrosis
8.	Radioopacity	28.	Good
9.	Periapical	29.	Poor
10.	Coronal	30.	Oral hygiene index (OHI)
11.	Coalesces	31.	Pus
12.	Pulpal	32.	Root surface instrumentation (RSI)
13.	Periodontum	33.	RCT
14.	Furcational	34.	Re-RCT
15.	Generalised	35.	Extraction
16.	Localised	36.	Periodontal surgery
17.	Dull	37.	Crestal
18.	Loss	38.	Combined lesions

Match the following:

BPE code	Clinical features	Treatment needs
0	(a) No calculus, no bleeding on probing	(1) OHI, eliminate plaque retentive factors, RSI
1	(b) No calculus, but bleeding on probing	(2) OHI, eliminate plaque retentive factors, Scaling and RSI
2	(c) No pockets more than 3 mm, supra or sub-gingival calculus, overhanging restoration	(3) OHI
3	(d) Probing depth greater than 3.5 mm but less than 5.5 mm	(4) Full periodontal assessment 6 ppt, mobility, recession and furcation involvement. Referral to specialist
4	(e) Probing depth greater than 5.5 mm	(5) No periodontal treatment required
*	(f) Furcation or total loss of attachment of 7 mm or more	(6) Complex treatment with/without flap, OHI, RSI and referral to specialist

Abbreviations: BPE-Basic periodontal examination; OHI-Oral hygiene index; RSI-Root surface instrumentation

CASE DISCUSSIONS

Case 1: Acute Necrotising Ulcerative Gingivitis (NUG)

- A 45-year old man attends your clinic complaining of bad taste in mouth and painful gums with recent onset. On examination, the patient has poor oral hygiene, yellow-grey ulcers of inter-dental papillae. Discuss likely diagnosis, risk factors and management of the patient
- In order to reach correct diagnosis, it is important to take history in patients own words—patient's complaint, history of complaint and history of pain including nature of pain, intensity and duration of pain, aggravating and relieving factors along with most recent medical and dental history. It should then be followed by extra-oral examination for swelling, injuries, facial symmetry and temporomandibular joint (TMJ) displacement, if any. Intra-oral examination is then followed by examining soft tissues and hard tissue examination for any pathology
- The diagnosis is NUG is based on the complaint and history of complaint. NUG is extremely painful condition and is characterized by painful ulcers of inter-dental papillae, clinically appearing as 'punched out'. The ulcers bleed readily on probing and patient often complains of metallic taste and foul smell in the mouth.

Risk Factors

- Poor oral hygiene
- Smoking
- Stress
- malnourished/immuno-compromised
- Persistent NUG in healthy adult can be associated with human immunodeficiency virus (HIV) infection.

Treatment

- Importance of good oral hygiene and plaque control to be discussed with patient
- Oral hygiene instructions to be reinforced
- Supra-gingival ultrasonic scaling under local anaesthesia. If not possible due to pain, can be done a week later
- Use of chlorhexidine mouth wash to irrigate and rinse necrotic slough
- Metronidazole 200–400 mg TDS for 3 days
- Smoking cessation and stress management advice
- Long-term management to include regular dental visits, maintenance of oral hygiene and manage risk factors.

Case 2—Perio-Endo Lesions.

- A patient presents to your clinic with pain in lower left permanent first molar (LL6), radiograph shows periapical radiolucency and bone loss in the above mentioned area. Discuss the likely diagnosis, treatment and management of this patient.
- In order to reach correct diagnosis, it is important to take history in patients own words—patient's complaint, history of complaint and history of pain including nature of pain, intensity and duration of pain, aggravating and relieving factors along with most recent medical and dental history. It should then be followed by extra-oral examination for swelling, injuries, facial symmetry and TMJ displacement, if any. Intra-oral examination is then followed by examining soft tissues and hard tissue examination for any pathology. After clinical examination, clinical investigation and special investigations are performed to aid diagnosis.

Look for:
- Pain as vitality
- Pain as percussion
- Pain as pocket.

Investigations

Periapical radiographs (LL6):
- Periodontal and periapical pathology can often co-exists which can result in diagnostic dilemma
- There is very little evidence to support the notion that periodontitis can lead to pulpal necrosis
- However, pulpal pathology can aggravate periodontal pathology.

Diagnosis	Primary periodontal pathology	Primary endodontic pathology
History	No history of toothache	History of toothache
Percussion	TTP mainly laterally	TTP vertically
Probing	Periodontal pocket always present	No pockets
Probing sinus	Can lead to pocket	Can lead to apex
Sinus drainage	Discharge through pocket	Discharge over apex
Swelling	Present mainly attached gingivae	Mainly at apex
Vitality test	Usually positive	Negative
Radiographs	Vertical bone loss	Apical radiolucency
Treatment	Periodontal therapy	Endodontic therapy
Abbreviation: TTP-Tenderness to percussion		

In order to reach accurate diagnosis, the general dental practitioner must take accurate history, conduct thorough clinical examination and investigations.

Both the lesions can co-exists, in that case resolve acute infection by drainage and antibiotics therapy. Follow with conventional RCT. The periodontal lesion should resolve over the period of few months. The worst prognosis is often due to extension of periapical pathology to periodontal pockets. This usually occurs when endodontic treatment fails to resolve the lesion of pulpal pathology.

Case 3: Furcation involvement.

- A 37-year-old man patient presents with grade II mobility of lower right permanent first molar (LR6). On examination, there is clinical evidence of furcation involvement. Discuss furcation involvement, treatment options available and management.
- In order to reach correct diagnosis, it is important to take history in patient's own words—patient's complaint, history of complaint and pain history including nature of pain, intensity and duration of pain, aggravating and relieving factors along with most recent medical and dental history. It should then be followed by extra-oral examination for swelling, injuries, facial symmetry and TMJ displacement, if any. Intra-oral examination is then followed by examining soft tissues and hard tissue examination for any pathology. After clinical examination, clinical investigations and special investigations are to be performed to aid diagnosis
- Periodontal disease when extends into the bifurcation or trifurcation of multi-rooted teeth is known as furcation involvement. Diagnosis is made by thorough clinical examination, by probing into the furcation, and radiographically. Radiographs show the degree and extent of alveolar bone loss both mesially and distally, and in the furcation area.

Classification

- 1st degree: Horizontal loss of support not exceeding 1/3 tooth width (**Fig. 4.1**)
  - ➢ Treatment: Scaling and root planning, possibly furcation plasty.
- 2nd degree: Horizontal loss of support exceeding 1/3 but not total width of furcation area (**Fig. 4.2**)
  - ➢ Treatment: May require furcation plasty and/or tunnel preparation, and/or root resection, and/or extraction.
- 3rd degree: Horizontal through and through destruction of the furcation area
  - ➢ Treatment: May require tunnel preparation, and/or root resection, and/or extraction.

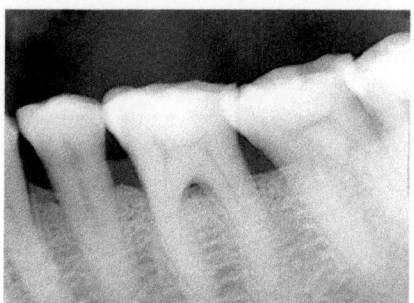
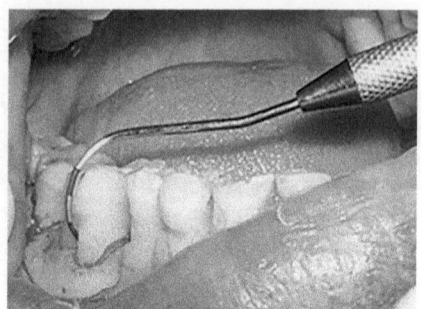

Fig. 4.1: 1st degree furcation involvement

Fig. 4.2: 2nd degree furcation involvement

Treatment Techniques

- **Scaling and root surface instrumentation:** Can only be successful, if patient keeps area clean post-treatment.
- **Furcation plasty:** A surgical procedure involving muco-periosteal flap to be raised for scaling and root planing and removal of tooth structure in the furcation to widen access for cleaning. Osseous recontouring may be required. Flaps are then repositioned and sutured. There is a potential risk of pulpal damage, caries and denture sensitivity post-operatively.
- **Tunnel preparation:** A surgical procedure similar to furcation plasty involving buccal-lingual flaps to be raised and exposing entire furcation area. The flaps are then sutured together intra-radicularly to expose large furcation. There can be increased risk of post-operative pulpal exposure, caries and dentine sensitivity. This is most valuable for lower molars in patients with excellent oral hygiene.
- **Root resection:** This involves amputation of one or two roots of a multi-rooted tooth leaving crown and root stump intact. The intact root needs to be treated endodontically with good periodontal support and should be restorable. Resection of the root is followed by smoothing, contouring and restoration of pulp cavity. This procedure can be difficult in maxillary molars.
- **Hemisection:** This involves division of two-rooted tooth in half for two smaller units with single root each. RCT is indicated pre-operatively and restoration of the crowns post-operatively.
- **Extraction:** Removal of periodontally affected tooth with poor prognosis.
- **Guided tissue regeneration (GTR):** It interposes a barrier to epithelial migration prior to treatment both surgically and non-surgically. This stimulates both bone and connective tissue deposition **(Fig. 4.3)**. The effectiveness of these techniques are currently under review. Examples: Millipore, PTFE, Goretex, Resolute, Tissue growth factor B2 and BMP.
- **Enamel matrix derivatives:** Helps in formation of acellular cementum and are locally applied on root surface. These substances like amelogenin are found in Hertwig's root sheath and induce root formation during development. Example: Endogain.

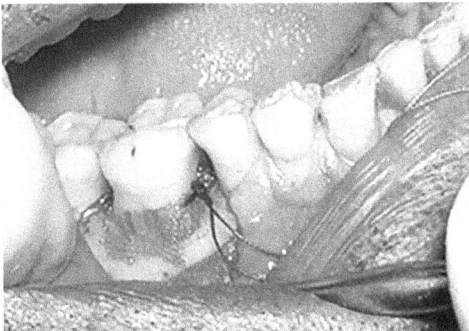

Fig. 4.3: Guided tissue regeneration technique

- It is extremely important for patient to maintain excellent oral hygiene in order to make these treatments successful.

Case 4: Localised aggressive periodontitis.

- A 12-year-old girl patient attends your clinic. Clinical examination reveals fair oral hygiene, drifted upper left permanent central incisor, pocketing around central incisors and first molar. What is the likely diagnosis? Discuss management and complication if any.
- In order to reach correct diagnosis, it is of paramount importance to take history in patient's own words—patient's complaint, history of complaint and pain history (including nature of pain, intensity and duration of the pain, aggravating and relieving factors) along with most recent medical and dental history. It should then be followed by extra-oral examination for swelling, injuries, facial symmetry and TMJ displacement, if any. Intra-oral examination is then followed by examining soft tissues and hard tissue examination for any pathology. After clinical examination, clinical investigations and special investigations are to be performed to aid diagnosis.
- Patient has localised aggressive periodontitis as per history and clinical examination. It is found in children and adolescents. Localised aggressive periodontitis is localized to upper and lower incisors and first molars. The gingivae around these affected teeth have normal appearance but deep periodontal pockets. The patients usually have fair oral hygiene but degree of destruction is out of proportion.
- *Aggregatibacter actinomycetemcomitans (AA)* is a major pathogen. Others include Eubacterium and bacteriodes like species. Prevalence of localised aggressive periodontitis is low approximately 0.2%, common in girls mainly Afro-Caribbean (2.5%) and often familial. These patients may have neutrophils abnormalities, macrophage chemotaxis and phagocytosis. These defects are usually inherited and therefore are familial.

Management
- Oral prohylaxis
- Scaling and root planing with/without access flap surgery
- Antibiotics: Systemic and local
    - Oxytetracycline 250 mgs QDS for 2-3 weeks
    - Doxycycline 100 mg OD for 2-3 weeks
    - Metronidazole 400 mg QDS for 7-14 days
    - Locally deposited slow release tetracycline (Dentomycin gel).
- Combination therapy—250 mg Amoxicillin TDS and Metronidazole 400 mg TDS for 7 days
- Host modulatory agents (Periostat 20 mg twice daily)
- Long-term maintenance with 3 month monitoring.

Risk
Tetracycline deposits in growing bone and teeth which results in staining and hypoplasia in permanent dentition therefore, tetracycline should be avoided in children under 12 years and during pregnancy.

Answers

1.	a.	T	b.	F	c.	F	d.	T		
2.	a.	T	b.	T	c.	T	d.	T	e.	T
3.	a.	F	b.	T	c.	F				
4.	a.	F	b.	F	c.	T	d.	T		
5.	a.	F	b.	T	c.	T	d.	F	e.	T
	f.	F	g.	F	h.	T				
6.	a.	T	b.	T	c.	T	d.	T	e.	T
	f.	F	g.	T						
7.	a.	T	b.	F	c.	T	d.	F	e.	F
8.	a.	F	b.	T	c.	F	d.	F	e.	T
9.	a.	T	b.	T	c.	F	d.	F	e.	T
	f.	T	g.	F	h.	T	i.	F		
10.	a.	F	b.	T	c.	F	d.	T	e.	F
	f.	F								
11.	a.	T	b.	T	c.	F	d.	T	e.	F
12.	a.	T	b.	F	c.	F	d.	F		
13.	a.	F	b.	T	c.	F	d.	F	e.	F
14.	a.	T	b.	T	c.	F	d.	T	e.	F
	f.	T	g.	F						
15.	a.	F	b.	T	c.	F	d.	F	e.	T
	f.	F	g.	F						
16.	a.	F	b.	T	c.	F	d.	T	e.	F
17.	a.	F	b.	F	c.	T	d.	F	e.	T
18.	a.	F	b.	F	c.	F				
19.	a.	F	b.	F	c.	T	d.	T	e.	F
20.	a.	T	b.	F	c.	F	d.	T	e.	F
21.	a.	T	b.	F	c.	F	d.	F	e.	T
22.	a.	T	b.	T	c.	F	d.	F	e.	F
23.	a.	F	b.	T	c.	F	d.	F	e.	T
24.	a.	F	b.	F	c.	T	d.	F	e.	F
25.	a.	F	b.	F	c.	F	d.	T	e.	F
26.	a.	F	b.	T	c.	T	d.	F	e.	F

27. a 28. b 29. b 30. a 31. a
32. a 33. a 34. a 35. a

36.	a.	1, 2	b.	4, 5	c.	3	d.	2	e.	1
	f.	1								
37.	a.	2	b.	3	c.	5	d.	6		
38.	a.	13	b.	2	c.	5	d.	9	e.	7
	f.	18	g.	33	h.	2	i.	3	j.	24
	k.	25	l.	31	m.	37	n.	33	o.	34
	p.	30	q.	35						
39.	a.	1	b.	16	c.	17	d.	6	e.	16
	f.	21	g.	22	h.	14	i.	32	j.	30
	k.	35								
40.	a.	27	b.	1	c.	4	d.	5	e.	26
41.	a.	11	b.	38	c.	23	d.	24	e.	29
42.	a.	5	b.	3	c.	2	d.	1	e.	6
	f.	4								

Chapter 5

Conservative Dentistry

Identify the following Statements as True (T) or False (F)

1. **With regards to anatomy of enamel:**
   a. Enamel is not prone to acid demineralisation from caries but only due to erosion
   b. Elastic dentine is required for good support
   c. The organic component is 86–95%
   d. The water component is 1–2%
   e. The rods and prisms are oriented at 45° angle to the external surface
   f. The aim of the restoration is to define aesthetics of the dentition.

2. **Properties of dentine:**
   a. Comprises 45–50% of organic matrix
   b. Comprises 30% of inorganic matrix
   c. Comprises 15–20% of water
   d. Peritubular dentine is the primary structure component
   e. Intertubular dentine is collagen free
   f. Peritubular dentine has hypermineralised tubular wall
   g. Intertubular dentine is filled with extended processes of odontoblasts
   h. Dentinal tubules forms interface between dentine and pulp.

3. **Dentine hypersensitivity:**
   a. All exposed dentine give rise to the symptoms of hypersensitivity
   b. There are specific nerve endings that lie within the tubules that cause dentine hypersensitivity symptoms
   c. Pain arises in response to thermal stimulus only
   d. Capillary expansion is related to hydrodynamic fluid movement
   e. Dentine hypersensitivity increases with age
   f. The treatment is to reduce permeability of dentinal tubules.

4. **Rubber dam:**
   a. Latex dental dam is available in assorted color and light shades
   b. Width of dental dam is 4 × 6 inches for successful use
   c. 5 × 6 inches width and is thin, medium, heavy, extra and special heavy weight or thickness
   d. 7 × 9 inches width is heavy, medium and light weight
   e. Dental rubber dam material is available in 5 × 5 inch (12.5 × 12.5 cm) or 6 × 6 inch (15 × 15 cm) sheets.

5. **Retraction cords facilitate:**
   a. Better accessibility
   b. Control gingival bleeding
   c. Control crevicular fluid seepage
   d. Provide anaesthetic effect.

6. **Basic instrument formula:**
   a. The basic instrument formula consists of three units whose measurements are based upon the metric system
   b. Fourth unit is placed in the third position of the formula, i.e. after length of blade
   c. Fourth unit is placed in the second position of the formula, i.e. before the length of the blade
   d. The third represents the angle which the blade forms with the axis of the handle. This angle is expressed in 100th of a circle or centigrades
   e. The instruments with their cutting edges at an angle other than right angle to the long axis of the blade, a fourth unit is added to basic three unit formula.

7. **Excavators:**
   a. It is to remove caries and to shape the walls, floor, line angle and point angle during cavity preparation by clearing, planning or lateral scraping
   b. According to Black's instrument nomenclature, hand-cutting instruments are of the order "excavator"
   c. Spoon excavator is a double plane instrument that is a modified hatchet
   d. The cutting edge of the spoon excavator is rounded.

8. **Rake angle:**
   a. Rake angle is the angle between the rake centre and the radial line
   b. Rake angle is the angle between the rake face and the radial line (line connecting the center of the bur and the blade)
   c. For cutting hard, brittle materials, a negative rake angle minimises fractures of the cutting edge there by increasing the tool life
   d. A rake angle is said to be negative when the rake face is ahead of the radius
   e. A rake angle is said to be negative when the rake face is behind the radius.

9. **Occlusion:**
   a. The term occlusion describes a functional complex which includes all of the components of the nervous and muscular system and the function or parafunction in which they are engaged
   b. The term occlusion describes a functional complex which includes all of the components of the masticatory system (teeth, periodontium, jaws, joints, nerves and muscles) and the function or parafunction in which they are engaged

c. Occlusion performs the function of bringing the jaws and teeth together during chewing, swallowing, other body movements, along with in parafunction, i.e. clenching and grinding of teeth
d. Centric occlusion is the position of maximum intercuspation of teeth which is in harmony with the neuromuscular mechanism
e. Centric relation refers to a retrusive opening and closing of the mandible on a hinge like axis, movement of about 25 mm.

10. **Carious lesion:**
    a. A carious lesion on the smooth surface of enamel is conical in shape with its broad base on enamel surface and the tip on the dentinoenamel junction
    b. The double inverted cone type of penetration is present, if carious lesion spreads laterally along the junction of dentine and pulp
    c. The carious lesion found in pits and fissures establish their initial penetration through the small enamel defect and broaden in area as the dentin is approached. At the DEJ, the lesion extends laterally at a somewhat more rapid rate that it does pulpally
    d. Smooth surface carious lesions on the proximal surfaces of teeth where normal contacts are present are readily detected by an explorer
    e. Peak rates for the incidence of new lesions occurs 5 years after the eruption of the tooth
    f. Dental caries is said to be extensive when distance between infected dentin and pulp is less than 1 mm.

11. **Patient evaluation:**
    a. Complete mouth examination requires 2 bitewing and 16 periapical films
    b. Recurrent caries at the cervical margin of restorations can frequently be observed from the posterior bitewing films
    c. Excavators are hand cutting instruments considered part of dental equipment
    d. 11 o'clock position provides access to all areas, except the more distal areas of the mandibular right quadrant and the cervical areas on the patient's right posterior quadrants. It is considered universal position for operator
    e. 12 o'clock position is utilised for the maxillary and mandibular interior segments
    f. Sizes of mouth mirror in common use are from the No.1 to the No.2.

12. **GV black classification:**
    a. Class II cavity are those cavities which occur on the proximal surface of bicuspids and molars
    b. Cavosurface angle is the angle formed at the junction of the dentin wall and enamel tooth surface
    c. Class I are pit and fissure cavities that occur in the occlusal surface of bicuspids and molars, the occlusal two-third of the buccal and lingual surface of the molar and the lingual surfaces of incisors

d. Class VI are cavities on the incisal edges of anterior or cusp tips of posterior teeth
e. By relating the carious lesions to their classic clinical location, GV black developed a cavity classification listing two classes as pits and fissures and three classes of smooth surface lesions.

13. **Dental caries:**
    a. The composition and thickness of dental plaque plays an important role in the development of carious lesion
    b. The composition and flow rate of saliva is important to maintain equilibrium between remineralisation and demineralisation
    c. Caries can be defined as progressive dissolution of dental hard tissue mediated by sugar intake
    d. Gingival inflammation cause demineralisation and remineralisation process
    e. Salivary flow rate does not modify caries development.

14. **Development of dental caries:**
    a. Caries in pits and fissures have wide area of origin
    b. Caries on smooth coronal surface are narrow at origin and wide at base
    c. Caries can develop as diffuse lesion
    d. The carious lesion progresses from white to brown spot to shadowing and surface breakdown
    e. Dentine caries progresses slowly due to increased resistance of dentine to acid dissolution
    f. Radiographs are best to diagnose occlusal caries
    g. Root caries are predominantly caused by gingival recession.

15. **Tooth wear:**
    a. Tooth wear can be exaggerated by xerostomia
    b. Erosion can only be caused by extrinsic acids
    c. This can be recorded as occupational hazard
    d. Attrition results due to parafunctional activities
    e. Reduction of posterior support may not lead to tooth wear
    f. Abrasion can only be caused by external sources
    g. Aetiology of tooth wear can also be due to eating disorders
    h. Management of tooth wear is limited to diet and oral hygiene advice only.

16. **With regards to restorations:**
    a. The primary indication of restorations is to restore aesthetics
    b. Cavity design is based on the principle of extension for prevention
    c. Tooth preparation should only be based on the requirements of the restorative material being used
    d. Unsupported enamel can be left if resin composite restoration is placed
    e. Margins should not be extended into the areas of cleaning and instrumentation

f. Resistance form is a cavity design used to resist any forces that will dislodge the restoration from the cavity
g. Dentin pins reduces amalgam's tensile and compressive strength
h. Friction grip is the most common dentin pin used in the present day.

17. **In adhesive dentistry:**
    a. In adhesive dentistry bonding occurs by strong Van der Waal forces
    b. Adequate surface wetting is required for increased surface tension
    c. Interatomic bonds to develop across tooth and restoration interface
    d. Quality of bond does not depend upon effect of repeated thermo-cycling
    e. Macro-tags during enamel bonding contributes mostly to the bond strength
    f. Rubbing is the preferred method of action for etching agent
    g. 1.6–3.5% oxalic acid can be used as dentine conditioning agent
    h. Air thinning is preferred to maintain sufficient film thickness
    i. Ceramic bonding agent results in area of macroporosity in expansion of ceramic surface area.

18. **Anterior restoration:**
    a. Cavity design is not important in anterior teeth
    b. Polymerisation shrinkage in composite can cause contraction forces of 4–7 MPa
    c. Glass ionomer cement have increased coefficient of thermal expansion than composites
    d. Desiccation in GIC causes shrinkage and crazing
    e. Compomer has increased compressive and flexural strength than composite.

19. **Posterior restorations:**
    a. Bevelling does not result in transverse cut enamel rod
    b. Gingival margin can be beveled below enamel-cement junction
    c. Occlusal bevelling is recommended where occlusal stops may be present
    d. High copper alloys result in elimination of strong gamma-2 phase
    e. Chemically cured resins polymerize towards the light source
    f. Lighter shades of composite cure better
    g. Onlays are preferred to amalgam restoration
    h. Polymerisation shrinkage does not occurs while placing indirect restorations
    i. There are no gaps in marginal fit of CAD-CAM restorations.

20. **Extra-coronal restorations:**
    a. Silane coupling agent provide strong chemical bond between silicone dioxide in porcelain and BIS-GMA polymer of composite
    b. Enamel reduction at gingival margin should be minimum 0.5 mm in the area (0.3 mm and 0.5 mm elsewhere)
    c. Occlusion in centric position is most important and should be assessed

d. A heavy chamfer is preferred for bevel for full gold veneer crown and metal ceramic crown
e. Shoulder bevel is used with inlay or onlay preparation only
f. Putty index can also used before tooth preparation.

21. **Crown and bridge:**
    a. The aim of the gingival cord is to displace gingival tissue laterally away from tooth than to force the cord into the depth of the sulcus
    b. Electrosurgery can also be used instead of retraction cord
    c. Polysulfides are the material of choice for crown and bridge impression
    d. Aluminium sulfate is incorporated in tissue management system by Ultradent
    e. Crown-lengthening surgery is not indicated
    f. Compatibility of impression material with disinfection solution and cast material is generally less important
    g. Putty and wash technique is used in custom tray.

22. **Bridgework:**
    a. Fixed movable bridge utilises only proprietary precision attachment between two parts of bridge
    b. Compound bridges is combination of fixed and cantilever element in single casting bridge
    c. Hybrid bridges are easy to place and is not technique sensitive
    d. Ridge lap is the most desirable pontic design
    e. Orthodontic uprighting can be indicated
    f. Use of facebow registration and semi-adjustable articulator is optional in crown and bridge work.

Identify the Single Best Answer for the following

23. **The teeth most commonly congenitally absent:**
    a. Mandibular 2nd bicuspids
    b. Mandibular lateral incisors
    c. Maxillary 1st bicuspids
    d. Mandibular primary 1st molar.

24. **The system to designate a tooth which is easy to communicate, simple to understand and teach is:**
    a. Zsigmondy system
    b. FDI/Two digit system
    c. Universal system
    d. None of the above.

25. **The term "occlusion" is used to define a functional complex that includes:**
    a. Teeth and the jaws
    b. Teeth, periodontium jaw joints
    c. Teeth, nerves and muscles
    d. All of above.

26. This represents a pit and fissure lesions:
    a. Apex of cone facing each other
    b. Base of cone facing each other
    c. Double inverted cone
    d. None of the above.

27. The most frequently used materials for restorative treatment are:
    a. Composite resin
    b. Alginate
    c. Amalgam and intermediate restorative material
    d. Dental gold alloy.

28. The most universal operating position for operator:
    a. 11 o'clock
    b. 3 o'clock
    c. 6 o'clock
    d. 12 o'clock.

29. The colour matching for composites when done in a dry state, would make the tooth appear:
    a. Same as of the adjacent teeth
    b. Lighter than the adjacent teeth
    c. Darker than that of the adjacent teeth
    d. Does not have any effect.

30. The purposes of cavity preparation is/are:
    a. Removal of all the defects of enamel, dentin and cementum
    b. Locate the margins of restoration as conservatively as possible
    c. Esthetic and functional placement of restorative material
    d. All of the above.

31. Who first described the mixture clove oil and zinc oxide forms a plastic mass:
    a. EJ Molnar
    b. JF Thomas
    c. EC Chisolm
    d. JK Avery.

32. Iontophoresis aids in:
    a. Reducing dentin sensitivity
    b. Mineralisation
    c. Demineralisation
    d. Increasing dentin permeability.

33. The radiolucent material is:
    a. Amalgam
    b. Some composite resin
    c. Calcium hydroxide
    d. Glass ionomer.

34. **This cement form chemical bond with the tooth structure:**
    a. Zinc polycarboxylate and zinc phosphate
    b. Zinc phosphate and glass ionomer
    c. Zinc polycarboxylate and glass ionomer
    d. Zinc polycarboxylate and eugenol.

35. **Cavity varnish indicated under amalgam restorations because:**
    a. Improves the marginal seal
    b. Prevents galvanic currents from reaching the pulp
    c. Is an effective thermal insulator
    d. None of the above.

36. **"Theta triangles" refer to:**
    a. Rubber dam retainers
    b. Cotton roll holders
    c. Absorbent wafers
    d. Cotton rolls.

37. **The easy and quick method of tooth separation is:**
    a. Grass line ligature thread
    b. Mechanical separation
    c. Chemical separation
    d. True separator.

38. **The material of hand-cutting instruments made up of:**
    a. Carbon stainless steel
    b. Gold
    c. Acrylic
    d. Porcelain.

39. **Most often used thickness of the matrix band is:**
    a. 0.015 inch
    b. 0.0015 cm
    c. 0.0015 inch
    d. 0.0028 mm.

40. **The term "universal precautions" means:**
    a. All patients are treated as infectious
    b. All patients and blood contaminated body fluids are treated as infectious
    c. High-risk group patients are only treated as infectious
    d. None of the above.

41. **The duration of dentinal pain is:**
    a. Greater than 5 minutes
    b. Less than 1 to 3 minutes
    c. About 4 minutes
    d. Less than 1 to 3 seconds.

42. The microhardness value of the reparative dentin is:
    a. 30 KHN
    b. 40 KHN
    c. 61 KHN
    d. 65 KHN.

Identify the Answers for Extended Matching questions

43. Regarding infection control:
    a. Best method for sterilising complex instruments and delicate materials
    b. Sterilisation method operates at 270°F (131°C) and 20 pounds of pressure
    c. An alternative means of sterilisation by chemical steam under pressure
    d. The most gentle method of sterilisation used for hand-pieces
    e. Carbon steel instruments and BURS are best sterilised.

    1. Ethylene oxide sterilisation
    2. Chemiclave
    3. Chemical vapor pressure steriliser
    4. Dry heat sterilisation.

44. Sterilisation method that readily achieved at temperatures above 160°C and 320°F. Regarding tooth preparation:
    a. The class V cavity preparation is
    b. Class VII division 2 cavity is
    c. Class VII division 1 cavity is

    1. Convex mesiodistally
    2. Convex mesiodistally
    3. Cavities on labial surface of anterior teeth in the region of incisal third without involving incisal edge
    4. Cavities in the middle third on the labial surface of anterior teeth
    5. Cavities on proximal surface of anterior teeth
    6. Cavities on cervical region on labial surface in anterior teeth
    7. Class II cavity
    8. Class I cavity
    9. Class V cavity

    d. Cavity occurring on the lingual fossa of incisors.

CASE DISCUSSION

Case 1

A 15-year-old girl attends your dental practice and is concerned about appearance of her front teeth. She has evidence of tooth surface loss on her anterior teeth. Please discuss management of this patient.

Tooth wear can also be called as non-carious tooth tissue loss or tooth surface loss. Physiological tooth surface loss is inevitable but unsatisfactory appearance, sensitivity and mechanical condition requires further investigation and treatment.

Types of Tooth Surface Loss

- **Abrasion:** Physical wear of a tooth caused by external agent. Toothbrushes can cause cervical notches on teeth. Abfraction lesions also caused due to flexure of teeth under excessive occlusal loading **(Fig. 5.1)**.
- **Erosion:** Tooth surface loss from non-bacterial chemical attack. Presence of acid results in demineralisation and tooth surface loss occurs in conjunction with abrasion, attrition or both. Dietary and gastrointestinal can cause tooth surface loss. Gastric reflux, vomiting (due bulimia or pregnancy), alcoholism will require referral **(Fig. 5.2)**.
- **Attrition:** Physical wear caused by movement of one teeth against another both interproximally and occlusally. Abrasive diet and bruxism causes attrition **(Fig. 5.3)**.

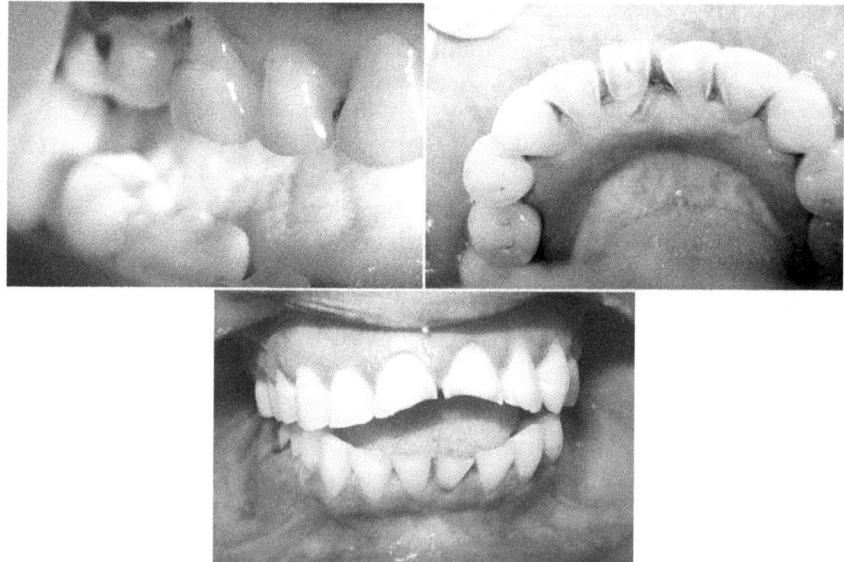

Fig. 5.1: Abrasion

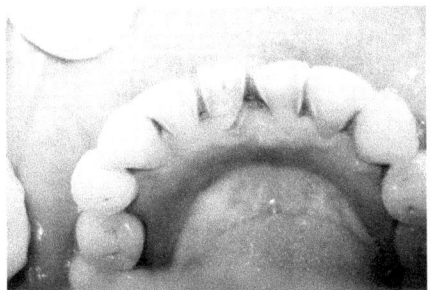

Fig. 5.2: Erosion

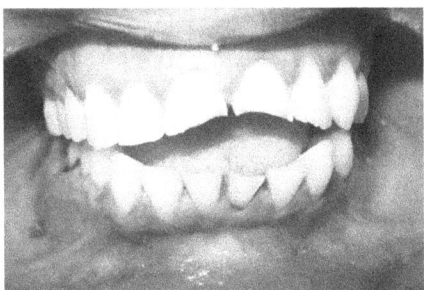

Fig. 5.3: Attrition

- Patient complaint: patient is unhappy and concerned about appearance of her anterior teeth
- History of complaint: Since what age or how long she has had this problem
- Comprehensive medical history should be taken including bulimia
- History of any pregnancy and Gastric reflux disease should also be included.
- Complete dental history including history of Bruxism, TMJ problems,
- Diet/Social history should include consumption of soda; Acidic drinks; Lemon vinegars; Alcohol.
- A complete extra-oral examination should be carried out including if patient is generally fit and well-induced TMJ examination.
- A thorough intraoral examination should include dental and restoration status, note any evidence of occlusal wear, evidence of tooth surface loss-labially, palatally or occlusally.

Diagnosis

- Dietary: Erosion on the labial surface of incisors are the first evidences.
- Gastric reflux and bulimia: Wear on palatal surface of upper incisors as gastric acid comes in contact with palatal surface first
- Attrition: Occlusal wear, usually caused by bruxism in conjunction with erosion and abrasion.
- Abrasion: Tooth wear caused by other surface like toothbrushes

Clinical Records
- Take clinical history, study models, photographs and toothwear indices to have baseline records prior to treatment.

Management
- Prevention: Discuss condition and its causes, removal of causative factors, referral of specialist of gastrointestinal (GI) problems and/or psychiatrist for eating disorder
- Monitor if not severe using baseline occlusal records
- GI or resin composite restoration to improve appearance and decreased sensitivity
- Excessive toothwear: Increase occlusal vertical dimension for aesthetic crown, acrylic overdentures are also an option but they are not aesthetically pleasing
- Referral to restoration specialist for complex restorative problem.

Case 2: Restorative Materials

A 45-year-old patient attends your dental practice and would like to know more about the direct restorative filling material options for restoring his lower left first molar permanent molar.
- Patient complaint: Patient complains about his current restoration on lower left first molar permanent molar is discoloured.
- History of complaint: Since when it has started bothering him? When was the restoration placed?
- Medical history: Any significant medical history/any sensitivity/any pain, etc.
- Dental history: Current restoration status of lower left first molar permanent molar—if it is vital, non vital, any endodontic treatment, direct or indirect restorations and extraction (**Fig. 5.4**).

Advantages of Composite
- Aesthically pleasing
- Conservative cavity preparation

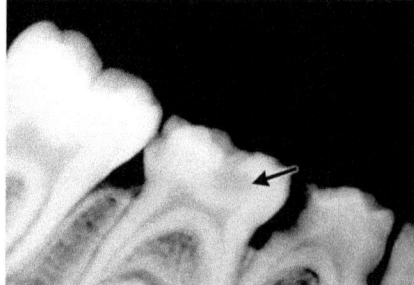

Fig. 5.4: Radiographic examination of lower left first molar permanent molar

- Conservative tooth tissue removal
- Provide insulation
- Decreased thermal conductivity
- Good bonding, retention, no staining, microleakage
- Can be repaired.

Disadvantages

- Polymerisation shrinkage
- Time consuming (isolation, etch, bond, and resin)
- Technique sensitive
- Finishing and polishing can be time consuming
- Difficult to maintain contact point
- Increased occlusal wear in increased occlusal stress
- Increased coefficient of thermal expansion.

Advantages of Amalgam

- Easy to use
- Increased compressive strength
- Wear resistance
- Less expensive than composite
- Not aesthetically pleasing
- No insulation
- Increased tooth substance removal, i.e. extensive preparation is required
- Weaken tooth structure
- Initial microleakage
- Difficult tooth/cavity design.

Bonded Amalgams

- Decreased microleakage
- Decreased staining
- Increased strength of remaining tooth structure
- Decreased post-operative sensitivity
- Retention benefit
- Technique sensitive.

Ask patient if they have any questions or if patient needs more information.

Case 3: Discoloured Dentition

A 23-year-old female patient attends your dental practice complaining of discolored teeth **(Fig. 5.5)**. Please discuss management of the patient.
- Patient complaint: Stained teeth and is unhappy with her appearance
- History: When did patient first noticed discolouration? Is the discolouration generalised or localised

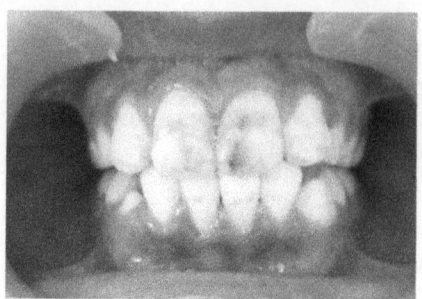

Fig. 5.5: Discolouration of teeth

- Medical history: Comprehensive medical history should be taken including history of any childhood illness, any medications taken in childhood or any treatments.
- Dental history:
  - Restoration status of the dentition should be noted whether dentition is mildly, moderately or heavily restored
  - if oral hygiene is good, average or poor.
- Extra-oral examination should include any history of trauma, trips, falls or accidents
- Intra-oral examination should include whether there is generalised or localised staining, oral hygiene, plaque index, or presence of calculus?

Causes of Tooth Discoloration

- Extrinsic staining:
  - Food and diet
  - Inadequate plaque removal
  - Poor oral hygiene, smoking habits.
- Intrinsic staining:
  - Amelogenesis or dentinogenesis imperfecta
  - Fluorosis
  - Tetracycline staining
  - Trauma
  - Hypoplasia
  - Age-related
  - Dental decay/root canal treatment.

Treatment Option

- Scaling and polishing should be sufficient if oral hygiene is poor
- Microabrasion with acid and pumice.

Bleaching or Whitening

- Vital bleaching: In surgery bleaching or chairside bleaching using 30–35% carbamide or hydrogen peroxide.

- Home bleaching: Custom made bleaching splints (10% carbamide 6-8 hrs/day (4-6 day).
- Non-vital bleaching: For endodontically treated anterior teeth—bleaching of deeper dentine.
- Direct restorations.
  - Composite resin veneer: Placing direct chairside composite veneer. Discoloured teeth may require bleaching first. Composite stains with time, it also shrinks and wears. However, it will require replacing every 4-5 years.
- Indirect Restorations
  - Porcelain veneer: This requires removal of 0.5 mm enamel on labial surface, etched and bonded. Porcelain veneer has much better aesthetic than composite, they are less plaque retentive than composite resin veneers and less destructive than crown
  - Porcelain crown: Porcelain crown has excellent aesthetic appearance, strong and retentive but destructive of tooth substance. It is not a good option if tooth is vital. However, it is good option for heavily restored tooth.

Answers

1.	a.	T	b.	F	c.	F	d.	F	e.	
	f.	F								
2.	a.	F	b.	F	c.	F	d.	F	e.	F
	f.	T	g.	F	h.	T				
3.	a.		b.	F	c.	F	d.	F	e.	F
	f.	T								
4.	a.	T	b.	F	c.	T	d.	F	e.	T
5.	a.	T	b.	T	c.	T	d.	F		
6.	a.	T	b.	F	c.	T	d.	T	e.	T
7.	a.	T	b.	F	c.	T	d.	F		
8.	a.	F	b.	T	c.	T	d.	T	e.	F
9.	a.	F	b.	T	c.	T	d.	T	e.	T
10.	a.	T	b.	F	c.	T	d.	F	e.	F
	f.	T								
11.	a.	F	b.	T	c.	F	d.	T	e.	T
	f.	F								
12.	a.	T	b.	F	c.	T	d.	T	e.	F
13.	a.	T	b.	T	c.	F	d.	F	e.	F
14.	a.	F	b.	F	c.	T	d.	F	e.	F
	f.	F	g.	F						
15.	a.	T	b.	F	c.	T	d.	T	e.	F
	f.	T	g.	T	h.	F				
16.	a.	F	b.	F	c.	F	d.	T	e.	F
	f.	F	g.	T	h.	F				
17.	a.	F	b.	F	c.	T	d.	F	e.	F
	f.	F	g.	T	h.	F	i.	F		
18.	a.	T	b.	T	c.	F	d.	T	e.	F

19.	a.	F	b.	F	c.	F	d.	F	e.	F
	f.	T	g.	F	h.	F	i.	F		
20.	a.	F	b.	F	c.	F	d.	F	e.	F
	f.	F								
21.	a.	T	b.	F	c.	F	d.	F	e.	F
	f.	F	g.	F						
22.	a.	F	b.	T	c.	F	d.	F	e.	T
	f.	F								
23.	a	24.	b	25.	d	26.	d	27.	c	
28.	a	29.	b	30.	d	31.	c	32.	a	
33.	c	34.	c	35.	a	36.	c	37	b	
38.	a	39.	c	40.	b	41.	b	42	b	
43.	a.	1	b.	3	c.	2	d.	1	e.	2
	f.	4								
44.	a.	2	b.	4	c.	3	d.	8		

CORRECT ANSWER FOR FALSE STATEMENTS

1. b. Elastic dentine is more liable to fracture and is brittle.
   c. Inorganic component is 86-95%.
   d. Water component of enamel is 4%
   f. The restoration should provide maximum strength for restoration and support tooth structure.
2. a. 45-50% Inorganic matrix
   b. 30% Organic Matrix
   c. 25% Water
   a. Intertubular dentine is primary structural component
   b. Peritubular dentine is collagen free
   g. Dentinal tubules is filled with extended processes of odontoblasts
3. c. Pain arises also due to capillary expansion, thermal expansion or diffusion
   a. Capillary expansion is related to thermal stimuli
   b. Dentine hypersensitivity decreases with age
   e. 3 years after eruption
   a. 4 bitewing and 18 periapical films
   c. Not considered part of dental equipment
   f. No.5 (1.0 inch diameter) to the No.2 (0.75 inch diameter)
3. b. Junction of the cavity wall and the unprepared tooth surface
   e. Cavity classification listing one class as pit and fissure and four classes of smooth surface lesions
   c. Caries can be defined as progressive dissolution of dental hard tissue mediated by Dental plaque.
   d. Gingival inflammation can cause plaque accumulation and toxin production but itself does not cause carious lesion.
   e. Salivary flow rate does affect caries development.
14. a. Small site of origin or inverted 'V'
    d. Carious lesion progress from shadowing to white spot lesion to brown spot lesion
    e. Dentine caries progress slowly due decreased resistance of dentine to acid dissolution.
    F. Radiographs are best to diagnose interproximal caries
15. a. Toothwear can be exaggerated by erosion
    b. Toothier is caused by both extrinsic and intrinsic acids
    e. Reduction of posterior support leads to rapid wear
    h. Management of toothwear includes diet counselling,OHI, occasionally psychiatric advice, protective appliances, adhesions restorations, topical fluoride applications.
16 a. To restore form, function and aesthetics.
    b. Cavity design should be based on minimum tooth tissue removal.

Conservative Dentistry

  c. tooth preparation should be based on morphology of the carious lesion
  e. Margins can be extended to avoid interference
  f. Retention form
  h. Self threading pin is the most common dentine pin used presently
17. a Bonding occurs by weak Van Der waal forces in adhesive dentistry
  b. surface wetting is required for decreased surface tension
  d. Quality of bond does depend upon effects of repeated thermocycling.
  e. Microtags contributes to bond strength during enamel bonding
  f. Agitation is preferred method of action for etching agent.
  h. Brush thinning is preferred to maintain film thickness.
  i. Results in area of microporosity in expansion of ceramic surface area.
18. c. GIC and composites have same coefficient of thermal expansion.
19 b. Gingival margins should be bevelled above ECJ
  c. Occlusal bevelling is not recommended
  d. High copper alloys results in elimination of weak gamma 2 phase
  e. Chemically cured resins polymerase towards the centre of the mass.
  g. Onlays are not preferred to amalgams due significant loss of occlusal tooth surface
  h. Polymérization shrinkage does occur in thin layer of luting cement while placing indirect restorations.
  i. There is about 125-175 micrometer gap in fit of CAD-CAM restorations.
20. a. Silane coupling agent provide weak chemical bond
  c. Occlusion in both centric and eccentric position is important
  d. Chamfer is preferred for bevel of full gold veneer crown and metal ceramic crown.
  e. Shoulder bevel should also be used for metal ceramic crown and porcelain jacket crown
21. b Electrosurgery can be used along with retraction cord.
  c. Polyvinyl siloxane or polyether rubber based material is used for crown and bridge impressions
  d. Ferric sulphate is used in tissue management system by ultradent
  e. Crown lengthening surgery can be done when clinical crown length is insufficient
  g. Putty and wash technique is used in stock trays
22 a. Fixed movable bridge utilizes both custom made or proprietary precision attachment.
  C. Hybrid bridges are complicated and operator's skill and experience is important.
  f. Facebow registration and semi adjustable articulator is mandatory in crown and bridge work.

Chapter 6

Endodontics

Identify the following Statements as True (T) or False (F)

1. **Pulpal and peri-radicular pathology:**
   a. May not result from irritation or inflammation
   b. Can develop without the absence of bacteria
   c. Can also be due to erosion and attrition
   d. Anachoresis does not cause pulpal pathology
   e. The aim of treatment is to seal the canal system
   f. Excessive orthodontic forces can cause peri-radicular and pulpal pathology
   g. Pulpal irritation may not result from conditioning materials
   h. Peri-radicular irritations occurs only due to the use of phenol-based medications.

2. **Reversible pulpitis:**
   a. Is a transient inflammation
   b. Pain occurs due to exposure to sweet
   c. No change in pain after stimulus is removed
   d. Can be localised fairly easily
   e. Normal radiographic appearance
   f. Teeth are tender to percussion
   g. Treatment involves dressing the tooth
   h. May lead to irreversible pulpitis.

3. **Irreversible pulpitis:**
   a. Can develop from reversible pulpitis
   b. Spontaneous pain gets worse during the day time
   c. Cold exaggerates the symptoms
   d. At later stages, cold eases the symptoms
   e. Pain remains after the removal of stimulus
   f. Is not sensitive to pressure
   g. Radiographic changes can be seen initially
   h. Extraction is usually treatment of choice
   i. Can also lead to hyperplastic pulpitis.

4. **Hard tissue response to inflammation:**
   a. Secondary dentine cannot occlude pulp chamber
   b. Tertiary dentine is not laid down in response to reparative dentine
   c. Reactionary dentine is laid in response to mild noxious stimuli

d. Reparative dentin is not deposited beneath the path of injured dentinal tubules
   e. "PINK SPOT" is a sign of dentino-clastic activity
   f. Internal resorption can be seen as punched out outline radiographically
   g. Root canal therapy (RCT) is the treatment of choice.

5. **Regarding peri-apical disease:**
   a. Acute peri-apical periodontitis can also be treated by occlusal adjustment
   b. Widening of periodontal ligament is not visible radiographically
   c. Negative response occurs to pulp sensitivity test in acute peri-apical periodontitis
   d. Positive response occurs to pulp sensitivity test in chronic apical periodontitis
   e. No tenderness over the apex of root in chronic periodontitis
   f. Condensing osteitis does not show decrease in trabecular bone
   g. Radiographically, condensing osteitis presents as radiolucent area around affected root
   h. Acute periapical pathology can also present as phoenix abscess
   i. Chronic apical abscess can communicate both as intra-oral and extra-oral sinus
   j. Primordial cyst can present as endodontic pathology
   k. Malignant lesions like squamous cell carcinoma (SSC) and osteosarcoma can present as endodontic lesion and associated with hard tissue destruction.

6. **The pulpal anatomy of root canal system:**
   a. The shape of canal does not necessarily reflect the outline of the crown and root
   b. Pulp morphology be can altered with irritants and abrasion
   c. Maxillary anterior can contain two root canals
   d. Apical anatomy does not varies with age
   e. Apical constriction can be detected by tactile sense
   f. Apical constriction is usually 1 mm short of apical foramina.

7. **Regarding accessing root canal system:**
   a. Coronal access preparation has convergent walls to hold temporary dressing between visits and preserving the tooth structure
   b. Radicular access preparation does not necessarily require curvature of the canal to be reduced
   c. Second canal may be present in maxillary lateral incisors in more than 40% of patients
   d. Maxillary first premolar can occasionally have third root/canal
   e. Maxillary molars mostly have two canals present in disto-buccal root
   f. Mandibular molar access is triangular in shape with base to mesial and apex to distal.

8. **Root canal preparation:**
   a. The principle of chemo-mechanical debridement is of utmost importance in root canal preparation
   b. The most popular irrigant is sodium hypochlorite 5% concentration
   c. The most effective way of delivering irrigation solution with 27 gauge needle
   d. Pre-enlargement of canals coronally is always necessary
   e. Temperature of irrigating solution is important for increased efficiency
   f. Apical constriction is 1–2 mm short of radiographic apex
   g. Patency filing is done by small and flexible instrument
   h. Patency filing is generally accepted technique.

9. **Root canals instruments:**
   a. Barbed broaches are used for exploring
   b. Reamers are widely used due to their flexibility with increased size
   c. Hedstrom file is made by twisting square metal blank
   d. K-flex-file is made by twisting a rhomboid shape blank
   e. Flex-o-file is made by twisting a rectangular metal blank
   f. Hedstrom file can be used with rotary action
   g. Rotary nickel titanium instruments can be used for canal negotiations
   h. Gates glidden burs are used for preparing coronal 1/3 of the canal.

10. **Root canal therapy materials:**
    a. Sodium hypochlorite is bacteriostatic and dissolves organic debris
    b. Ethylenediaminetetraacetic acid (EDTA) is only used for the removal of smear layer
    c. Phenolic compounds are recommended during RCT
    d. Non-setting calcium hydroxide (hypocal) should not be used in infected canal
    e. Ledermix should not be used for hyperaemic pulp
    f. Gutta-percha is extracted from tropical trees
    g. Hypocal is used as inter-appointment medication
    h. Calcium hydroxide can be used in the management of perforations.

11. **Root canal filling materials:**
    a. Should be able to absorb moisture
    b. Should expand on setting
    c. Should be difficult to remove
    d. Should not stain the teeth
    e. Should be radiolucent
    f. Should seal root apically and coronally
    g. Should be bactericidal.

12. **The acceptable root canal obturation techniques:**
    a. Single point gutta-percha is widely used technique
    b. Warm lateral condensation is used for denser root filling

c. Thermo-mechanical compaction can be used to plasticise and condense gutta percha
d. Silver points can be used
e. Vertical condensation requires good apical stop
f. Thermoplasticised injectable gutta-percha is useful for irregular canal defects
g. Coated carriers can be excellent.

13. **Regarding endodontic problems:**
    a. Acute periapical abscess always require drainage through the tooth and antibiotics
    b. Phoenix abscess can occur occasionally
    c. Recurrent symptoms always require surgical intervention
    d. In sclerosed canals, elective RCT can be performed
    e. Fractured instruments can be removed by Masseran trepan with ultrasonic vibrations
    f. Apical silver points may not require apicoectomy
    g. Non-setting calcium hydroxide can be considered as retrograde filling
    h. Lateral perforation in middle one-third can be sealed by using lateral condensation technique
    i. Perforation in apical one-third usually can be managed with vertical condensation technique.

14. **In surgical endodontics:**
    a. It is preferable to treat acute infection with antibiotics than to establish drainage
    b. Cortical trephination have to be performed
    c. Peri-radicular surgery is also used for obtaining tissue for a biopsy
    d. Lateral pathology does not indicate root re-treatment instead of root resection
    e. Luebke-Ochsenbein flap design are preferable
    f. Approximately 3 mm of root is required to be resected in root end resection procedure
    g. Super ethoxybenzoic acid is preferred material of choice for retro fillings
    h. Extraction with subsequent replantation is method of choice in surgical endodontics.

15. **Restoration of endodontically treated teeth:**
    a. Resistance and retention form is of primary importance while restoring endodontically treated teeth
    b. Amalcore can be used on molar teeth
    c. Screw post are recommended due to added retention
    d. Post length should ideally be half of the root length
    e. Post with wider diameter are preferred
    f. Post diameter is of more significance than post length
    g. Parallel posts are more retentive than tapered post
    h. Coronal preparation should have maximum 2 mm of ferrule effect.

Identify the Single Best Answer for the following

16. The nerve fibres responsible for pulpal pain transmission:
    a. A beta and A delta nerve fibres
    b. A alpha and A delta nerve fibres
    c. A beta and C nerve fibres
    d. A delta and C nerve fibres.

17. The structure rich in proprioceptors is:
    a. Periapical area
    b. Dental pulp stroma
    c. Dentine layer
    d. Odontoblastic layer.

18. The instrument used to find pulp horns is:
    a. Hedstrom file
    b. Small round burr
    c. A file with a curved tip
    d. Briault probe.

19. The most successful indirect pulp capping technique occurs in:
    a. Extensive carious teeth
    b. Attrited teeth
    c. Young patients
    d. Young patient with diminished pulp vascularity.

20. Cracked tooth syndrome is characterized by:
    a. Sharp pain following application of cold
    b. Severe pain while eating
    c. Sharp pain following application of heat
    d. All of the above.

21. The use of calcium hydroxide as a pulp capping agent is:
    a. Providing a good thermal insulation
    b. Providing a mild irritant action on pulp
    c. Providing a soothing action on pulp
    d. All of the above.

22. The greatest curvature in the root canal of mandibular first molar is present in:
    a. Distal canal
    b. Mesiolingual canal
    c. Mesiobuccal canal
    d. None of the above.

23. Predominant organisms observed in infected root canals are:
    a. *Candida albicans* and *Spirochetes*
    b. *Lactobacillus* and *Staphylococcus*
    c. *Staphylococcus* and *Lactobacillus*
    d. *Staphylococcus* and *Streptococcus*.

Endodontics 107

24. The most important test in differentiating between an apical abscess and a periodontal abscess is:
    a. Anesthetic test
    b. Pulp vitality test
    c. Palpation
    d. Percussion test.

25. The access preparation for root canal in a maxillary central incisor most bear a resemblance with:
    a. Circle
    b. Square
    c. Triangle
    d. Trapezoidal.

26. Biomechanical preparation of root canal causes:
    a. Creation of ledge
    b. Debridement of root canal
    c. Perforation of apical foramen
    d. All of the above.

27. The use of 5% sodium hypochlorite solution for irrigation of root canal is due to its potential as:
    a. Bacteriocidal
    b. Solvent for pulp tissue and debris
    c. Lubricant for instruments within canals
    d. All of the above.

28. Death of pulp is:
    a. Necrosis
    b. Apoptosis
    c. Atrophy
    d. Aplasia.

29. What is localised collection of pus at the apex of root with spread of infection into periapical tissue following death of pulp in alveolar bone region known as?
    a. Acute periapical pericementitis
    b. Phoenix abscess
    c. Acute apical pericementitis
    d. All of the above.

30. A 8-year-old patient has been reported with fleshy, reddish pulpal mass in the pulp chamber. No history of pain but persistent bleeding is present. Radiographically, it appears as a large open cavity with direct acess to pulp. Histopathologically, granulation tissue is highly vascular connective tissue containing inflamed polymorphonuclear neutrophils, lymphocytes and plasma cells. The pulp tissue is evident. What can be probable diagnosis?

a. Internal resorption
b. Pulp stones
c. Chronic hyperplastic pulpitis
d. Irreversible pulpitis.

31. An active inflammatory radiation exacerbating on an existing chronic lesion for, e.g. cyst or granuloma is called as:
    a. Phoenix abscess
    b. Alveolar abscess
    c. Periapical abscess
    d. Periodontal abscess.

32. An inflammation in a closed gravity, filled with semi-solid material or fluid; particularly proteinaceous in nature found at the apex of tooth. Radiographically, loss of continuity of lamina dura is evident. The radiolucent area is round or may be flattened or oval in shape, if it is located close to an adjacent tooth. Histopathologically, cavity is lined with stratified squamous epithelium. The surrounding connective tissue is infiltrated by plasma cells, polymorphonuclear neutrophils and lymphocytes. Cholesterol clefts, macrophages, presence of debris and eosinophilic material may be evident. What can be probable diagnosis?
    a. Condensing osteitis
    b. Radicular cyst
    c. Infected granuloma
    d. Dentigerous cyst.

33. A method that involves induction of development of root apex in pulpless, immature tooth with the formation of bone like tissue or osteocementum. In this method, irrigation of the periapical tissue with sodium hypochlorite is done. Name this method?
    a. Apexification
    b. Apexogenesis
    c. Pulpotomy
    d. Pulpectomy.

34. Which among the following are used in cold sterilization of instruments against vegetative bacteria and tubercle bacilli?
    a. Ethyl alcohol
    b. Isopropyl alcohol
    c. All of above
    d. None of above.

35. The diameter of size of glass beads as substitution of salt in hot-salt sterilizer is?
    a. 5 mm
    b. 2 mm
    c. 7 mm
    d. 1 mm.

36. Average length of maxillary central incisor:
   a. 21.8 mm
   b. 22.0 mm
   c. 21.7 mm
   d. 20.9 mm.

37. Which instrument is used to remove the lingual roof and lingual shoulder of an anterior tooth pulp chamber?
   a. Round bur No. 4
   b. Round bur No. 2
   c. Gates Glidden drill No. 4
   d. Gate Glidden drill No. 2.

38. Which among the following are used for shaping in root canal treatment?
   a. Reamers and files
   b. Reamers and pluggers
   c. Files and spreaders
   d. Files and spreaders.

39. A rhomboidal or diamond-shaped blanks are twisted and used to produce a file. This file is very efficient for removal of debris. Name the instrument?
   a. K-flex
   b. K-Instrument
   c. H-file
   d. Reamer.

40. This technique is used for preparation of root canal. In this method, larger root canal instrument is used consecutively for shaping the wall of root canal. This instrument is placed short of the apex, once the size of canal has been enlarged to No. 25 or 30 instrument in the apical-third of the tooth.
   a. Step-down method
   b. Step-back method
   c. Hybrid technique
   d. Roanes technique.

41. A non-toxic, mild irritating, highly stable, soluble, metal chelate used as a chemical aid to instrumentation?
   a. Ethylenediaminetetraacetic acid (EDTA)
   b. Calcium hydroxide
   c. Ammonium chelate
   d. Cetavlon.

Identify the Answers for Extended Matching Questions

42. **Regarding pulpal pathologies:**
    a. An acute painful inflammation of the pulp characterized by abscess formation upon the surface or within the pulp
    b. An excessive accumulation of blood in the pulp resulting from vascular congestion
    c. Formation of an ulcer on the surface of the pulp in the region of an exposure
    d. An acute inflammation of the dental pulp characterized by intermittent paroxysm of pain.

    1. Acute serous pulpitis
    2. Acute suppurative pulpitis
    3. Hyperaemia
    4. Chronic ulcerative pulpitis
    5. Reversible pulpitis

43. **The pain of a tooth which disappears at once when stimulus is removed is a characteristic of regarding endodontic anatomy:**
    a. The root canals most likely to share a common apical opening
    b. Group of teeth which exhibit the least number of anomalies
    c. The apex of the mandibular central incisor most closely approaches.

1. Mesiobuccal and distobuccal root canals of maxillary first molar	5. Maxillary anteriors
2. Mesial and distal root canals of maxillary second bicuspids	6. Lingual cortical plates
3. Mesiobuccal and mesiolingual root canals of mandibular first molars	7. Mandibular anteriors
	8. Labial cortical plates
	9. Mandibular lateral incisor
4. Mesial and distal root canals of mandibular bicuspids	10. Mandibular central incisor

44. **The anterior tooth most likely to display two canals. Regarding obturation:**
    a. Most common solid-core filling material
    b. Technique of filling lateral and accessory canals
    c. Technique in which guttapercha cone is fitted to instrumented main canal
    d. Chemically plasticised gutta percha
    e. Used to fill root canals
    f. A rapid setting hydrophilic material, a root canal sealer without use of core
    g. Root canal cement.

h. Polyvinyl resin used as root canal cement
i. Root canal cement which hardens slowly at body-temperature in 36–48 hours.
j. AH-26

1. Gutta percha	7. Vertical condensation
2. Zinc Oxide ZnO-resin cement	8. Chlorpercha
3. Diaket	9. Hydron
4. Lateral condensation	10. Calcium hydroxide cement
5. Eucapercha	11. Amalgam
6. Silver cone method	

45. Regarding treatment of traumatized tooth:
a. Vital pulp, exposure more than 1 mm, less than 24 hours
b. Necrotic pulp, pulp has died in the developing tooth with incomplete root formation
c. Clinical crown is extensively fractured, pulp exposed in fully developed tooth
d. Emergency treatment for luxated tooth
e. Crown that is needed to restore extensively fractured tooth.
f. Treatment of choice for incompletely developed root apex or one with fractured root.

1. Endodontic treatment	9. Root resection
2. Pulpotomy	10. Apicoectomy
3. Apexification	11. Periapical curettage
4. Pulpectomy	12. Implantation
5. Application of cold	13. Transplantation
6. Apexogenesis	14. Trephination
7. Post-core crown	15. Root submergence
8. Concussion	

CASE DISCUSSION

Case 1: Acute Irreversible Pulpitis.

A 25-year-old female complaints of sharp pain at night that increases with intake of hot fluids. Discuss and advice approach for management of possible underlying condition?

History of Presenting Complaint

Several weeks of history of sharp, spontaneous and severe pain in right mandibular region. The pain got aggravated with hot fluids and relieved by cold water in respect to lower right permanent second premolar (LR5) (Fig. 6.1).

Previous Dental History

Patient had been given soft bite guard and prescribed course of antibodies, though no details for prescribed medication. There was no record of hands on treatment.

Medical History

No history of depression or mental illness.

Social History

- No evidence of illicit drug use
- Drinks alcohol socially.

Clinical Examination

- Mouth opening: Normal
- No evidence of temporomandibular joint problems

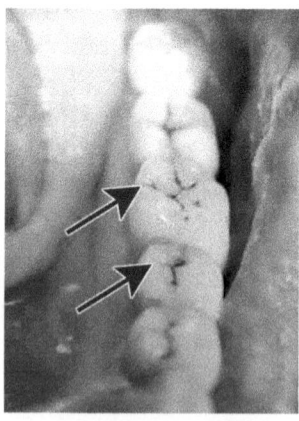

Fig. 6.1: Carious lesion in lower posterior teeth (Second premolar and first molar)

- Multiple amalgam filling in posterior teeth
- Lower right permanent second premolar was restored with disto-buccal amalgam
- Tender on percussion was present in affected tooth, hypersensitivity to heat was also present
- Caries was present in upper right permanent first molar UR6 and lower left first permanent molar.

Investigations
Bitewing and periapical films; confirmatory diagnosis for extensive caries.

Diagnosis
Acute irreversible pulpitis.

Treatment
- Lower right permanent second premolar was extirpated immediately, under local anaesthesia
- Symptoms reduced with treatment
- Endodontic treatment completed for lower right permanent second premolar
- Restorative treatment of upper right permanent first molar and lower right permanent second premolar done
- Advised for plaque control, diet counseling and use of fluoride.

Case 2: Management of Dental Caries.

A 35-year-old male complaints of food lodgment mandibular molar tooth. Discuss and advice approach for management of dental caries?

History of Presenting Complaint
There was food lodgment from two weeks in right mandibular region. The pain gets aggravated with cold, food and fluids.

Previous Dental History
There was no history of hands on treatment. The patient had no previous record.

Medical History
No confirmation of medical history.

Social History
- No evidence of illicit drug use
- Drinks alcohol socially.

Investigations

Periapical radiograph; confirmatory diagnosis **(Fig. 6.2)**.

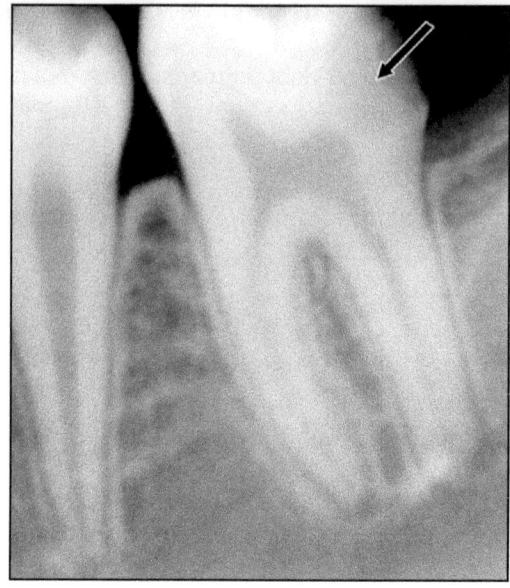

Fig. 6.2: Carious lesion extending up to enamel, dentin and pulp horn

Treatment

Preventive measures of optimal caries

Various approaches that can be practiced for preventive measures are as follows:

Measurements	Effectiveness
1. Fluoride agents	
1.1 Community-based methods	Water fluoridation: Decreases carious lesions in children and adults. Salt fluoridation: More effective in caries prevention as compared to tooth without fluoride exposure. Milk fluoridation: No much evidence on effectiveness
1.2 Professional-based methods	Fluoride gels and varnish aid to reduce incidence of dental carious lesions
1.3 Individual methods (toothpaste, mouthwash)	Fluoride toothpaste and mouthwashes are effective in caries prevention
1.4 Silver diamine fluoride (SDF)	There is lack of evidence showing that SDF is as effective as a caries control agent in non-cavitated lesion.

2. NON-FLUORIDE AGENTS	
2.1 Sugar substitutes	Xylitol and sorbitol are the most fre-quently used sugar substitutes. The use of sugar-free dental chewing gum had proved to be effective for carious lesion control on school premises
2.2 Chlorhexidine	Evidence regarding chlorhexidine gel and varnish for carious control and prevention is inconclusive
2.3 Casein phosphopeptide amorphous calcium phos-phate	A short-term remineralisation effect and a promising caries control effect for long-term clinical use
2.4 Ozone therapy	No reliable evidence available
2.5 Infiltration resin	Infiltration of non-cavitated lesions has been considered as a promising therapy to avoid carious lesion progression in enamel and dentine
2.6 Pit and fissure sealants	It is an effective measure for both carious prevention and arresting non-cavitated carious lesions

Restorative Therapy

- Atraumatic restorative treatment (ART)
- **Hall technique:** A prefabricated metal crown is cemented over the cavitated tooth, using a low-viscosity glass-ionomer cement, after removing debris but without removal of decomposed carious dentine.

Non-restorative Therapy

- Carious lesions in anterior teeth should preferably be restored using a proven anterior resin composite because of its superior aesthetic performance
- The buccal and cervical carious lesions in the posterior area are best restored using a (resin-modified) glass-ionomer, while three-step etch-and-rinse adhesive and a resin composite is the second best restorative material
- The use of a hand excavator for removing decomposed carious tissues near the gingival margin may cause less bleeding than the bleeding occurs by the use of a rotary instrument and this in turn may increase the survival rate of the restoration
- Restoring multiple-surfaces in posterior teeth is best done using amalgam or resin composite materials following 'the box only' cavity design.

Answers

1.	a.	F	b.	F	c.	T	d.	F	e.	F
	f.	T	g.	T	h.	F				
2.	a.	T	b.	T	c.	F	d.	F	e.	T
	f.	F	g.	T	h.	T				
3.	a.	T	b.	F	c.	F	d.	T	e.	T
	f.	F	g.	F	h.	F	i.	T		
4.	a.	F	b.	F	c.	T	d.	F	e.	T
	f.	T	g.	T						
5.	a.	T	b.	F	c.	F	d.	F	e.	F
	f.	T	g.	F	h.	T	i.	T	j.	T
6.	a.	F	b.	T	c.	F	d.	F	e.	F
	f.	F								
7.	a.	F	b.	F	c.	F	d.	T	e.	F
	f.	F								
8.	a.	T	b.	F	c.	F	d.	F	e.	T
	f.	T	g.	T	h.	F				
9.	a.	F	b.	F	c.	F	d.	T	e.	F
	f.	F	g.	F	h.	F				
10.	a.	F	b.	F	c.	F	d.	F	e.	F
	f.	T	g.	T	h.	T				
11.	a.	F	b.	F	c.	F	d.	T	e.	F
	f.	F	g.	F						
12.	a.	F	b.	T	c.	T	d.	F	e.	T
	f.	T	g.	T						
13.	a.	F	b.	T	c.	F	d.	F	e.	T
	f.	F	g.	F	h.	T	i.	T		

14.	a.	F	b.	F	c.	T	d.	F	e. F
	f.	T	g.	T	h.	F			
15.	a.	T	b.	T	c.	F	d.	F	e. F
	f.	F	g.	T	h.	F			
16.	d	17.	a	18.	d	19.	c	20.	b
21.	b	22.	c	23.	d	24.	b	25.	c
26.	b	27.	d	28.	a	29.	d	30.	c
31.	a	32.	b	33.	a	34.	c	35.	d
36.	a	37.	c	38.	a	39.	a	40.	b
41.	a								
42.	a.	2	b.	3	c.	4	d.	1	e. 5
43.	a.	3, 4	b.	5	c.	6	d.	9	
44.	a.	2	b.	8	c.	5	d.	6	e. 7
	f.	10	g.	3,1,11	h.	4	i.	2, 6	
45.	a.	2	b.	3	c.	4	d.	5	e. 7
	f.	6							

CORRECT ANSWER FOR FALSE STATEMENTS

1. d Anachoresis can cause Pulpal Pathology
   e. The aim of the treatment is also to eliminate the bacteria
   h. Periradicular irritations can also occurs due use of irrigation solutions or extrusion of filling materials.
2. c. Pain subsides when stimulus is removed
   d. Pain cannot be localised as pulp does not contain proprioceptive fibers
   f. Teeth are not TTP unless there is occlusal trauma
3. b. Pain is worse during the night time.
   c. Heat usually exaggerates the symptoms of irreversible pulpitis.
   g. Radiographic changes can be seen at later stages of infection.
   h. Root canal therapy (RCT) or extraction is treatment of choice
4. a Secondary dentine can decrease size of the pulp chamber with age
   b Tertiary dentine is laid down in response to reparative dentine which is formed by a odontoblast directly affected by noxious stimulus.
   d Reparative dentine is deposited beneath the path of injured dentinal tubules.
5. c. In Acute Periapical Periodontitis there is positive response to pulp sensitivity test.
   d. There is negative response to pulp sensitivity test in Chronic Apical Periodontitis
   e. TTP and tenderness is present over apex of the root.
   g. Radiographically, Condensing Osteitis presents as radiopaque area around the affected root.
6. a The shape of canal does reflect the outline of crown and root.
6. f. Apical constriction occurs 0.5–0.7 mm short of foramina.
7. c. Second canal may be present in Mandibular lateral Incisors
   e. Maxillary molars mostly have two canals present in mesio-buccal root.
   f. Mandibular molar access is Trapezoid in shape.
8. b. Sodium Hypochlorite 2.5% concentration.
   c. Ultrasonic handpiece effective delivers irrigation solution.
9. a. Smooth broaches are used for exploring
   b. Reamers are rarely used due to their inflexibility.
   c. K-type file is made up of twisting square metal blank
   e. Flex-o-file is made by twisting a triangular metal blank.
   f. Hedstroem file should not be used with rotary action as it can fracture.

- g. Rotary Nickel titanium instruments are used for canal enlargements.
- h. Gates Glidden burs are used for preparing coronal ⅔ of the canal
10. a. Sodium Hypochlorite is Bactericidal.
    b. EDTA also has demineralising action.
    e. Ledermix should be used for hyperaemic pulp as it reduces inflammation.
11. e. Root Canal filling material should be Radiopaque.
    f. Root Canal filling material should also laterally.
    g. Root Canal filling material should be bacteriostatic.
13. a. Antibiotics should not be prescribed in the absence of cellulitis.
    c. Recurrent symptoms requires re-treatment.
    g. Mineral trioxide aggregate (MTA) should be used as retrograde filling
14 D Lateral pathology indicate root retreatment rather than root resection
14 e Luebke- Ochsenbein flap design is not prefered due to limited visibility for root and crestal bone.
14. h. Orthograde or surgical approach is method of choice in surgical endodontics
15. d. Post length should be 2/3 of root length.
    e. Post with same diameter as of canal is prefered.
    h. Coronal preparation should have minimum 2 mm of ferrule effect.

Chapter 7

Prosthodontics

Identify the following Statements as True (T) or False (F)

1. Patient seek prosthetic replacement of missing teeth to:
   a. Improve speech
   b. Restore form
   c. Restore function
   d. Improve oral health
   e. Space maintenance
   f. Also prepares patient for complete denture.

2. Partial denture assessment should include:
   a. History of tooth loss
   b. Denture history
   c. Medical history
   d. Social history
   e. Any emergency treatment
   f. Clinical and radiographic assessment of remaining teeth
   g. Oral hygiene and periodontal health
   h. Patient expectations.

3. Treatment planning for complete denture:
   a. Relief of pain and dental history
   b. Emergency treatment if required
   c. Dental history
   d. Medical history
   e. Rebase/copy existing denture
   f. Removal of pathological abnormality
   g. Patient expectations
   h. Discussion with patient regarding limitation of dentures.

4. With regards to components of removable partial denture:
   a. Saddles are entirely made of acrylic
   b. Rests provide support and prevent overeruption
   c. Wrought rests are preferred for strength and fit
   d. Cast cobalt-chrome can be used for occlusally approaching clasps on premolar teeth
   e. Cast cobalt–chrome clasp can engage in 0.5 mm undercut
   f. Cast cobalt-chrome clasp cannot be cast as integral part of denture framework

- g. Stainless steel clasps are more flexible and easily adjusted than wrought gold clasps of similar length
- h. Lingual bars can be used if lower incisors are retroclined
- i. Sublingual bar is more rigid than lingual bar
- j. Lingual bar contributes to indirect retention
- k. Connectors only join parts of denture together, they do not contribute to support and retention
- l. Buccal bars are indicated when lower incisors are proclined
- m. Dental bars are useful for teeth with long clinical crowns.

5. **With regards to copy denture:**
   - a. Is useful for elderly patients with long-term successful denture wearing experience
   - b. Can be used for recurrent fractures of denture base
   - c. No loss of retention
   - d. Incorrect placement of anterior teeth
   - e. Replacement of immediate dentures
   - f. Patient requiring spare set of dentures
   - g. Only two clinical stages
   - h. Only three laboratory stages are involved
   - i. Record blocks are required
   - j. To correct zone of adaptation
   - k. To correct position of teeth in the neutral zone.

6. **Immediate replacement dentures:**
   - a. It involves total or partial replacement
   - b. Helps in maintaining soft tissue contour of the face
   - c. Can cause formation of abnormal mandibular movements
   - d. Existing occlusion can be used for jaw registration procedure
   - e. Does not control haemorrhage
   - f. Prevents alveolar bone resorption
   - g. Reduced cost
   - h. Advisable for single tooth replacement in anterior region
   - i. Patient at risk of tooth movement, if replacement unit not placed after extraction
   - j. Patient losing upper second molar tooth
   - k. Flanged dentures are prone to loss of aesthetics as resorption continues
   - l. Socket fit dentures are easier to add flange
   - m. Socket fit dentures have good retention
   - n. Temporary recline may be required at first week of review appointment
   - o. A replacement denture is made using the copy denture technique at 6 month review appointment.

7. **With regards to overdenture:**
   - a. Can be partial or complete denture
   - b. Indicated for cleft palate and surgical defects

c. Preservation of proprioception
d. Additional retention is not possible in overdentures
e. Reduced masticatory force
f. Less maintenance for both patient and dentist
g. Over dentures are useful for upper removable partial denture or free end saddles
h. Root canal therapy may be required
i. Maintenance of alveolar bone
j. Preference for abutment teeth are molars and premolars
k. May require preparation of crown for thimble/telescopic gold coping
l. Existing implants in edentulous area can be used with precision attachment
m. Patient with over dentures shows decreased caries prevalence.

8. **With regards to clinical technique for complete denture:**
    a. The preliminary impressions are taken using close fitting custom trays
    b. Upper trays should be closely fitted for silicone impressions
    c. Spaced tray is required when extensive undercuts are present
    d. Special trays should not be modified
    e. Special trays are perforated
    f. Dentures made with muco-compressive impression technique are not retained well at rest
    g. Lower master impression are recorded in silicone or alignate and upper master impression by using zinc oxide eugenol (ZOE) or alignate
    h. Wax bases are suitable for upper rims
    i. Post dam on upper cast is not required if permanent acrylic bases are requested from laboratory.

9. **With regards to neutral zone technique:**
    a. Can be used for maxilla
    b. Requires upper trial denture in place
    c. Is used for recording neutral zone of patients with limited natural retention of lower removable partial denture
    d. Patient is asked to swallow and purse lips
    e. Helps to determine the pre-extraction position of the natural dentition
    f. Does not require use of laboratory stents to locate teeth
    g. Records second impression and occlusion.

10. **Occlusion for complete denture:**
    a. A freeway space of the denture should be determined
    b. Horizontal jaw relationship is recorded
    c. Position of occlusal plane increases with age
    d. At rest, the tongue should rise just above occlusal plane anteriorly
    e. Artificial teeth should be placed labial and buccal to the ridge
    f. Posterior teeth should be wider to increase masticatory efficiency

Prosthodontics

g. Patient's age, facial appearance and characteristics, patient's opinion must be considered
h. A head posture does not affect freeway space
i. Heat cured base plates may provide increased stability
j. The tooth shade is selected at this stage
k. The centre line is marked
l. Facebow registration of upper rim can be used for accurate location of the cast on the articulator in the laboratory.

11. **Trial insertion of complete denture:**
    a. Dentist only must be satisfied before dentures are processed in acrylic
    b. To check extension, stability and position of the teeth relative to soft tissues
    c. Examine vertical dimension, occlusion, aesthetics and phonetics with both the dentures in mouth
    d. Shape of polished surfaces and peripheral extension is examined
    e. Appearance, shade, mould, position of anterior teeth and contour of labial flanges in natural appearance
    f. Gingival colour should be included before laboratory prescription
    g. Post dam is prepared
    h. Patient satisfaction with the appearance should be recorded in the notes.

12. **Fitting complete denture:**
    a. Adjustment of fitting surface may be required
    b. On an average, 1 mm increase in facial height occurs following processing
    c. Upper palatal and lower buccal cusps should be adjusted while checking occlusion
    d. Cusp tips rather than fossa should be ground off
    e. Removing any interferences to protrusive movements
    f. Balancing contacts are essential
    g. Patient to be reviewed 1-2 weeks after fitting
    h. Ask patient to wear denture 24 hours before review appointment if experiencing pain or soreness
    i. Written and verbal instructions should be given for their new dentures
    j. Tooth paste can be used to clean dentures
    k. Immersion cleaner is recommended.

13. **Denture maintenance:**
    a. Regular annual maintenance increases the likelihood of early detection of oral pathology
    b. Lack of aftercare of full denture can lead to loss of retention and stability
    c. Movement of denture in function can result in predisposition to candidal infection

d. Ill-fitting denture can also cause inflammatory papillary hyperplasia of the palate
e. Relining of denture involves addition of a material to the fitting and polished surface of the denture
f. Rebasing increases the thickness of the palate
g. Relining can be temporary
h. Self-cure acrylic is material of choice for rebasing
i. Tissue conditioners gives even distribution of load
j. Soft linings are indicated following hemimaxillectomy.

14. **Denture problems and complaints:**
    a. Generalised discomfort over denture bearing areas can be caused by decreased occlusal face height
    b. Collapsed face is caused by lack of facial support
    c. Denture induced hyperplasia is caused by overextension
    d. Pressure on superficial mental nerve can cause pain in lower premolar region
    e. Pain from cheek and tongue is caused by irregularities on fitting surface
    f. Denture displacement on opening or in speech is caused due to overextension/underextension of border
    g. Teeth meet too soon is due to decreased occlusal face height
    h. Denture stomatitis is caused by increased free monomer
    i. Nausea due to dentures is caused by lack of tongue space
    j. Midline fracture is not caused by teeth set excessively off the ridge.

Identify the Single Best Answer for the following

15. The distal extension partial denture is also called as:
    a. Kennedy class I
    b. Kennedy class IV
    c. Kennedy class II
    d. Applegate class VI.

16. The width of the palatal bar is:
    a. >8 mm
    b. <8 mm
    c. 1.8
    d. >8.8 mm.

17. The primary denture support area for a mandible complete denture is:
    a. Buccal shelf
    b. Vestibule
    c. Frenum
    d. Palatophayrngeal fold.

18. The impression technique used for a patient with a sharp mandibular ridge:
    a. Minimum pressure impression technique
    b. Excessive pressure impression technique
    c. Selective pressure impression technique
    d. Any of the above.
19. The position of upper occlusal rim in the articulator is adjusted by:
    a. By using a facebow
    b. Arbitrary means
    c. Need not to be adjusted
    d. By adjusting inter-condylar distance.
20. The position of the patient while recording the rest position is:
    a. Head should be supported by the head rest
    b. Neck should be extended
    c. Head and neck can be in position
    d. Head should be upright and supported.
21. Bulkiest portion of a proximal minor connector is towards its:
    a. Inferior
    b. Lingual
    c. Buccal
    d. Centre.
22. All are contraindications for sublingual bar, *except*:
    a. Lingual
    b. Large tongue
    c. High lingual frenum
    d. High elevation of the floor of the mouth.
23. Marginal ridge for a rest seat should be reduced by a least:
    a. 1 mm
    b. 2 mm
    c. 1.5 mm
    d. 3 mm.
24. The advantage of internal occlusal rest is:
    a. Provides retention
    b. Provides support
    c. Provides stabilisation
    d. Eliminates visible clasp arm.
25. Kennedy classification is determined by:
    a. The first tooth to be lost
    b. The largest tooth in the space
    c. The most anterior tooth missing
    d. The most posterior tooth missing.

26. When designing palatal major connector, relief should be given for:
    a. Elevated mid suture line
    b. Rugae area
    c. Palatal torus
    d. Ridge area
    e. Gingival area.

27. The distance between the implant and the superior aspect of the inferior alveolar canal should be:
    a. 1 mm
    b. 2 mm
    c. 3 mm
    d. 5 mm
    e. 6 mm.

Identify the Answers for Extended Matching Questions

28. Select single most appropriate component or function of component of partial denture that matches the statement. Each option can be used once/more than once or not at all:
    a. Resistance to vertical forces directed towards mucosa
    b. Resistance to horizontal forces providing by rigid components of denture
    c. Join together components of denture
    d. Resist displacement of denture
    e. Covers edentulous area and corners artificial teeth and gum work
    f. Resistance to rotation through hinge axis of the clasps tips
    g. Dentures tends to rock where saddles are loaded
    h. Resistance to horizontal tooth movement during clasps engagement
    i. On abutment teeth to limit path of insertion and improve retention and stability
    j. Maximum bulbosity of a tooth lies in plane of path of withdrawal
    k. Tissue-borne partial denture that can Sink
    l. Allows movement between saddle and remaining unit of partial denture.

1. Saddle	7. Survey line	12. Bracing
2. Connector	8. Stress breaker	13. Stability
3. Indirect retention	9. Support	14. Reciprocation
4. Retainers	10. Occlusal rest	15. Clasps
5. Fulcrum axis	11. Retention	16. Gum stripper
6. Guide planes		

29. With regards to classification of RPD — Select single most appropriate classification that matches the statements.
    a. This describes patterns of tooth loss.

b. Patient with upper right 1st and 2nd molar and premolar and upper left canine, central and lateral incisor, 1st and 2nd molar and premolar present
c. Unilateral bound saddle
d. Patient with lower right 1st and 2nd premolar, canine, lateral incisor present and lower left canine, premolars, first and second molar teeth present
e. Patient with upper right 54321 and upper left 12345 present
f. Patient has bilateral free-end saddles and anterior saddle
g. Patient with lower right 76521 and lower left 12367 teeth present would be described as
Mucosa and tooth borne denture type
Unilateral free end saddle
Anterior bound saddle
Mucosa borne denture type
Tooth borne denture type
This describes the type of denture.

1. Kennedy classification	5. Kennedy class III	10. Class I modification 1
2. Craddock classification	6. Kennedy class IV	11. Class I modification 2
3. Kennedy class I	7. Craddock I	12. Class II modification 1
4. Kennedy class II	8. Craddock II	13. Class III modification 1
	9. Craddock III	

30. **Speech problems with denture:**
    a. Difficulty with 'f' sound
    b. Difficulty with 'v' sound
    c. Difficulty with 'd' sound
    d. Difficulty with 's' sound
    e. Difficulty with 't' sound
    f. 's' becomes 'th'
    g. Whistling
    h. Clicking teeth.

1. Incisor too far palatally	7. Lack of retention
2. Alteration of palatal contour	8. Over extension
3. Incorrect overjet and overbite	9. Decrease freeway space
4. Palate too thick	10. Under extension
5. Palate vault too high behind incisors	11. Decrease occlusal vertical dimension
6. Increased occlusal vertical dimension	12. Increase freeway space

CASE DISCUSSIONS

Case 1: Removable Partial Denture (RPD) Design.

A 60-year-old patient presents to your clinic requesting new lower partial denture. The present partial denture has become loose and unstable and has

upper intact dentition $\quad\dfrac{6\,5\,4\,3\,2\,1\,|\,1\,2\,3\,4\,5\,6}{4\,3\,2\,1\,|\,1\,2\,3\,4}$

- Discuss the treatment options possible to restore missing teeth
- Discuss principles of RPD design
- Discuss design problems in class I and its solution.

History of Complaint

Since when the denture has become uncomfortable to the patient.

Medical History

Any relevant medical history like hypertension, diabetes, history of bleeding disorder, medications, etc.

Dental History

- Denture history, loss of dentition
- Restoration status of remaining dentition—heavily restored or minimally restored
- Any tooth wear, periodontal health status.

Social History

- Is patient Smoker
- Is he an? alcoholic?
- What is the occupation?

Examination

- Extra-oral examination:
  - Look for lipseal, symmetry, lymph nodes, temporomandibular joint (TMJ).
- Intra-oral examination:
  - Number of teeth present
  - Restoration status—heavily/minimally restored
  - Periodontal status—basic periodontal examination (BPE)/plaque score/6 point pocket chart (6 PPc)
  - Any tooth wear—palatal, labial or incisal.

Treatment Options to Restore Missing Teeth

Implant supported bridges:
- Mandible has sufficient bone present for implant

- Check for the bone density and quality to support implant using CT scans and to check relationship of inferior dental canal
- In this case, three implant fixtures will be necessary and is required to be placed more mesially than distally
- Mesial implants would likely to achieve optimum length of 10–12 mm whereas distal implants may only be able to approach 8 mm optimal length.

However, this implant retained option should be discussed with patient and let patient decide, if he would consider implant retained bridge option or partial denture.

Partial Denture

- Acrylic lower removable partial denture
- Cobalt-chromium (Co-Cr) Lower removable partial denture.

If patient already have acrylic dentures, the problem of support and retention may not be solved and Co-Cr RPD can provide better comfort and retention. However, both the options are discussed with patients including the cost to help the patient make informed decision.

Principles of RPD Design

Removable partial denture design should be carried out after thorough clinical assessment of the patient including any previous denture history.
- Outline saddles:
  - Outline the edentulous area and use Kennedy and Craddock classification. In the case, it is Kennedy classification I modification 1 and the RPD is both tooth and tissue-borne support (s).
- Plan support:
  - Occlusion rests
  - As teeth can withstand occlusal loading and support will not be compromised following resorption. The concept of RPI mesial rest, distal guide plate, gingivally approaching I-bar clasp is selected in the mandible. The lower RPD should conform to existing occlusal relationship and there should be sufficient depth for rest seat.
- Retention:
  - Direct:
    Clasps
    Guide plane
    Soft tissue undercuts
    Precision attachments
    Clasps are most commonly used and three clasps to be placed as far away from each other as possible
    Common clasp design should be occlusally and gingivally approaching
    Guide planes establishes path of insertion and withdrawal and requires 2–3 mm in length.

- Indirect:
    - It is derived by placing components of denture to resist displacement from rotational forces. This is planned around direct retainers by the position of clasps, rests and type of connector.
- Bracing:
    - Bracing required should be assessed in RPD design process. Bracing is provided by the connector, maximum saddle extension and reciprocal arms of clasps. Bracing arm allows the force applied to the tooth to activate clasps, otherwise clasps will not activate without bracing component.
- Connect the denture:
    - Is there a space in the occlusion to accommodate the connector? The lower partial denture is connected along lower anterior teeth by lingual plate, lingual bar or sublingual bar.
- Reassess:
    - For form and function
    - Aesthetics.

Removal Partial Denture: Design Problems and Solution

Class I presents problems due to lack of tooth support and retention distally, small saddle area in comparison to increased force applied from opposing dentition and distant leverage on abutment tooth in function can cause increased resorption.
- Maximize indirect retention by placing rests and clasps mesially on abutment tooth and use plate design
- Muco-compressive impression technique (for saddle area) to reduce tissue displacement in function
- The altered cast technique to improve support of distal extension saddles dentures
- Maximise base extension and use smaller and fewer teeth
- RPI system for distal abutments—Mesial rest, distal guide plane and mid-buccal I-Bar.

Case 2: Over-dentures.

A 60-year-old male patient presents to your practice complaining difficulty with chewing food. He is concerned about progressively worn teeth and would like this to be addressed. Patient has history of gastric reflux disease but has not sought medical advice.
- Discuss the management of this patient.
- What are the treatment options available?

History of Complaint

Since how long patient is experiencing difficulty chewing food, history of tooth surface loss.

Medical History

Here patient has gastric reflux disease which is the likely cause of tooth wear. Patient should be directed towards his general medical practitioner or gastroenterologist for investigations and medications for regurgitation problem.

Dental History

Restorative state of dentition, pattern of tooth surface loss, regular attender or not? If any parafunctional habits are there.

Social History

- Ask if the patient is smoker?
- If the patient consumes alcohol?
- Does he consumes acidic drinks?

Examination

- Extra-oral examination:
- Look for lipseal, symmetry, lymph nodes, TMJ, etc. Teeth visible at rest.
- Intra-oral examination: In this case intra-oral examination may reveal
  - Teeth worn to the gingival margin
  - Complete loss of clinical crowns in maxilla
  - More tooth wear in maxilla than mandible
  - Little or no loss of occlusal vertical dimension.

Causes of Tooth Wear

- Dual aetiology: In this case, cause of tooth wear are erosion and attrition
- Regurgitation of stomach has dissolved the enamel and dentine, and has been exacerbated by parafunctional habit
- The fact that maxilla is affected more than mandible shows erosion as the major cause. If attrition was the main reason, tooth wear would be equal in both mandible and maxilla
- There is a induced compulsory alveolar eruption which maintain occlusal vertical dimension. Therefore, there are short clinical crowns and no room for restorations.

Treatment Options Available

- Occlusal adjustment:
  - Simple and cost-effective option, depends on existing occlusal relationship. It may require extensive tooth preparation to create anterior space.
- Full mouth rehabilitation:
  - Immediate results, composite build-up (conservative treatment); full conventional crowns coverage, but not conservative of tooth tissue and is very costly.

- Dahl appliance:
  - Conserves vitality of tooth
  - Reposition gingival margins to original position
  - Reversible
  - Long process
  - Laboratory fees involved
  - Not for partially dentate
- Surgical crown lengthening:
  - Maintain existing vertical dimension
  - Reposition gingival margin apically
  - Uncomfortable, invasive, poor interdental appearance
  - Increased risk of root treatment
  - Possibility of pulp exposure.
- Elective devitalisation:
  - Useful for excessive worn teeth with little crown height, loss of vitality, increased risk of root fractures (more important with attrition).
- No treatment and monitoring study cast:
  - When unsure regarding restorations
  - It has to be balanced as to regarding when restorations are needed, and if delayed too long restorations may not have sufficient tooth tissue remaining for restoration
  - Over denture derives support from one or more abutment teeth by completely enclosing them beneath its fitting surface
  - It can be partial or complete dentures.
- Over dentures:
  - Retains the teeth
  - Preserve alveolar bone
  - Improved retention stability and support.

Advantages

- Preservation of proprioception via periodontal ligament
- Increased masticatory force
- Improved crown to root ratio reduces damaging lateral forces.

Disadvantages

- Root canal therapy may be required
- In the region of retained tooth, denture base may need to be thinned, therefore increased risk of fracture
- Increased caries and periodontal breakdown
- Increased maintenance for both patient and general dental practitioner (GDP)
- Parafunctional habit increases risk of fracture of base plate.

Clinical Procedure

- Clinical assessment—Examination, study models, radiographs
- Root canal therapy if required

- Preparation of abutment teeth—precision attachment, gold coping, if required
- Primary impression of denture design
- Secondary impression
- Record occlusion
- Anterior set-up—to record position of incisal edge of the teeth, midline and lip support
- Try-in of metal bases
- Try-in and fit of denture
- Review and reassess
- Regular maintenance 6 monthly for increased success.

Case 3: Edentulous maxilla.

A 65-year-old patient attends your clinic for his unstable upper full denture. The patient had his maxillary teeth extracted 10 years ago and was provided with immediate fixed denture. The upper denture was replaced twice since. The patient has sound caries-free lower dentition 3-3 and lower RPD causing ulceration. Patient is fit and healthy.

Discuss the treatment option and management of this patient.

The upper denture instability is related to fibrous edentulous ridge that has developed as the result of lower natural dentition. Due to this patient often complains problem with support and stability. However, problem of retention can also be present.

- The extension of the existing denture should be assessed
  - The denture should ideally be fully extended into buccal sulcus or around maxillary tuberosities. If not then retention of upper full denture can be compromised
  - Post dam should be examined to see if the upper full denture extends up to vibrating line
- The recurrent oral ulceration of lower ridge is due unretentive and unstable lower RPD caused by extensively resorbed lower edentulous ridge
- There will be height discrepancy between the occlusal plane and residual ridge
- Denture base overlying fibrous ridge needs to be well supported and the buccal flange should be made to the full depth of the sulcus
- The management of an unsupported flabby ridge can use either muco-compressive or mucostatic impression technique for recording flabby ridge
  - Severe cases—2 stage technique using special tray with window cut over flabby ridge
  - Impression is recorded in the tray with zinc oxide eugenol or silicone impression material
  - Impression than reseated
  - Lower viscosity elastomer or impression plaster placed into the window to complete impression
  - Flabby ridge can also be removed surgically.

Treatment Options for Upper Arch
- Well fitted replacement complete Fixed Denture
- Implant supported overdenture with 2 implants placed in canine region
- Fixed-fixed with 4–6 fixtures.

Treatment Option for Lower Arch
- New replacement lower partial denture
- Extraction of remaining dentition and provide patient with Fixed
- RCT of lower left and right canine and used stud attachment to retain Fixed denture. The stud retainers will stop the movement of lower denture, therefore eliminating ulceration.

Answers

1. a. T b. T c. T d. F e. T
   f. T
2. a. T b. T c. T d. T e. T
   f. T g. T h. T
3. a. T b. T c. T d. T e. T
   f. T g. T h. T
4. a. F b. T c. F d. F e. F
   f. F g. F h. F i. T j. F
   k. F l. F m. T
5. a. T b. F c. F d. F e. T
   f. T g. F h. F i. F j. T
   k. T
6. a. T b. T c. F d. T e. F
   f. F g. F h. T i. T j. F
   k. F l. F m. F n. F o. F
7. a. T b. T c. T d. F e. F
   f. F g. T h. T i. T j. F
   k.   l. T m. F
8. a. F b. F c. T d. F e. F
   f. T g. F h. F i. F
9. a. F b. T c. T d. T e. T
   f. F g. T
10. a. T b. T c. F d. F e. T
    f. F g. T h. F i. T j. T
    k. T l. T
11. a. F b. T c. T d. T e. T
    f. T g. T h. T

12.	a.	T	b.	F	c.	F	d.	F	e.	T
	f.	F	g.	T	h.	T	i.	T	j.	F
	k.	T								
13.	a.	T	b.	T	c.	T	d.	T	e.	F
	f.	F	g.	T	h.	F	i.	T	j.	T
14.	a.	F	b.	F	c.	T	d.	T	e.	F
	f.	T	g.	F	h.	T	i.	T	i.	F
15.	a	16.	b.	17.	a	18.	a	19.	a	
20.	d	21.	b	22.	c	23.	b	24.	a	
25.	d	26.	c	27.	c					
28.	a.	9	b.	12	c.	2	d.	4	e.	1
	f.	3	g.	5	h.	14	i.	6	j.	6
	k.	16	l.	8						
29.	a.	1	b.	6	c.	5	d.	12	e.	3
	f.	10	g.	13	h.	9	i.	4		
30.	a.	1	b.	1	c.	2, 3	d.	2, 3	e.	2, 3
	f.	3, 4	g.	5	h.	6				

CORRECT ANSWER FOR FALSE STATEMENTS

4. a. Saddle can also be made of metal framework overlaid by acrylic.
   C. Cast clasps are preferred for strength and fit
   D. Cast Co-Cr occlusally approaching clasp should not be used as they are too stiff
   e. Cast cobalt chrome can engage in 0.25 mm undercut
   f. Co-cr can be cast as integral part of denture framework
   h. Lingual bars are not to be used if lower incisors are retroclined.
   J. Lingual bar does not contribute to indirect retention.
   K. Connectors do contribute to support and retention.
   L. Buccal bars are indicated when lower incisors are Retroclined.
5. c. Copy denture can be indicated when there is loss of retention but otherwise favourable denture.
   g. There are three clinical stages in copy denture.
   h. There are two laboratory stages involved
   i. Record blocks are not required as copy of old appliances are used as substitute for record blocks and special trays.
6. c. Immediate replacement denture prevents abnormal mandibular movements.
   f. Increases rapidly alveolar bone resorption
   g. Increased cost as relines, rebases and new dentures are required later.
   l. Not easy to reline/rebase/add flange.
   n. Temporary reline may be required at 1 month review appointment.
   o. Replacement denture at 12 months review appointment.
7. d. Additional retention is possible using retention attachments.
   e. Increased masticatory forces.
   f. Increased maintenance for both patient and dentist
   J. Canines and molars are preferred abutment teeth.
   m. Increased caries prevalence.
8. a. Preliminary impressions are taken using Stock trays.
   b. Upper tray should be closely fitted for ZOE impressions.
   d. Special trays can be modified by using any over extensions and addition of greenstick tracing compound.
   e. Special trays are Non-perforated.
   e. Upper master impression are recorded using silicone or alginate whereas lower master impression are recorded using ZOE or alginate.
   h. Wax bases are never suitable for upper rims.
   i. Post dam is required and indicates position of palatal relief.

10. c. Position of occlusal plane decreases with age.
    d. At rest, the tongue should rise just above occlusal plane posteriorly.
    f. Posterior teeth should be narrow to increase masticatory efficiency.
    h. Position of head does affect Freeway Space
11. a. Dentist and Patient both must be satisfied before dentures are processed in acrylic.
12. b. 0.5 mm increase in facial height occurs following processing.
    c. Upper palatal and lower buccal cusps should not be adjusted as they maintain vertical dimension of dentures
    d. Fossae should be adjusted rather than cusps tip
    f. Balancing contacts are desirable.
13. e. Rebasing of dentures involves addition of a material to the fitting and polished surface of the denture.
    f. Relining increases the thickness of the palate.
    h. Heat cured acrylic is preferred material for rebasing.
14. a. Generalised discomfort over denture bearing areas is caused by increased occlusal facial height.
    b. Decreased occlusal facial height causes collapsed face.
    e. Pain from teeth and tongue is due to teeth not set in neutral zone.
    g. Premature teeth contact is due to increased occlusal face height.e

Chapter 8
Oral Medicine and Pathology

Identify the following Statements as True (T) or False (F)

1. **Bacterial infection of the mouth:**
   a. Bacterial infection of oral mucosa are common
   b. Scarlet fever causes upper respiratory tract infections
   c. A later stages of scarlet fever, dorsum of tongue becomes smooth and red–the strawberry tongue of scarlet fever
   d. Oral lesions of tuberculosis occurs secondary to open pulmonary infection
   e. Oral manifestation of tuberculosis commonly affects posterior palate
   f. Mycobacteria can be revealed by Ziehl-Neelsen stains
   g. The causative organism of syphilis is *Borrelia burgdorferi*
   h. The primary syphilis lesions is usually found on palate
   i. The secondary lesions of syphilis develops several years after primary lesion
   j. Tertiary lesion of syphilis is marked by mucosal snail track formations
   k. Focal necrosis can lead to perforation of palate
   l. Hutchinson incisors and mulberry molars are presentation of congenital syphilis.

2. **Viral infection of mouth:**
   a. Herpetic gingivostomatitis is caused by human herpes virus 2 (HHV-2)
   b. HHV-1 can cause herpetic encephalitis
   c. 'Lipschutz Bodies' presence can confirm diagnosis of herpes labialis
   d. HHV-1 can remain dormant in trigeminal ganglion
   e. Varicella zoster is RNA virus
   f. Shingles always presents as unilateral lesion
   g. Herpangina is caused by cox virus A 22
   h. Hand foot and mouth disease is caused by Epstein-Barr virus
   i. Gingivae is commonly involved in Coxsackie A virus
   j. Human papilloma virus associated with squamous cell papillomas and condyloma accuminatum
   k. Human papilloma virus 16 and 18 can causes oropharyngeal carcinoma
   l. Koplik spots are seen in patients with glandular fever
   m. Petechial haemorrhages at the junction of hard and soft palate are pathognomonic of infectious mononucleosis

n. Infectious mononucleosis is commonly caused by cytomegalovirus
o. Mononuclear spot test is used for diagnosis of infectious mononucleosis caused by Epstein-Barr virus
p. Increased erythrocyte sedimentation rate and leucocytosis can present in Reiter's disease
q. Reiter's disease predominantly affects orders males and is associated with HLA B27 in most of the patients
r. Mitral stenosis is associated with tertiary syphilis.

3. **Human immunodeficiency virus:**
   a. Kaposi's sarcoma is caused by cytomegalovirus
   b. Hairy leucoplakia can be caused by proliferation of human herpesvirus 4
   c. In AIDS patients, hairy leucoplakia can be due to increased CD4 T lymphocyte count
   d. Erythematous candidiasis is uncommon in HIV patient
   e. Severe alveolitis and osteomyelitis with sequestration of teeth can be presented in HIV patients
   f. Bacillary angiomatosis is oral manifestation of HIV infection
   g. HIV infection may result in salivary gland lesion.

4. **Fungal infection:**
   a. Acute pseudomembranous candidiasis can affect infants
   b. Acute erythematous candidiasis is caused by continuous wearing of acrylic denture
   c. Chronic atrophic candidiasis is caused by smoking
   d. Chronic hyperplastic candidiasis is associated with decreased CD4 cell counts
   e. Erythematous candidiasis does not cause linear gingival erythema
   f. Angular cheilitis is combined staphylococcal, streptococcal and candidalinfection
   g. Epithelial hyperplasia with neutrophils in parakeratin layer is found in chronic hyperplastic candidiasis
   h. Candidalhyphae invade parakeratin layer in chronic hyperplastic candidiasis
   i. Skin and mouth lesion occurs in isolation with endocrine abnormalities in chronic mucocutaneous candidiasis
   j. Candida carriage rate is higher in smokers than in non-smokers.

5. **Recurrent aphthous stomatitis:**
   a. Recurrent aphthous stomatitis affects up to 10% of the population
   b. Minor recurrent aphthous stomatitis affects keratinised mucosa
   c. Minor recurrent aphthous stomatitis heals within 5–10 weeks
   d. Minor recurrent aphthous stomatitis is associated with tissue destruction and scarring
   e. Can presents as oral manifestation of Crohn's disease
   f. Major recurrent aphthous stomatitis are usually 5 mm diameter
   g. Recurrent aphthous stomatitis is always related to underlying folate and B_{12} deficiency

Oral Medicine and Pathology

    h. Herpetiform ulcers may involve hard palate
    i. Herpetiform ulcers are caused by herpes virus
    j. Recurrent aphthous stomatitis is major diagnostic criteria in Behcet's disease
    k. Recurrent aphthous stomatitis is accompanied by genital ulceration, erythema uveitis and erythema nodosum in Behcet's disease
    l. Behcet's disease is a disease of adults over the age of 50 years.

6. **Pemphigus—vesiculo-bullous lesions:**
   a. Is a sub-epithelial blister
   b. Is an autoimmune disorders
   c. Is most prevalent in males
   d. Prevalent in middle aged Mediterranean women
   e. A positive Nikolsky's sign is only found in Pemphigus vulgaris
   f. It is characterised by loss of intercellular adherence of supra-basal spinous cells
   g. Ocular involvement may lead to blindness
   h. Diagnosis is made by direct immunofluorescence on fresh biopsy
   i. Treatment is by topical antibiotics
   j. Lesions last 1–3 days before they burst
   k. Benign chronic pemphigus is a disease of young adults.

7. **Vesiculo-bullous lesions—mucons membrane pemphigoid:**
   a. Mucons membrane pemphigoid onset is in 3th/4th decade
   b. It is characterised by deposits of immunoglobulins and complements components in the basement membrane
   c. Pemphigoid is an intraepithelial lesion
   d. Mucons membrane pemphigoid is most common cause of desquamative gingivitis
   e. Ocular involvement may lead to scarring
   f. Prompt fixation of a mucosal biopsy is required for indirect immunofluorescence testing
   g. May be a 'marker' of internal malignancy.

8. **With regards to vesiculo-bullous lesions:**
   a. Angina bullosa haemorrhagica commonly presents in buccal mucosa
   b. Dermatitis herpetiformis is associated with gluten sensitivity
   c. Dermatitis herpetiformis is common in middle-aged females
   d. Epidermolysis bullosa is dystrophic autosomal dominant
   e. Erythema multiforme in severe form is seen in Steven-Johnson syndrome
   f. Oral lesions of erythema multiforme can mimic primary herpetic gingivostomatitis.

9. **Lichen planus:**
   a. Histologically shows hyperkeratosis, elongated rete ridges with saw tooth appearance
   b. Affects males more than females

c. It is an inflammatory condition
d. Is typically associated with subepithelial band of infiltrating B-lymphocytes
e. Oral lesions are bilateral and posterior in the buccal mucosa
f. Common oral lesion is in the form of plaque like pattern
g. Papular lichen planus has greatest malignant potential
h. Caldwell spots are cutaneous lesion of lichen planus
i. Lichen planus can be solely diagnosed clinically
j. Improve clinically with topical corticosteroid therapy.

10. **Granulomatous disorders—mucosal manifestation of gastrointestinal disease:**
    a. Granuloma are typically caseating
    b. Orofacial granulomatosis can be associated with benzoates and cinnamaldehydes
    c. Crohn's disease affects terminal two-thirds of the ileum
    d. Oro-facial granulomatosis is most prevalent in 18–30 years age group
    e. In Gardner's syndrome the facial swelling is associated with fissured tongue and facial palsy
    f. Oral lesions in sarcoidosis presents as sub-mucosal nodules and granular gingival patches
    g. Anti-neutrophil cytoplasmic antibodies can be detected in circulation in Wegener's granulomatosis
    h. Celiac associated recurrent oral ulceration can be detected by testing α-gliadin autoantibodies
    i. Pystomatitis vegetans is a manifestation of ulcerative colitis.

11. **White patches:**
    a. White sponge naevus is autosomal recessive disorder
    b. White sponge naevus is restricted to oral mucosa
    c. White sponge naevus histologically shows hyperplastic epithelium, intraepithelial oedema and basket weave appearance
    d. Frictional keratosis can be seen as self-mutilation in psychiatric disorders
    e. Smoker's keratosis only affects buccal mucosa
    f. Stomatitis nicotina mainly affects tongue.

12. **Tongue:**
    a. Can show migratory glossitis as an indicator of systemic disease
    b. Can become enlarged in amyloidosis
    c. Can develop lozenge shape red patch on the dorsum of the tongue as a result of candidiasis
    d. Can become smooth and red in sickle cell anaemia
    e. Black hairy tongue by pigmented hyperkeratotic filiform papillae in haemochromatosis.

13. **Pigmented lesion of the mouth:**
    a. Amalgam tattoos are most common mucosal pigmentation
    b. Ephelis is formed in response to chronic trauma

c. Pigmented naevi are common on vermilion border of lips and palate
d. Can be seen in Peutz-Jeghers syndrome
e. Oral contraceptives does not cause mucosal pigmentation
f. Nelson disease can be associated with pigmented lesion of the mouth
g. Haemosiderin deposits cause hyperpigmentation.

14. **Epulis:**
    a. Should always be radiographed
    b. Fibrous epulis is associated with hormonal changes in puberty
    c. Vascular epulis is pathological equivalent of pyogenic granuloma
    d. Giant cell epulis shows foci of osteoclasts like multinucleated giant cell
    e. Giant cell epulis is similar to central giant cell granuloma.

15. **Premalignant conditions:**
    a. Oral submucous fibrosis is related to using betel nuts
    b. Submucous fibrosis produces thickening of buccal mucosa and soft palate resulting in limited mouth opening
    c. Is a hereditary disorder
    d. Risk of developing oral carcinoma is about 15%
    e. Biopsy shows sub-epithelial band of fibrillar collagen in lamina propria
    f. Atrophic oral epithelium
    g. Risk of oesophageal carcinoma in Paterson-Brown-Kelly syndrome
    h. Erosive LP can be malignant
    i. Dyskeratosis congenita does not have premalignant potential.

16. **Pre-malignant lesions:**
    a. Proliferative verrucous leucoplakia is a high risk oral lesion
    b. Homogeneous leucoplakia are plaque like lesions with increased risk of malignant transformation
    c. Non-homogenous leucoplakia shows leaping of keratin nodularity and ulceration
    d. Risk of malignant transformation is greater in smokers
    e. Floor of mouth and ventral surface of tongue are likely to undergo malignant change
    f. Candidal leucoplakia have decreased risk of malignant changes
    g. Biopsy is guided by toluidine blue staining
    h. Erythroplakia is carcinoma-in-situ mostly
    i. Erythroplakia shows drop shaped rete processes, nuclear pleomorphism and minimal keratinisation.

17. **Malignant lesions—carcinoma of the lip:**
    a. Is equally common in both upper and lower lip
    b. Main aetiological factor in cancer of lip is smoking
    c. Risk of developing lip cancer doubles every 250 miles nearer the equator

d. Excess alcohol and tobacco consumption can show synergistic effect
e. Usually arises in angular cheilitis
f. Has better prognosis than intra-oral lesions
g. Often arises in a field of dysplastic change
h. Can spread via sub-mandibular nodes.

18. **With regards to squamous cell carcinoma:**
    a. Can be caused by irritation from poor restoration on the lingual aspect of the teeth
    b. Can be caused by pooling of carcinogens in the floor of mouth
    c. Can present as leucoplakia
    d. Non-human papilloma virus carcinoma have better prognosis than human papilloma virus positive carcinomas
    e. Tongue deviate to the side of oropharyngeal tumour on protrusion
    f. Can metastasise on both sides of the neck
    g. Infiltration of the submandibular duct can cause symptom of obstructive sialadenitis
    h. Can late spread via blood stream
    i. Referred otalgia can be a manifestation of oral cancer.

19. **The TNM classification findings:**
    a. Is a system used for regarding histopathological grading
    b. Primary carcinoma in floor of mouth can spread directly to level IV nodes
    c. Infiltration of adjacent structures by primary carcinoma without spread into neck indicates stage IV disease
    d. Metastasis in lymph nodes is indicator of poor prognosis
    e. Stage I squamous cell carcinoma have 80%, 5 year survival rate
    f. Overall mortality rate in 50%.

20. **Sialadenitis:**
    a. Viral sialadenitis is caused by Epstein-Barr virus
    b. Orchitis occurs in around 30% of affected males
    c. In adults, it may involve central nervous system, pancreas, testes and ovaries
    d. Unilateral parotid involvement is more common than bilateral
    e. In bacterial sialadenitis, there is involvement of unilateral parotid gland
    f. Reduced flow is predisposing factor in chronic bacterial sialadenitis than acute bacterial sialadenitis
    g. Infecting organism in bacterial sialadenitis are *Streptococcus pyogenes, Staphylococcus aureus, Haemophilus* species and black pigment bacteriodes
    h. Recurrent chronic sialadenitis is an indication of removal of the gland
    i. There is acinar atrophy and progressive fibrous replacement in radiation sialadenitis.

Oral Medicine and Pathology

21. **Xerostomia:**
    a. Can be caused by reduced salivary flow, i.e. less than 5 mL/min
    b. Can be a feature of cystic fibrosis
    c. Can be caused by hyperbaric oxygen treatment of osteoradionecrosis
    d. Predisposes mouth, salivary glands and pharynx to infection and caries
    e. It is uncommon side effects of drugs
    f. Can be caused by state of anxiety
    g. Carboxymethylcellulose can be used for treatment of xerostomia.

22. **Sjogren's syndrome:**
    a. It is characterised by polyconal T-cell proliferation as result of loss of B-cell regulation
    b. Primary Sjogren is associated with xerostomia and an autoimmune connective tissue disorder
    c. Secondary Sjorgen is associated with xerostomia and xerophthalmia
    d. There is 25% risk of malignant lymphomatous transformation of the affected gland
    e. Fatigue syndrome is associated with Sjogren syndrome
    f. Antibodies against extractable nuclear antigens particularly Sjogren's syndrome antigens-A and sjogren's syndrome antigens-B are sensitive and specific indicator
    g. Progressive lymphocytic infiltrate with acinar destruction and proliferation of residual duct results in myoepithelial islands can be seen in labial gland biopsy
    h. Increased erythrocyte sedimentation rate.

23. **Salivary gland tumours:**
    a. Pleomorphic adenoma is commonly encountered neoplasm accounts for 60% of salivary gland tumour
    b. In major salivary glands, pleomorphic adenoma presents as rubbery nodule
    c. Carcinoma in pleomorphic salivary adenoma has better prognosis than mucoepidermoid carcinoma
    d. Contains myxoid and chondroid stroma
    e. Can arise in maxillary sinus and nasal septum
    f. Occurs in superficial lobe of parotid gland
    g. Pleomorphic adenoma is removed by superficial parotidectomy
    h. Warthin's tumour—adenolymphomas affects young men
    i. Adenolymphomas arises exclusively in submandibular glands
    j. Adenolymphomas presents bilaterally in 40% of cases
    k. Histologically, Warthin's tumor have eosinophilic ductal cells supported by lymphoid stroma
    l. Smoking is aetiological factor.

24. **Malignant salivary gland tumours:**
    a. Adenoid cystic carcinoma affects elderly patients
    b. Does not invade or spread along nerve pathways

c. It is rapidly growing tumour
d. Histopathologically shows 'Swiss cheese' appearance
e. Can arise in paranasal sinuses
f. Has poor prognosis and worse survival rate
g. Mucoepidermoid carcinoma affects elderly patient
h. Shows mucous and squamous differentiation
i. Acinic cell carcinoma is low-grade and slowly progressive
j. Polymorphous low-grade adenocarcinoma is malignant tumour
k. Polymorphous low-grade adenocarcinoma occurs in maxillary sinus
l. Polymorphous low-grade adenocarcinoma has got good prognosis despite its infiltrative growth patterns
m. Haemangiomas are common tumours found in salivary gland in children.

25. **Bilateral parotid swelling can be a feature of:**
    a. Sarcoidosis
    b. Warthin tumour
    c. Primary Sjogren syndrome
    d. Secondary Sjogren syndrome
    e. Sialadenitis
    f. HIV
    g. Chronic lymphocytic leukaemia.

26. **Sialoliths:**
    a. Causes xerostomia
    b. Occurs commonly in sublingual gland
    c. Occurs commonly in parotid gland
    d. Forms due to bacterial sialadenitis
    e. Can result in submandibular saliva being supersaturated with calcium and phosphate ions
    f. May be forced into submandibular gland from anterior duct during removal under local anaesthesia
    g. Is asymptomatic
    h. Is always visible on radiograph.

27. **Salivary gland cysts:**
    a. Occurs commonly in major salivary glands
    b. Mucous extravasation mucocele occurs frequently in upper labial mucosa
    c. Has granulation tissue capsule
    d. Contains foamy macrophages
    e. May undergo spontaneous resolution
    f. Tends to relapse
    g. Mucous retention mucocele is found in buccal mucosa (upper labial mucosa)
    h. Mucous retention cysts contains clear fluid with minimal inflammatory reaction
    i. Surgical removal is treatment of choice for both mucous extravasation and retention cyst.

28. **Facial pain— trigeminal neuralgia:**
    a. Mainly affects less then 50
    b. Presence in young patient is suggestive of multiple sclerosis
    c. Is normally treated with carbamazepine
    d. Usually crosses midline of the face
    e. Occurs in response to touching trigger point
    f. Does wake patient up from sleep
    g. Can last for hours
    h. Prevalent in males more than females.

29. **Glossopharyngeal neuralgia:**
    a. Causes dull pain on swallowing
    b. May be a referred otalgia
    c. Carbamazepine is drug of choice
    d. Presence in young patient can be suggestive of intracranial neoplasm
    e. Occurs in response to eating and drinking.

30. **Giant cell arteritis:**
    a. Occurs commonly in men
    b. Usually under 50 year
    c. Pain is bilateral and affects temples
    d. Temporal artery is only affected
    e. Slightly elevated ESR
    f. Can be treated with systemic steroids
    g. Can cause blindness
    h. May cause tongue necrosis.

31. **Post-herpetic neuralgia:**
    a. More common in males
    b. Is intermittent in nature
    c. Is only type of facial pain associated with herpes zoster infection
    d. Is well controlled by carbamazepine
    e. Is not accompanied by facial palsy
    f. Is a consequence of herpes-zoster infection.

32. **Atypical facial pain:**
    a. Mainly affects mandible than maxilla
    b. There are initiating and exacerbating factors
    c. Bilateral pain crossing anatomical boundaries
    d. Is strongly associated with depression than anxiety
    e. May be alleviated by simple reassurance
    f. May be caused by anaemia
    g. Is a diagnosis of exclusion.

33. **Temporomandibular joint—the following are the muscles that opens mouth?**
    a. The masseter muscle
    b. Temporalis muscle

c. Lateral pterygoid muscle
d. Mesial pterygoid muscle
e. Digastric muscle
f. Stylomandibular muscle.

34. Disorders of joint:
a. Prevalence is more in males than females
b. Joint sounds with headache are diagnostic of TMJ pain/dysfunction
c. Abnormalities can be apparent on radiograph
d. Anterolateral displacement is the most common internal derangement
e. Clicking on opening and closing is clinically presently features. Disc displacement with reduction
f. Transient jaw deviation on opening and closing is clinical feature of disc displacement without reduction
g. Disc displacement without reduction can present pain in front of the ear
h. Treatment is usually reassurance and explanation to the patient.

35. Deviation to the left side on opening could be caused by:
a. Right temporomandibular joint anterior displacement without reduction
b. Left temporomandibular joint anterior or displacement without reduction
c. Right temporomandibular joint effusion
d. Left temporomandibular joint effusion
e. Bony ankylosis.

36. Condylar hyperplasia:
a. Is a development disorder
b. Is an inflammatory disorder
c. Can be assessed during radioisotope imaging
d. Is self-limiting
e. May have anterior open bite
f. Treatment—orthognathic surgery
g. Associated with ankylosis
h. Is common in females.

37. Erosion of condyle may occur in:
a. Pain
b. Dysfunction
c. Synovial chondromatosis
d. Internal derangement
e. Psoriasis
f. Dislocation.

38. Imaging methods can be used to measure joint spaces:
a. Panaromic radiographs
b. Transpharyngeal radiographs
c. Transcranial oblique lateral radiograph

    d. Transorbital radiograph
    e. Computed tomography.
39. **Systemic lupus erythematosus:**
    a. Common in males
    b. Skin lesions shows classic malar rash
    c. Oral muscosal lesions includes ulceration and purpura
    d. Anti-nuclear antibodies are uncommon
    e. Systemic lupus erythematosus can progress to discoid lupus erythematosus
    f. Anaemia is frequent presentation is systemic lupus erythematosus
    g. Systemic lupus erythematosus has specific double stranded DNA anti-nuclear antibody in serum
    h. Lip lesion in discoid lupus erythematosus can be premalignant.
40. **Ameloblastomas—odontogenic tumours:**
    a. Is equally prevalent in male and female
    b. Occurs most commonly between 25–40 years
    c. Usually found in anterior mandible
    d. Plexiform ameloblastoma is most common type
    e. It is multilocular
    f. It does metastasise
    g. Peripheral type is least aggressive
    h. Polycystic shows tendency to invade surrounding tissues
    i. Unicystic can be enucleated provided rim of enclosing bone is removed.
41. **With regards to odontogenic tumours:**
    a. Adenoameloblastoma tends to occur in posterior maxilla in females
    b. Pindborg tumour shows radiolucency on X-ray with scattered radio-opacities
    c. Myxoma does not invade surrounding tissues
    d. Ameloblastic fibroma causes painless expansion of the jaw
    e. Complex odontomes are multiple small teeth in fibrous sac.
42. **Cysts—radicular cysts:**
    a. Mostly prevalent in males
    b. Discovered due to obvious swelling
    c. Commonly affect maxillary wisdom teeth
    d. Tooth associated is vital tooth
    e. Root sheath of Hertwig proliferates to form radicular cysts
    f. It is derived from reduced enamel epithelium
    g. Fat is frequently found in these cysts
    h. Stratified squamous epithelium makes up cyst lining
    i. Most appropriate treatment is extraction of affected tooth
    j. Expansion of the cyst is by hydrostatic pressure
    k. Necrotic pulp is stimulus.

43. Dentigerous cysts:
   a. Is an inflammatory cyst
   b. It is usually found in under 18 years age group
   c. Mandibular wisdom teeth are commonly affected
   d. Arises from rests of malassez
   e. Forms around the root of unerupted permanent tooth
   f. Treatment is excision and extraction
   g. 40% of dentigerous cysts makes up proportion of all dental cysts.

44. Odontogenic keratocysts:
   a. Predominantly prevalent in females
   b. Is lined by stratified squamous epithelium
   c. Arise from reduced enamel epithelium
   d. Commonly found in mandibular posterior region
   e. Treatment is enucleation
   f. Is associated with Larsen's syndrome
   g. Usually these replaces missing tooth.

45. Multiple myeloma:
   a. Prevalent in males of Caucasian origin
   b. Mostly presents in age group 35–60 years
   c. Pepper-pot skull is classical finding on radiograph
   d. Is a tumour of epithelial cell
   e. There is presence of Bence-Jones protein in urine
   f. Patients presents with symptoms of hypercalcaemia.

46. Fibrous dysplasia:
   a. Is equally prevalent in males and females
   b. Commonly found in 10–20 years age group
   c. Most commonly found in mandible
   d. Classic radiographic appearance is of snow storm
   e. Patient usually complains of painful hard swelling
   f. Histologically, there is fibrous replacement of bone with osseous trabeculae
   g. Can be a feature of Albright's syndrome.

47. Paget's disease:
   a. Can present bilaterally in jaws
   b. Present in 30–50 year age group
   c. Mandible is frequently affected than maxilla
   d. Commonly affects long bones
   e. Biochemistry shows increase alkaline phosphatase
   f. Disease is usually active for 3 year
   g. X-rays shows hair-on-end appearance
   h. Prophylactic antibiotics are not required for extraction
   i. Bisphosphonates and calcitonin are used for treatment
   j. Aetiology unknown but measles and respiratory syncytial virus has been implicated.

48. **Osteosarcoma:**
    a. Commonly affects older males
    b. Mainly affects mandible
    c. Metastasis occurs to the kidneys
    d. Five year survival rate is 60%
    e. Tumour consists of abnormal fibroblasts
    f. Radiographically seen as ragged areas of radiolucency and radiopacity with no defined pattern.

49. **The following are features of osteopetrosis:**
    a. Maxillary sinus may be obliterated on occipitomental radiography
    b. Osteomyelitis is a recognised complication
    c. Osteoclastic activity is normal
    d. Anaemia is uncommon
    e. Dense bone fills the medullary cavities, increasing bone strength.

50. **Chronic osteomyelitis:**
    a. Is associated with sickle-cell disease
    b. Is an appropriate term to describe 'dry socket'
    c. The most common source of infection is blood-borne Streptococci
    d. May produce bony sequestra, involucrum and chronic sinus tract
    e. May lead to amyloidosis.

51. **Giant-cell lesions of jawbones:**
    a. May occur in renal osteodystrophy
    b. May be treated by direct calcitonin injection
    c. Can be feature of primary hyperparathyroidism
    d. Contains cells with histological and functional feature of osteoclasts
    e. May perforate alveolus.

52. **Trigeminal neuralgia:**
    a. Neuralgia of fifth cranial nerve
    b. It affects the first division of trigeminal nerve
    c. Pain distribution is unilateral
    d. The common trigger zones are vermilion border of lips, alae of nose, cheeks and around eyes
    e. Pain is not accompanied by brief facial spasm or tic.

53. **Ectodermal dysplasia:**
    a. Inherited disorder that involves more than one ectodermal derivatives
    b. Commonly involved tissues are skin, hair, nails, eccrine glands and teeth
    c. Clouston syndrome is most common phenotype in this group
    d. Saddle nose, frontal bossing are not characteristic features
    e. Conical or pegged teeth, anodontia or oligodontia in both permanent and deciduous teeth is seen.

54. Keratocystic odontogenic tumour:
   a. It has low recurrence rate
   b. Scalloping border typically corrugated, rippled or wrinkled parakeratinized surface is a histologic feature
   c. Lumen of keratocyst is filled with thin straw colored fluid or with thicker creamy material
   d. It is a malignant neoplasm
   e. It manifests as multilocular radiolucent odontogenic keratocyst radiographically.

55. Nasopalatine duct cyst:
   a. It is most common nonodontogenic cyst
   b. It is developmental cyst, non-neoplastic in nature
   c. It affects midline anterior maxilla
   d. Females are more commonly affected
   e. It is an inflammatory cyst.

56. Enamel hypoplasia:
   a. Hutchinson's teeth are anterior teeth in enamel hypoplasia due to congenital syphilis
   b. Turner's hypoplasia involves maxillary incisors or maxillary or mandibular premolars
   c. Mottled enamel is a type of enamel hypoplasia
   d. Mulberry molars are not present in enamel hypoplasia
   e. Hypocalcemia is one of the cause of enamel hypoplasia.

57. Oral Naevi:
   a. It is non-developmental malformation
   b. Blue naevus is true mesodermal structure that consist of dermal melanocytes
   c. The most common mucosal type is blue naevus
   d. Blue naevus is more common on skin than in mouth
   e. Intradermal naevus is most common lesion of skin.

Identify the Single Best Answer for the following

58. Oral ulcerations in immunosuppressed patients is caused by this organism:
   a. Cytomegalovirus
   b. Varicella-zoster virus
   c. Herpes simplex virus
   d. Coxsackie virus.

59. The first structure to show evidence of destruction in an early carious lesion is:
   a. Cuticle
   b. Enamel prism
   c. Inter-prismatic substance
   d. Dead tracts.

60. All the developmental cysts of the jaws present as radiolucent lesions, *except*:
    a. Nasolabial cyst
    b. Epidermoid cyst
    c. Median palatal cyst
    d. Globulomaxillary cyst.

61. Koplik's spot are seen as an oral manifestation in:
    a. Varicella
    b. Rubella
    c. Mumps
    d. Acquired immunodeficiency syndrome.

62. Corticosteroids are contraindicated in:
    a. Primary herpes
    b. Pemphigus
    c. Lichen planus
    d. Erythema multiforme.

63. Non-keratotic white lesions is:
    a. Linea alba
    b. Focal epithelial hyperplasia
    c. Uremic stomatitis
    d. Stomatitis nicotina palate.

64. All have precancerous potential, *except*:
    a. Keratosis follicularis
    b. Actinic keratosis
    c. Dyskeratosis congenital
    d. Erythroplakia.

65. Café au lait pigmentations are found in:
    a. Gardner's syndrome
    b. Xanthomatosis
    c. Neurofibromatosis
    d. Peutz-Jeghers syndrome.

66. Cysts involving hair follicles, sweat glands and sebum are called as:
    a. Follicular cyst
    b. Teratomas
    c. Epidermoid cyst
    d. Stafne's cyst.

67. The complication of a radiation therapy is:
    a. Micrognathia
    b. Trismus
    c. Parotitis
    d. Candidiasis.

68. **Strawberry tongue is a classical sign of:**
    a. Salmonella typhi
    b. Herpes simplex virus
    c. Capnocytophaga
    d. Streptococcus pyogens.

69. **Which is most common malignant epithelial tumor?**
    a. Epidermoid carcinoma
    b. Basal cell carcinoma
    c. Rodent ulcer
    d. Malignant melanoma
    e. Squamous acanthoma
    f. Lipoma.

70. **Ulcerative gingivostomatitis with sore mouth is common clinical finding:**
    a. Herpetic stomatitis
    b. Aphthous stomatitis major
    c. Minor aphthous stomatitis
    d. Gonococcal stomatitis
    e. Allergic stomatitis.

71. **Syphilitic rhagades are present near angle of mouth in:**
    a. Tertiary syphilis
    b. Primary syphilis
    c. Secondary syphilis
    d. Congenital syphilis.

72. **Hemophilia A is caused due to:**
    a. Deficiency of Christmas factor
    b. Deficiency of antihemophilic factor
    c. Excessive production of Christmas factor
    d. Deficiency of Stuart factor
    e. Deficiency of Hageman factor
    f. Increased antihemophilic factor.

73. **Disseminated intravascular coagulation can be treated by administration of:**
    a. Intravenous heparin
    b. Subcutaneous heparin
    c. Dicumarol
    d. All of the above
    e. None of the above.

74. **Which clinical tests are used to evaluate primary hemostasis?**
    a. Platelet count
    b. Bleeding time
    c. All of the above
    d. None of the above.

75. Which among the following is associated with the occurrence of Burkitt's lymphoma?
   a. Varicella-zoster virus
   b. Cytomegalovirus
   c. Epstein-Barr virus
   d. Coxsackie virus
   e. Herpes simplex virus.

76. AIDS patients becomes susceptible to infections when T4 lymphocytes count is below:
   a. 100 mm^3
   b. 150 mm^3
   c. 75 mm^3
   d. 50 mm^3.

77. The recommended dose of epinephrine for treatment of anaphylaxis in adults is:
   a. 0.2 ml intravenously
   b. 0.5 ml subcutaneously
   c. 0.5 ml intravenously
   d. 0.3 ml subcutaneously
   e. 0.6 ml intravenously.

78. Micrognathia and anterior open bite are present in:
   a. Septic arthritis
   b. Juvenile rheumatoid arthritis
   c. Psoriatic arthritis
   d. Rheumatoid arthritis.

79. Dosage of intraductal erythromycin in chronic nonspecific bacterial sialadenitis treatment is:
   a. 25 mg/ml for 7 days
   b. 25 mg/ml for 5 days
   c. 15 mg/ml for 7 days
   d. 15 mg/ml for 5 days
   e. 5 mg/ml for 7 days.

80. Salt and pepper appearance of salivary glands, in MRI suggests:
   a. Sialadenosis
   b. Sarcoidosis
   c. Necrotising sialometaplasia
   d. Sjogren's syndrome.

81. What is the most common site for carcinoma of tongue?
   a. Dorsum of tongue
   b. Base of tongue
   c. Anterior two-third of tongue
   d. Ventral surface of tongue.

Identify the answers for the following Extended Matching questions

82. Syndromes:

a. Oral ulceration, genital ulceration and Uveitis-clinical diagnosis can be made on finding two of these three. It is multisystem disease of immunological origin. Affects young adults, especially males and there is association with HLA-B5

b. This comprises of a group of disorders characterised by hyper-flexibility of joints, increased bleeding and bruising and hyper-extendable skin. There appears to be an underlying molecular abnormality of collagen

c. This syndrome consists of facial paralysis, facial oedema and a fissured tongue. It is a variant of orofacial-granulomatosis

d. Consists of a constricted pupil, drooping eyelid and unilateral anhydrosis on the face and occasionally enophthalmos. It is caused by an interruption of the sympathetic nerve at cervical ganglion secondary to a tumour

e. A condition in which gustatory sweating and flushing of the skin occurs. It follows trauma to the salivary glands and is thought to be caused by crossover of the sympathetic and parasympathetic innervation to the gland and the skin

f. Consists of polyostotic fibrous dysplasia, patchy skin pigmentation and an endocrine abnormality. Facial asymmetry affects upto 25% of cases

g. This comprises of multiple osteomas, multiple polyps of the large intestine, epidermoid cysts and fibromas of the skin. It shows autosomal dominant inheritance

h. Malformation syndrome caused by trisomy of chromosome 21. Patient has macroglossia, delayed eruption of teeth, small nose, brachycephaly, midface retrusion, upward sloping palpebral fissures

i. Multiple neurofibromas with skin pigmentation, skeletal abnormalities, central nervous system involvement and predisposition to malignancy. Autosomal dominant

j. Severe version of erythema multiforme, a mucocutaneous disorder autoimmune, precipitated classically by drugs. Classic lesions are target lesions, concentric red rings which especially affects hands and teeth

k. A lower motor neuron facial palsy with vesicles on the same side in the pharynx, external auditory canal and on the face. May lead to deafness caused by herpes zoster

l. The occurrence of dysphagia, microcytic hypochromic anaemia, koilonychias and angular cheilitis. The dysphagia is due to post-cricoid web, usually a membrane on the anterior oesophageal wall which is premalignant. Affect middle aged women

m. Consist of multiple basal cell naevi, multiple odontogenic keratocysts, calcified falx cerebri, cleidocranial dysostosis.

1. Albright syndrome	8. Harmer's syndrome
2. Behcet's syndrome	9. Down's syndrome
3. Ehlers-Danlos syndrome	10. Gorlin-Goltz syndrome
4. Frey's syndrome	11. Paterson-Brown-Kelly syndrome
5. Gardner's syndrome	12. Ramsay-Hunt syndrome
6. Graves' disease	13. Stevens-Johnson syndrome
7. Melkersson-Rosenthal syndrome	14. Von Recklinghausen syndrome

83. **Cysts:**
    a. A midline cyst of the anterior maxilla with lining of squamous and/or ciliated columnar epithelium. There may be neurovascular bundle and sometimes salivary acini found in cyst wall
    b. A developmental cyst which forms in anterior maxilla between lateral incisor and canine. Both teeth are vital. The cyst has fibrous wall which may be squamous columnar or columnar ciliated.
    c. Rare soft tissue cyst external to the alveolar ridge below ala nasi. It occurs from the remnants of the lower end of the nasolacrimal duct. Peak incidence 40-50 year
    d. Solid may be benign odontogenic tumour. Second decade occurrence. It has fibrous walls with lining of squamous epithelium but basal layer may be columnar and ameloblast like in appearance. Abnormal keratinisation of spinous cells produces ghost cells. Patchy calcification is also found
    e. A possible developmental defect or result of bleeding into or vascularisation of pre-existing lesion such as giant cell granuloma
    f. Almost invariably occur in the mandible. The cavity and radiolucency can extend through callus bone and arch up between the roots of teeth but rarely expands the bone. The cyst cavity may contain serosanguineous fluid or may be empty.

    1. Aneurysmal bone cyst
    2. Calcifying odontogenic cyst
    3. Globulomaxillary cyst
    4. Nasopalatine cyst
    5. Residual cyst
    6. Solitary bone cyst

84. **Oral manifestation of endocrine disease:**
    a. Enlargement of lips and tongue, spacing of teeth, increase jaw size particularly mandible resulting in class III malocclusion
    b. Melanotic brown pigmentation of the oral mucosa, commonly cheek
    c. The appearance of a 'moon face' and oral candidiasis
    d. Congenital form of this disease is associated with puffy enlargement of lips and delayed tooth eruption
    e. Increase susceptibility of periodontal disease, xerostomia. Some patient complaint of oral dysaesthesia
    f. Endocrine disorder causes radiographic changes in the mandible causes loss of lamina dura, ground glass appearance of bone, cystic lesion which are indistinguishable from a brown tumour.

1. Acromegaly	6. Hyperthyroidism
2. Addison disease	7. Hypoparathyroidism
3. Cushing's syndrome	8. Hypothyroidism
4. Diabetes	9. Sex hormones
5. Hyperparathyroidism	

85. **Burning mouth syndrome:**
    a. Which sex is mainly affected by burning mouth syndrome?
    b. In which age group does this condition presents?
    c. Common site affected.
    d. Which systemic condition must be ruled out in patients with burning mouth syndrome?
    e. Which vitamin is most commonly low in these patients?
    f. Which bacteria are commonly associated with this condition?

1. Male	11. HIV
2. Female	12. Diabetes
3. 18–30 years	13. Crohn's Disease
4. 30–45 years	14. Vitamin A
5. 45–60 years	15. Vitamin B6
6. Above 60 years	16. Vitamin B12
7. Lips	17. Vitamin E
8. Tongue	18. *Staphylococcus aureus*
9. Floor of mouth	19. *Streptococcus pyogenes*
10. Pharynx	20. *Candida albicans*.

86. **Addison's disease:**
    a. Which gland is atrophic in Addison's disease?
    b. What substance is absent or decreased in this disease?
    c. What lesion is present on gingivae and skin?
    d. What is the colour of these lesions?
    e. Diagnosis of this condition is by
    f. Treatment of Addison's disease.

1. Hypothlamus	10. Raised polypoid lesions
2. Anterior pituitary	11. Lichenoid reaction
3. Post-pituitary	12. Hyperpigmentation
4. Adrenal gland	13. Thyroxine (T4) blood test
5. Thyroid	14. Thyroid-stimulating hormone (TSH)
6. Thyroxine	15. Adrenocorticotropic hormone (ACTH) test
7. Corticosteroids	16. Red
8. Calcitrol	17. Brown
9. Ulcers	18. White

87. **Kaposi sarcoma:**
    a. Mostly prevalent in which sex
    b. Causative organism
    c. Causative virus organism it is associated with?
    d. Colour of the lesion in the mouth
    e. From which tissue this tumour originates
    f. Mean survival time from diagnosis to death.

1. Male	8. Red	15. Muscle
2. Female	9. Yellow	16. 6 months
3. Equally prevalent	10. Pink	17. 1 year
4. HIV	11. Purple	18. 2 years
5. HPV	12. Epithelial	19. 5 years
6. Paramyxovirus	13. Endothelial	20. Lifelong
7. HHV	14. Bone	

88. **Histology of caries:**
    a. Zone closest to advancing edge of enamel caries
    b. Zone 2nd closet to advancing edge of enamel caries
    c. Zone 3rd closest to advancing edge of enamel caries
    d. Outermost to advancing edge of enamel caries
    e. Zone closest to advancing edge of dentinal caries
    f. Zone 2nd closest to advancing edge of dentinal caries
    g. Zone 3rd closest to advancing edge of dentinal caries
    h. Zone outermost to advancing edge of dentinal caries.

1. Body of lesion	5. Zone of bacterial invasion
2. Dark zone	6. Zone of demineralisation
3. Surface zone	7. Zone of destruction
4. Translucent zone	8. Zone of sclerosis

89. **Squamous cell carcinoma:**
    a. The classical histopathologic alterations present are.
    b. What type of neoplasm?
    c. Which chromosomes have been detected with genetic mutations in squamous cell carcinoma?
    d. Which tissue has been associated with its origin?

1. Malignant	12. Nervous
2. Benign	13. Muscle
3. Male	14. Keratinisation
4. Female	15. Non-keratinised
5. Chromosome 3p	16. Bone
6. Chromosome 4q and 11q	17. Red
7. Epithelial	18. White patch
8. Squamous epithelium	19. Increased nuclear/cytoplasmic ratio
9. Mesenchyme	20. Hyperchromatic and enlarged nuclei
10. Metastasis	21. Dyskeratotic and increased/aberrant mitotic activity
11. Spindle cells	

90. **Epithelial dysplasia:**
    a. The diagnosis and grading of epithelial dysplasia is based on which features?
    b. The most severe form of epithelial dysplasia
    c. Which features are the criteria for moderate dysplasia?
    d. Mild dysplasia is diagnosed based on which features?
    e. Which features help to distinguish severe dysplasia?

1. Carcinoma in situ	13. Marked pleomorphism with abnormal nuclei and prominent apoptotic bodies
2. Architectural	
3. Cytological	
4. Combination of architectural and cytological	14. Deep abnormal keratinisation and absence of stratification
5. Proliferation of basal and parabasal layers	15. Bulbous rete pegs
	16. Loss of rete pegs
6. Does not extend beyond lower third of epithelium	17. Normal stratification
	18. Decreased nuclear/cytoplasmic ratio
7. Mitosis not prominent	
8. Slight cytological atypia	19. No epithelial atrophy
9. Extend into middle one-third of epithelium	20. Mesenchyme
	21. Lymph nodes
10. Mitosis prominent	22. Metastasis
11. Cytological changes are more severe	23. Primary tumor
12. Abnormal proliferation from basal layer into upper third of epithelium	24. Epithelial atrophy

91. **Dentin dysplasia:**
    a. Which is more common?
    b. What are different types of dentin dysplasia?
    c. Which dentition is affected in coronal?
    d. Which dentition is affected in radicular?
    e. What type of dentine is present in coronal type?
    f. The lava flowing around boulders is histopathological feature of which type?
    g. What is characteristic radiographic feature of coronal type?

1. Deciduous	8. Abnormal dentine
2. Permanent	9. Radicular
3. Autosomal dominant	10. Thistle tube
4. Autosomal recessive	11. Coronal
5. Opalescent teeth	12. Atubular dentine
6. Rootless teeth	13. Pulp stones
7. Normal enamel	

CASE DISCUSSIONS

Case 1: Recurrent Aphthous Stomatitis (RAS)

Patient aged 16 years female attends your surgical clinic with a complaint of recurrent oral ulcers. Please give this patient advice on aphthous ulcers.

Minor RAS

- Recurrent aphthous ulceration is a common mucosal disorder (~ 25% of population)
- It is more common in females and have a familial tendency (~ 45%)
- No single causative factor—Autoimmune?
- Associated with reduced levels of iron, folic acid or vitamin B12 which are found in up to 20% of patients. Therefore, correction of these deficiencies results in resolution of the symptoms of the patient.

Predisposing Factors

- Hypersensitivity to foodstuff, benzoate preservatives E210–219
- Cessation of smoking
- Psychological factor—stress
- Injury to mucosa
- Other diseases—manifestation of Crohn's disease ulcerative colitis or gluten enteropathy.

Biopsy

- Usually not needed
- Blood test to exclude haematinic deficiencies
- If patient is associated with gastrointestinal symptoms like:
- Heavy menstrual blood loss
- vegan
- Full blood count (FBC), levels of vitamin B12, whole blood folate and ferritin levels

Diagnosis

- Diagnosis is based on history and clinical presentation
- Usually appears as a group of 1-6 ulcers at a time
- Variable size 2-5 mm diameter
- Occurs on non-keratinised mucosa
- Heals within 1-2 week without scarring
- Prodromal discomfort may precede painful ulcers.

Treatment

- Treatment is based on identifying predisposing factors and treating them followed by symptomatic relief
- Avoid food containing benzoate preservatives
- Avoid chips and chocolate.

Symptomatic Relief

- Mouthwashes:
  - Chlorhexidine
  - Sodium bicarbonate
  - Benzydamine
  - Tetracycline (250 mg QDS in water 7 days)
  - Doxycycline
- Topical steroid:
  - Hydrocortisone
  - Triamcinolone
  - Beclometasone
  - Betamethasone.

Systemic Treatment

- When severe—to be prescribed only by specialist
  - Prednisolone
  - Monoamine oxidase inhibitors
  - Levamisole
  - Thalidomide
  - Dapsone.

Major RAS

Seen in 10% of RAS patients.

Clinically Features

- Large ulcers >10 mm
- Last for 5-10 weeks on keratinised mucosa
- Associated with tissue destruction and scarring
- Any site of the mouth (Figs 8.1A and B)
- Oropharynx may be affected
- Higher association between major aphthae and gastrointestinal and haematological disorder
- Also seen in Aquired immune deficiency syndrome (AIDS).

Treatment

Application of topical steroid along with systemic steroid.

Herpetiform Ulcers

Least common form of ulcers.

Clinical Features

- Manifest as a crop of small but painful ulcers which usually last 1-2 weeks
- Commonest site being floor of mouth, lateral margins and tip of tongue

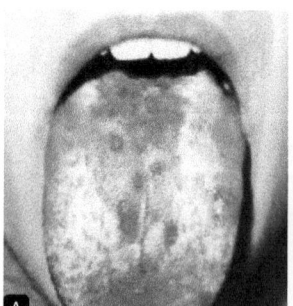 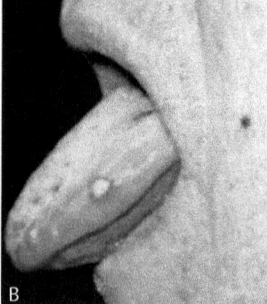

Figs 8.1A and B: (A) Multiple lesions on surface of tongue. (B) Solitary lesion on lateral border of tongue

- They heal without scarring
- May occur on keratinised and non-keratinised mucosa
- Rarely, merge to form large ulcer which heals with scarring.

Treatment
- Same as minor aphthae ulceration.

Case 2: Lichen Planus

Lichen Planus is common condition affecting 1% of the population and involves skin and mucous membranes. Peak incidence is in 3-6th decades of life more prevalent in females.

Clinical Features
- Bilateral, affects buccal mucosa, lateral tongue (Fig. 8.2)
- May also manifist as desquamative gingivitis
- Atypical distribution suggests lichenoid reaction, may be systemic lupus erythematosus SLE.

Types of Oral Lesion
- Reticular lesions: Linear white bands
- Plaque lesions: White patches
- Papular lesions: Small white spots
- Atrophic: Diffuse red areas
- Annular: Circular array of white lines
- Erosive: Extreme atrophy leading to ulceration
- Bullous: Blood filled blisters.

Skin Lesions
- Volacious, itchy macules and papules on flexure surface
- Wickham striae—may be more widespread on trunk
- Fingernails may be ridged or atrophied

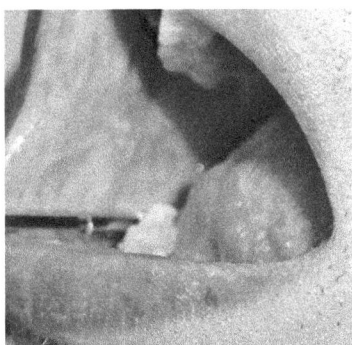

Fig. 8.2: Lichen planus on the buccal surface of oral mucosa.

- Scalp involvement (may be hair loss)
- In female—vulva and vagina may be affected.
- Skin lesions tends to be transitory
- White oral lesions are persistent

Predisposing Factors
- Drugs, e.g. anti-malarial, anti-diabetic drugs, NSAIDs, gold salt, anti-hypertensive
- Dental restorative material (e.g. amalgam and gold)
- Graft versus host disease
- Hepatitis C and chronic liver disease.
- Alcohol and smoking may be contributory factors

Treatment
- To alleviate symptoms, but will not cure the condition which may persists for several years
- Modification of diet (avoid spicy, acidic and salty food)
- Analgesic mouthwash/spray-benzydamine hydrochloride
- Topical steroids:
  - Paste—Triamcinolone dental paste
  - Lozenges—Hydrocortisone lozenges
  - Soluble tablets for mouthwash—Betamethasone, sodium phosphate
  - Inhaled sprayed onto the affected areas (Beclometasone dipropionate)
  - Specialist oral medicine opinion should be sought prior to prescription
  - Choice of medication is determined by disease severity and site involved
  - Localised lesions—Triamcinolone paste
  - Generalised lesions—Steroid mouthwash
  - Severe cases—systemic medication–systemic steroids in combination with immunosuppressant azathioprine (presented by hospital-based specialist).

Case 3: White Patches

A 36-year old patient attends your surgery complaining white patch in his mouth. He is concerned about it:
- What is the differential diagnosis of the lesion?
- What steps would you take to reach diagnosis?

Diagnosis

History of presenting complaint under the following headings.

a. Medical History
- Drugs—Antibiotics, immunosuppressants, steroids
- Underlying disease predisposing to *Candida* infection
- Syphilis—Rare cause of a white patch.

b. Dental History
- Restorations causing lichenoid reactions
- Cheek biting and trauma
- Chemical burns.

c. Social History
- Alcohol/smoking habits
- High-risk group of keratosis, Squamous cell carcinoma.

Clinical Examination
- Extra oral—nodal involvement, angular cheilitis
- Intra oral—soft and hard tissue examination
- Character of patch:
  - Is it fixed or does it rub off (e.g, Candida)
  - Is it uniform or striated—lichen planus, hairy leucoplakia, lupus, etc.

Site of Patch
- Unilateral—Idiopathic leucoplakia, squamous cell carcinoma
- Bilateral—LP, Fordyce spots, white sponge naevus, cheek biting, *Candida*, submucous fibrosis
- Localised or widespread at different site (Figs 8.3A and B)
- Sublingual—sublingual keratosis.

Local Cause
- Friction from teeth
- Restorations—intact or fractured
- Blood tests
- Swabs for Candida
- Incisional biopsy for definitive diagnosis
- Reassure patient.

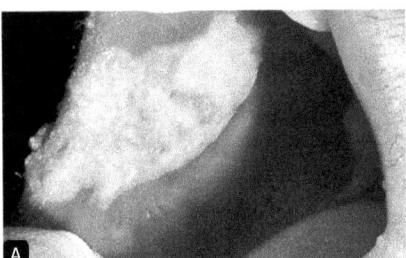 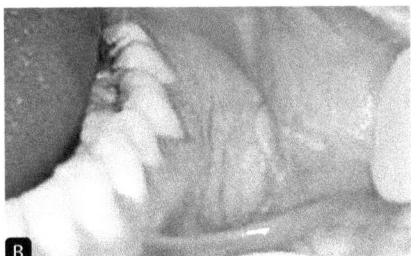

Figs 8.3A and B: (A) White patch on buccal mucosa. (B) White patch angle of mouth and buccal vestibule

Differential Diagnosis
- Neoplastic and potentially malignant disease:
  - Leucoplakia
  - Carcinoma
  - Keratosis.
- Inflammatory:
  - Infective disease—Candidiasis
  - Hairy leucoplakia
  - Papilloma
- Non-infective conditions:
  - Lichen planus
  - Lupus erythematosus
- Congenital:
  - White sponge nevus
  - Fordyce spots
  - Leukoedema
- Others:
  - Cheek biting/burns/grafts
  - Smoker's keratosis.

Case 4: Sjogren's syndrome.

You are seeing patient with dry mouth in oral medicine clinic. You suspect Sjogren's syndrome. Discuss aetiology, treatment for this patient.
- Sjogren's syndrome is autoimmune chronic inflammatory disease involving the salivary and lacrimal glands
- Characterised by polyclonal B-cell proliferation as a result of loss of T-cell regulation
- Lymphocytic infiltrate and destruction of glandular parenchyma
  - Primary Sjogren—associated with xerostomia and xerophthalmia
  - Secondary Sjogren—associated with both xerostomia, xerophthalmia and autoimmune connective tissue disorder
- Including nasal and vaginal dryness
- Fatigue syndrome
- Rheumatoid arthritis most commonly associated disorder.

Clinical Features
- Seen mostly in middle aged females
- Sjogren like features can also be seen in T-cell dysfunction including HIV, graft versus host disease, therapeutic immunosuppression
- Patient complain about difficulty in eating dry food, tongue adhering to palate
- Symptoms worsen during night/disturbed sleep
- Difficulty swallowing/speaking/wearing dentures
- Glazed oral mucosa, lobulated and beefy red tongue (Fig. 8.4)
- Oral candidiasis can be present

- Enlargement of salivary glands—may result in obstruction, acute infections and transformation to malignant lymphoma.

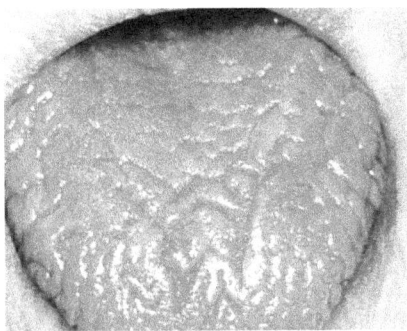

Fig. 8.4: Clinical presentation of tongue in Sjogren's syndrome

Diagnosis

- Sialometry test—to measure rate of production of saliva in the mouth
- Lacrimal gland flow rate by Schirmer's test, tear production reduces when salivary flow rate is decreased. It involves placing piece of filter paper under a lower eyelid for 5 minutes and measuring how far moisture travels along the paper; less than 5 mm is indicative of reduced production of tears
- Labial gland biopsy—sample of salivary gland from the lower lip
- Sialography—involves injecting radiopaque dye into salivary gland duct and then taking radiograph of the gland and the duct. It shows architecture of gland, stones or filling defects along with functional abnormalities
- Scintigraphy—IV injection of radioactive isotope (technetium-99 m pertechnetate). Uptake of radioactive isotope is then assessed using gamma camera to visualise functional salivary gland tissue
- Blood tests—are carried out as there can be systemic involvement. Full blood count, erythrocyte sedimentation rate, SSA (RO), SSB (LA), IgA immune complex, rheumatoid factor.

Management

- By multidisciplinary team:
  - Dry mouth can be treated
  - Salivary stimulants if there is residual salivary function
  - Sucking sugar-free pastilles (Salivix), sugar-free chewing gum
  - Salivary substitutes
    - Carboxymethylcellulose based (lubriant)
    - Mucin based, e.g. Saliva Orthana
    - Gel containing enzymes presents in saliva (Bioxtra)
  - Preventing advice related to increased caries risk and periodontal diseases
  - Use of fluoride mouthwash
  - Xerostomia residual salivary gland function is present on stimulation, pilocarpine can be prescribed which benefits in radiation induced xerostomia and Sjogren's syndrome.

Answers

1.	a.	F	b.	T	c.	F	d.	T	e.	F
	f.	T	g.	F	h.	F	i.	F	j.	F
	k.	T	l.	T						
2.	a.	F	b.	T	c.	F	d.	T	e.	F
	f.	T	g.	T	h.	F	i.	F	j.	T
	k.	T	l.	F	m.	T	n.	F	o.	T
	p.	T	q.	F	r.	F				
3.	a.	F	b.	T	c.	F	d.	F	e.	F
	f.	T	g.	T						
4.	a.	T	b.	F	c.	F	d.	F	e.	F
	f.	T	g.	F	h.	T	i.	F	j.	F
5.	a.	F	b.	F	c.	F	d.	F	e.	T
	f.	F	g.	F	h.	T	i.	F	j.	T
	k.	T	l.	F						
6.	a.	F	b.	T	c.	F	d.	T	e.	F
	f.	T	g.	F	h.	T	i.	F	j.	F
	k.	T								
7.	a.	F	b.	T	c.	F	d.	F	e.	T
	f.	F	g.	T						
8.	a.	F	b.	T	c.	F	d.	F	e.	T
	f.	T								
9.	a.	T	b.	F	c.	F	d.	F	e.	T
	f.	F	g.	F	h.	F	i.	F	j.	T
10.	a.	F	b.	T	c.	F	d.	F	e.	F
	f.	T	g.	T	h.	F	i.	T		
11.	a.	F	b.	F	c.	T	d.	T	e.	F
	f.	F								

Oral Medicine and Pathology

12. a. F b. T c. T d. F e. F
13. a. T b. F c. T d. T e. F
    f. T g. T
14. a. T b. F c. T d. T e. F
15. a. F b. F c. F d. F e. T
    f. T g. T h. F i. F
16. a. T b. F c. T d. F e. T
    f. F g. T h. T i. T
17. a. F b. F c. T d. T e. F
    f. T g. T h. F
18. a. F b. T c. T d. F e. T
    f. T g. F h. T i. T
19. a. F b. T c. T d. T e. T
    f. T
20. a. F b. F c. T d. F e. T
    f. F g. T h. T i. F
21. a. F b. T c. F d. T e. F
    f. T g. T
22. a. F b. F c. F d. F e. T
    f. T g. F h. T
23. a. F b. F c. F d. T e. T
    f. T g. T h. F i. F j. F
    k. T l. T
24. a. T b. F c. F d. T e. T
    f. T g. F h. T i. F j. T
    k. F l. T m. T
25. a. T b. T c. T d. T e. F
    f. T g. T
26. a. F b. F c. F d. F e. T
    f. T g. T h. F

27.	a.	F	b.	F	c.	T	d.	T	e.	T
	f.	T	g.		h.	T	i.	T		
28.	a.	??	b.	T	c.	T	d.	F	e.	T
	f.	F	g.	F	h.	F				
29.	a.	F	b.	T	c.	T	d.	T	e.	T
30.	a.	F	b.	F	c.	T	d.	F	e.	F
	f.	T	g.	T	h.	T				
31.	a.	F	b.	F	c.	F	d.	F	e.	F
	f.	F								
32.	a.	F	b.	F	c.	T	d.	T	e.	T
	f.	F	g.	F						
33.	a.	F	b.	F	c.	T	d.	F	e.	T
	f.	F								
34.	a.	F	b.	F	c.	F	d.	F	e.	T
	f.	F	g.	T	h.	T				
35.	a.	F	b.	T	c.	F	d.	T	e.	F
36.	a.	T	b.	F	c.	T	d.	T	e.	F
	f.	T	g.	F	h.	F				
37.	a.	F	b.	F	c.	T	d.	T	e.	T
	f.	F								
38.	a.	F	b.	F	c.	T	d.	F	e.	T
39.	a.	F	b.	T	c.	T	d.	F	e.	F
	f.	T	g.	F	h.	T				
40.	a.	F	b.	F	c.	F	d.	F	e.	T
	f.	F	g.	F	h.	T	i.	T		
41.	a.	F	b.	T	c.	F	d.	T	e.	F
42.	a.	F	b.	F	c.	F	d.	F	e.	F
	f.	F	g.	F	h.	T	i.	F	j.	T
	k.	T								

43.	a.	F	b.	F	c.	T	d.	F	e.	T
	f.	T	g.	F						
44.	a.	F	b.	F	c.	F	d.	T	e.	F
	f.	F	g.	T						
45.	a.	F	b.	F	c.	T	d.	F	e.	T
	f.	T	g.	T						
46.	a.	T	b.	T	c.	F	d.	F	e.	F
	f.	T	g.	T						
47.	a.	T	b.	F	c.	F	d.	F	e.	T
	f.	F	g.	F	h.	F	i.	T	j.	T
48.	a.	F	b.	T	c.	F	d.	F	e.	F
	f.	T								
49.	a.	T	b.	T	c.	F	d.	F	e.	F
50.	a.	T	b.	F	c.	F	d.		e.	T
51.	a.	T	b.	T	c.	T	d.	T	e.	T
52.	a.	T	b.	F	c.	T	d.	T	e.	F
53.	a.	T	b.	T	c.	F	d.	F	e.	T
54.	a.	F	b.	T	c.	T	d.	F	e.	F
55.	a.	T	b.	T	c.	T	d.	F	e.	F
56.	a.	T	b.	T	c.	T	d.	F	e.	T
57.	a.	F	b.	T	c.	F	d.	F	e.	T
58.	c	59.	c	60.	a	61.	b	62.	a	
63.	c	64.	a	65.	c	66.	c	67.	c	
68.	d	69.	a	70.	a	71.	d	72.	b	
73.	a	74.	c	75.	c	76.	d	77.	c	
78.	b	79.	d	80.	d	81.	c			
82.	a.	2	b.	3	c.	7	d.	8	e.	4
	f.	1	g.	5	h.	9	i.	12	j.	13
	k.	12	l.	11	m.	10				

83.	a.	5	b.	3	c.	4	d.	2	e.	1
	f.	6								
84.	a.	1	b.	2	c.	3	d.	8	e.	4
	f.	5								
85.	a.	2	b.	6	c.	8	d.	12	e.	16
	f.	20								
86.	a.	4	b.	7	c.	12	d.	17	e.	16
	f.	7								
87.	a.	1	b.	7	c.	4	d.	11	e.	13
	f.	19								
88.	a.	4	b.	2	c.	1	d.	3	e.	8
	f.	6	g.	5	h.	7				
89.	a.	18, 19, 20	b.	1, 7	c.	5, 6	d.	8		
90.	a.	4	b.	1	c.	9, 11, 17, 10	d.	6, 7, 8, 17	e.	12, 13, 14, 15, 24
91.	a.	9	b.	9, 11	c.	1, 2	d.	1, 2	e.	12
	f.	9	g.	10						

CORRECT ANSWER FOR FALSE STATEMENTS

1. a. Rare
   c. Raspberry tongue of scarlet fever
   e. Oral manifestation of TB commonly affects Posterior aspect of dorsum of the tongue
   a. Treponema pallidum
   b. Tongue
   c. 2-4 months after primary lesion
   d. Tertiary lesions of syphilis are marked by Gumma formation.
2. a. HHV-1.
   c. Herpetic gingivostomatitis.
   e. Neurogenic DNA virus.
   a. Cox-A virus A16.
   b. Rarely.
   l. Measles.
   n. EBV and less commonly by CMV.
   a. Young males.
   b. Aortic aneurysm.
3. a. HHV-8.
   a. Decreased CD4.
   b. Frequent manifestations.
   c. Patient with advanced acquired immune deficiency syndrome (AIDS).
4. b. Caused by prolonged use of wide spectrum antibiotics.
   a. Poor denture hygiene and continuous wear of acrylic denture.
   b. Erythematous candidiasis
   c. Does cause linear gingival erythema
   g. Median rhomboid glossitis
   a. Occur in conjunction
   b. Also in pregnancy and denture wearers
5. a. 20–25%.
   a. Non-keratinised
   b. Major RAS.
   c. Major RAS.
   a. >10 mm diameter.
   b. 25% of RAS patients
   l. Young adults below 50 years.
1. a. Intra-epithelial
   c. Females

e. Also in mucous membrane pemphigoid (MMP) and other vesiculo-bullous disorders.
g. Pemphigoid.
a. Systemic corticosteroids.
b. less than 24 hrs.
2. a. >60 years age group.
  a. Sub-epithelial
  b. Lichen planus (LP) but can also be caused by MMP, pemphigus, plasma cell mucositis.
  f. Perilesional mucosa is required and tissue must be snap frozen.
3. a. Posterior hard and soft palate.
  a. Common in middle age Males.
  b. Autosomal Recessive.
4. c. Autoimmune.
  d. T-lymphocytes.
  a. Retricular pattern.
  b. Erosive Lichen Planus.
  c. Wickham's striae.
  d. Must be biopsied to differentiate from other lesions, lichenoid reaction or cancer.
5. a. Non-caseating.
  a. Terminal ⅓ of the ileum
  b. Under 18 years
  c. Melkersson – Rosenthal syndrome
  h. Replaced by testing for endomysial or tissue transglutaminase antibody
6. b. Anogenital region, nose and oesophagus
  a. Also tongue and palate
  b. Mainly affects Palate
7. a. Migratory Glossitis is not linked to any systemic disease
  a. Haematinic deficiency
  b. Not associated.
8. b. Freckle of oral mucosa.
9. b. Vascular epulis is associated with hormonal changes
10. a. Areca nuts
  b. Fibrous bands develops in buccal mucosa resulting in limited opening and swallowing.
  d. 5%.
  a. Erosive lichen planus is Premalignant.
  b. White plaque have premalignant potential

11. b. Decreased risk.
    d. Non-smoker.
12. a. Vermilion border of lower lip
    b. Sun exposure—ultraviolet B
    h. Can spread via Submental nodes.
18. a. Remove source causing irritation
    d. HPV positive carcinoma-response better to chemotherapy and radiotherapy.
19. a. Tumour staging
20. a. Paramyxovirus.
    b. 20%.
    d. Bilateral parotid involvement in viral sialadenitis
    f. Common in both chronic and acute bacterial sialadenitis
    i. Acinar damage in radiation sialadenitis
21. a. 0.1mL/min—Lower limit of normal resting salivary flow.
    c. Does not cause, patient may have dry mouth following radiotherapy.
22. a. B-cell proliferation and loss of T-cell regulation.
    b. Secondary Sjorgen.
    c. Primary Sjorgen.
    d. ~5%.
    g. Only major glands show these changes.
23. a. 80–90%.
    b. Minor salivary glands.
    h. Affects older men.
    i. Parotid gland
    j. 10%.
24. c. Slow growing tumour.
    g. Young and middle aged patient
    i. Aggressive.
    k. Palate.
27. a. Minor salivary glands.
    b. Lower labial mucosa.
    g Upper labial mucosa
28. a. >50's.
    g. Last few seconds
    h. M = F
29. a. Sharp shooting pain
30. a. Females.
    b. >50 years.
    c Unilateral Pain

d. Retinal arteries
   e. Grossly elevated ESR
31. a. Females.
   b. Continuous pain
   c. Also preherpetic neuralgia and development of vesiculo-bullous lesions
   d. Tricyclic Antidepressants (TCA)
   e. Ramsey Hunt syndrome
32. f. Variable incidence, increased age, F>M.
   g Does not have characteristics features to contribute to its diagnosis.
33. a. Closes mouth.
34. b. Closes mouth.
   d. Closes mouth
   e. Disc replacement with reduction
35. e. No movement due to true ankylosis.
36. e. Posterior open bite.
39. h. Males.
   a. SLE common in Females.
   e. Progresses from DLE to SLE.
40. g. DLE
   a. Males
   b. Above 40 years.
   c. Posterior Mandible
   d. Follicular ameloblastoma is common type
41. a. Unicystic
   b. Anterior maxilla.
   c. Invades extensively.
42. e. Compound odontmes.
   b. Incidental finding.
   c. Maxillary incisors
   d. Non vital.
   e. Rests of malassez.
   f. Root sheath of hertwig.
   g. Cholesterol.
43. i. Enucleation.
   a. Developmental.
   b. 18–30 years.
   d. Reduced enamel epithelium.
   e. Crown.

44. g. 15–20%.
    a. Males.
    b. Parakeratinised epithelium.
    c. Glands of Serres.
    e. Enucleation with curettage.
45. f. Gorlin-Goltz syndrome.
    a. Afro-caribbean.
    b. Above 60 years.
46. d. Plasma cells.
    c. Maxilla.
    d. Ground glass.
47. e. Painless swelling causing disfigurement or malocclusion.
    b. Above 50 years.
    d. Pelvis.
    f. 5 year.
48. g. Cotton wool appearance.
    a. Young males.
    c. Metastasis to Lungs.
    d. 40%.
49. e. Osteoblasts.
    c. Defective osteoclast function.
    d. Is common and may require bone marrow transportation
50. e. Bones are fragile.
    b. Osteitis.
    c. Staphylococcus.

Chapter 9

Oral Radiology

Identify the following Statements as True (T) or False (F)

1. **Ionising radiation:**
   a. The use of ionising radiation in medicine and dentistry is governed by Ionising Radiation Regulation (1999) and Ionising Radiation Medical Exposures regulation (2000)
   b. Ionising Radiations include X-ray, gamma rays, microwaves and radiowaves
   c. They are long wavelength high frequency radiations
   d. Compton interaction occurs at the atomic level when X-ray interact with matter
   e. Coherent scatter results in absorption of all or part of X-ray photon energy and ionisation of an atom.

2. **Somatic and genetic effects of X-ray:**
   a. The irradiation of cells results in genetic effects
   b. Somatic effects are those occurring in germ cells
   c. Genetic effects are those occurring in the irradiated somatic cells of an individual
   d. Somatic effects can only have stochastic effects
   e. Everyday risks to patient having radiographs taken during their course of dental treatment include genetic stochastic effects
   f. The risk from dental radiography is for stochastic effects.

3. **The principle of international commission of radiation protection:**
   a. Screening
   b. Justification
   c. Limitation
   d. Optimisation
   e. Personal dosimeter monitoring.

4. **Dose and risk in dental radiography:**
   a. Periapical X-rays have effective dose 2-10 microsievert
   b. The risk of cancer from bitewing radiograph is 0.06-0.7 per million
   c. Lateral cephalogram have estimated effective dose of 3 msv
   d. The risk of cancer from dental panoramic tomographs is 0.21-1.9/million
   e. CBCT scan has risk of developing cancer in <10/per million
   f. CT scan of mandible for implantology has estimated effective dose ranging from 480-3300 msv.

Oral Radiology

5. **Radiation protection:**
   a. X-ray examination can be done routinely
   b. Radiographic screening is acceptable
   c. When periodontal probing depths exceed 5 mm, vertical bitewing radiographs are required
   d. Pre-extraction radiographs are indicated
   e. Working length estimation radiographs are not recommended
   f. Radiographs prior to preparation of tooth for a crown and bridge retainers is usually uncommon
   g. For most dental diagnosis, panoramic radiographs are best imaging technique
   h. Orthopantomogram (OPG) is useful in orthodontic assessment.

6. **Dose limitation—dose in dental radiography can be minimised by:**
   a. Use of optimal kilovoltage 70 KV
   b. Use of aluminium filters
   c. Rectangular collumination
   d. F-speed films
   e. Using DC generation of X-rays
   f. Use of digital systems
   g. Lead shielding of patients.

7. **Staff protection:**
   a. For intraoral radiography, only patient should be in the controlled area
   b. Control area extends above and below the patient and X-ray set
   c. Ceiling and floor material provide an adequate barrier to limit the controlled area
   d. Radiation dose monitoring for anyone performing >100 intraoral radiographs per week
   e. Dental practice should have set of local rules for radiation safety
   f. Guideline on the safe use of radiation is produced by the National Institute of Care and Excellence.

8. **Administration of radiation protection:**
   a. Employer has legal responsibility to ensure that regulations are followed
   b. It is the duty of referer to supply adequate clinical information to justify examination
   c. The practitioner is qualified to justify radiological examination
   d. Dental therapist can carry out radiological examination
   e. Radiation practitioner supervisor takes role of checking legal requirement and good practice
   f. All general dental practice must appoint radiation protection advisor to ensure regulations and good practice is maintained. Usually this is dentist.

9. The following are everyday risk to patients in dental radiography:
    a. Deterministic effects
    b. Somatic stochastic effects
    c. Genetic stochastic effects
    d. Salivary gland cancer
    e. Cataract formation.

10. The dose of radiation from a panoramic radiograph is:
    a. The same as 1 to 4 days of background radiation
    b. Much less than the dose from chest radiograph
    c. Equivalent to that from a set of posterior bitewing radiographs
    d. Always 7–26 μsv
    e. Associated with a risk of cancer typically higher than that from lateral cephalogram.

11. Radiographic features which suggest that patient is at high risk of suffering from damage to inferior dental (ID) nerve during removal of lower third molar are:
    a. Loss of tramlines of inferior dental canal
    b. Deviation of tramlines of inferior dental canal
    c. Widening of tramlines of inferior dental canal
    d. Narrowing of tramlines of inferior dental canal
    e. Radiopaque band across root
    f. A radiolucent band across the root.

12. Processing radiographs:
    a. Developer is an acidic solution
    b. Developer is oxidised by air and is changed daily
    c. If the film is left in developer too long, it will become pale
    d. The lower the temperature of developer, the faster the process will occur
    e. Fixation involves unsensitised silver halide crystals being removed to reveal the white areas of the film.

13. Stages of processing radiographs films are:
    a. Fixation, washing, development, washing, drying
    b. Washing, development, washing, fixation, drying
    c. Washing, fixation, washing, development, drying
    d. Washing, development, fixation, washing, drying
    e. Development, washing, fixation, washing, drying.

14. The annual dose limits under ionising radiation regulation 1999 are:
    a. General public 2 msv
    b. Non-classified workers 5 msv
    c. Non-classified workers 6 msv
    d. Classified workers 20 msv
    e. Classified workers 40 msv
    f. Classified worker 60 msv.

15. **Film faults:**
    a. Film too dark can be due to underdevelopment
    b. Film too pale can be due to increased temperature
    c. Poor contrast could be due to over development
    d. Poor definition is due to inadequate fixations
    e. White blotches on the film are due to developer splashes.

16. **Regarding thermoluminescent dosimeters:**
    a. They are used for monitoring radiation dose of the whole body
    b. They provide permanent record of dose received
    c. They use a materials that absorb radiation and then releases the energy in the form of light
    d. The monitor should be replaced after 1-3 months
    e. Should be worn outside the clothes at the level of reproductive organs
    f. Should be replaced every 6 months
    g. They do not need to be replaced so frequently like film badges.

17. **Advantages of the paralleling technique of periapical radiography over bisecting angle technique are:**
    a. Accurate and reproducible radiographs
    b. Does not require film holders
    c. Held in place by patient's finger
    d. No coning off
    e. Beam is directed at right angles to the tooth and film
    f. The image produced shows little or no magnification.

18. **Indications for taking lower occlusal radiographs:**
    a. To detect salivary calculi in parotid duct
    b. To detect salivary calculi in submandibular gland duct
    c. To assess buccolingual position and unerupted maxillary teeth
    d. To assess fractures in anterior body of mandible
    e. To assess buccolingual position of unerupted mandibular third molar
    f. To assess pathological lesions in anterior mandible.

19. **The following presents as multilocular radiolucency lesions of the mandible:**
    a. Ameloblastoma
    b. Calcifying epithelial odontogenic tumours
    c. Odontogenic keratocyst
    d. Odontogenic myxoma
    e. Aneurysmal bone cyst.

20. **The following are unilocular radiolucent lesions of the mandible:**
    a. Dentigerous cyst
    b. Ameloblastoma
    c. Ameloblastic fibroma

d. Residual cyst
e. Stafne's bone cavity.

21. The following lesions appear as radiolucent lesion in the mandible on dental panoramic tomography:
    a. Calcifying epithelial odontogenic tumour
    b. Complex odontoma
    c. Compound odontoma
    d. Odontogenic fibroma
    e. Odontogenic keratocyst
    f. Cemento-osseous dysplasia
    g. Submandibular gland calculus.

22. X-ray beam:
    a. Current flows from cathode to anode
    b. The unwanted X-rays are absorbed from surrounding lead
    c. High voltage between anode and cathode accelerates the electrons
    d. X-rays are electromagnetic radiation made up of electrons
    e. X-rays radiations are visible to eyes.

23. Hyperparathyroidism:
    a. Pepper-pot appearance is observed
    b. There is generalized skeletal bone resorption
    c. Osteopenia is present
    d. There is decreased level of parathyroid hormone
    e. Bone has overall stippled pattern.

24. Collimator:
    a. Most commonly used is tubular collimator
    b. It is metallic barrier with an aperture in the middle to reduce the size of X-ray beam
    c. It improves image quality
    d. Rectangular collimator limits the size of X-ray to size of the film
    e. It deflects the scattered radiation.

25. Osteomyelitis:
    a. Areas of radiolucency appears as ragged, patchy or moth eaten areas
    b. The outline of area of destruction is regular and clearly defined
    c. Osteomyelitis is defined as inflammation of bone and its marrow contents
    d. Condensing osteitis is acute focal sclerosing osteomyelitis
    e. Radiographically, cotton-wool appearance is seen in chronic diffuse sclerosing osteomyelitis.

Identify the Single Best Answer for the following

26. The unit of measurement of radiation exposed to the patient during radiograph is:
    a. Rad
    b. Roentgen

c. Curie
d. Rem.

27. Removal of less penetrating X-rays during radiography is known as:
   a. Beam attenuation
   b. Filtration
   c. Collimation
   d. None of the above.

28. "Cotton wool" appearance on radiograph is evident in:
   a. Fibrous dysplasia
   b. Paget's disease
   c. Osteoradionecrosis
   d. Osteomyelitis.

29. The following radiographs show best views of fractures, *except*:
   a. Occipitomental view for nasal septum
   b. Submentovertex view for the calvarium
   c. Lateral view for the nasal bone
   d. Towne's view for the base of skull.

30. Cervical burnout is visible in periapical and bitewing view of:
   a. Root caries in molars
   b. Cervical abrasion
   c. Intact proximal root surface of premolars
   d. Hypercementosis.

31. The use of sodium sulphite in the developer is:
   a. Restrainer
   b. Hardener
   c. Preservative
   d. Activator.

32. Out of the following options, all are the radiographic feature of thalassemia, *except*:
   a. Cotton-wool appearance
   b. Widened diploic space
   c. Hair-on-end appearance
   d. Ground glass appearance.

33. Radiograph showing small roots and obliterated pulp chamber of a permanent teeth in is suggestive of:
   a. Achondroplasia
   b. Cleidocranial dysostosis
   c. Amelogenesis imperfecta
   d. Dentinogenesis imperfecta.

34. The radiograph used for best view of the maxillary sinus:
   a. Occipitomental view
   b. Lateral skull view

c. Lateral oblique view
d. Submentovertex.

35. **The radiograph with onion-skin effect is indicative of:**
    a. Squamous cell carcinoma
    b. Chondrosarcoma
    c. Ewing's sarcoma
    d. Fibrosarcoma.

36. **Punched out radiographic outline is suggestive of:**
    a. Outline showing no peripheral bone reaction
    b. Outline blending with the normal anatomy
    c. Non-uniform radiographic boundary
    d. Ragged and invasive appearance.

37. **A bilateral, asymptomatic, cyst-like radiolucent lesions in the bone at the angles of the mandible is observed in 8-year-old child. The provisional diagnosis is:**
    a. Cherubism
    b. Static bone cavities
    c. Latent bone cysts
    d. Embryonic cysts.

38. **A radiolucent shadow at the apex of the maxillary left central incisor is seen in periapical radiograph. Lamina dura is continuous and the tooth responds normally to the pulp tester. No clinical signs or symptoms are present. What is the likely diagnosis?**
    a. Periapical pathology of unknown etiology
    b. Nutrient canal
    c. Infection
    d. Normal anatomic landmark.

39. **A periapical radiograph of a right maxillary lateral incisor reveals a sharp right angle bend in the apical one-third of the root. The probable diagnosis is:**
    a. Dens in dente
    b. Concrescence
    c. Dilacerations
    d. Gemination.

40. **Among the following, numerous areas of radiolucency in bones are common, *except*:**
    a. Multiple myeloma
    b. Albers-Schonberg disease
    c. Metastatic tumors of bone
    d. Hyperparathyroidism.

41. **The function of an aluminum disk in the primary X-ray beam:**
    a. Reduces long wavelength radiation
    b. Increases density of exposed film

c. Reduces the diameter of the primary beam
d. Reduces the developing time.

42. **Tooth vitality is determined radiographically by:**
    a. Closeness of caries to pulp
    b. The presence of secondary dentine
    c. Periapical involvement
    d. None of the above.

43. **An occlusal radiograph of maxillary arch shows a relatively large radiolucent area between the right lateral incisor root and the right canine root. The roots are displaced laterally. What is the most likely diagnosis?**
    a. Nasoalveolar cyst
    b. Globulomaxillary cyst
    c. Incisive canal cyst
    d. Nasoalabial cyst.

44. **What is the function of lead foil in a film packet?**
    a. To enhance the contrast of image
    b. To absorb secondary radiations
    c. To reduce exposure time
    d. To reduce developing time.

45. **Why is 'oil' circulated around the X-ray tube?**
    a. Disinfect the target
    b. Dissipate the heat
    c. Produce the heat
    d. All of the above.

46. **What produces hard radiations?**
    a. Metals of high atomic weight
    b. Metals of low atomic weight
    c. Noble metals
    d. Metals of specific atomic weight.

47. **Secondary radiations:**
    a. Are reduced by increasing the grid ratio
    b. Are reflected from object
    c. Reduce the contrast of the image
    d. All of the above are correct.

48. **The tissue is most susceptible to radiation:**
    a. Muscles and skin
    b. Blood forming cells
    c. Bones
    d. Nervous tissue.

49. **Fluorescence is:**
    a. Emission of light by crystal after activating source has ceased
    b. Emission of visible light by a crystal when subjected to an activating form of energy
    c. Emission of light by a crystal when subjected to a bending of a crystal
    d. None of the above.

50. **The technique based on geometrical theorem:**
    a. Le' masters technique
    b. None of the above
    c. Bisecting technique
    d. Paralleling technique
    e. All of the above.

51. **X-rays were discovered in:**
    a. 1909
    b. 1895
    c. 1890
    d. 1906.

52. **Radiology is:**
    a. Study and evaluation of a radiograph
    b. Science and art of production of X-rays, and their applications to medicine and dentistry
    c. Science and art of marking permanent records of an object
    d. All of the above.

53. **Cathode in a X-ray tube is made up of:**
    a. Copper
    b. Tungsten
    c. Aluminium
    d. Lead.

54. **Which of the following statement is correct**
    a. Wavelength is inversely proportional to applied voltage
    b. Wavelength is directly proportional to applied voltage
    c. Wavelength is directly proportional to the square of applied voltage
    d. Wavelength is inversely proportional to the square of applied voltage.

55. **The stage in which foetus is most susceptible to the radiation-hazards:**
    a. Stage of organogenesis
    b. Stage of morphodifferentiation
    c. Growth and development stage
    d. All of the above.

56. **The disinfectant is used for infection control during radiography:**
    a. Chlorines
    b. Iodophors
    c. Phenols
    d. All of the above.

57. **Soft X-rays:**
    a. Possess less energy
    b. Have little penetrating power
    c. Have larger wavelength
    d. All of the above.

58. **This radiographic view aids to confirm the diagnosis of multiple myeloma:**
    a. Lateral skull view
    b. Occipitomental view
    c. Anteriorposterior view
    d. None of the above.

59. **The maxillary sinus can be best viewed in this radiographic view:**
    a. Water's view (or occipitomental view)
    b. Lateral skull view
    c. Submentovertex
    d. Lateral oblique view.

60. **Cervical burnout is seen in periapical and bitewing view of:**
    a. Root caries in molars
    b. Cervical abrasion
    c. Intact proximal root surface of premolars
    d. Hypercementosis.

61. **Mostly commonly used collimator is:**
    a. Oval
    b. Square
    c. Rectangular
    d. Any shape.

Identify the answers to the following Extended Matching questions

62. **Radiograph of odontogenic keratocyst (Fig. 9.1):**
    a. What is the diagnosis?
    b. Proportion of odontogenic cysts they form
    c. Direction of expansion
    d. Lesions appears
    e. Usually occurs in which age group
    f. Associated with syndrome
    g. Associated with cancer
    h. The epithelial remnant it develops from.

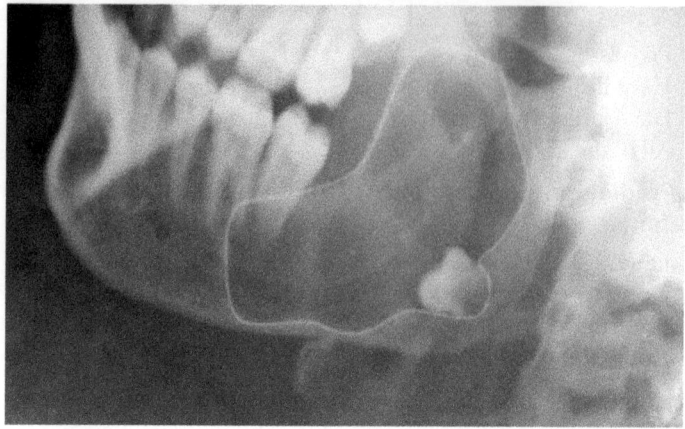

Fig. 9.1: Radiograph illustrating odontogenic keratocyst

1. Dentigerous cyst	12. Mesio-distal
2. Radicular cyst	13. Medio-lateral
3. Odontogenic keratocyst	14. Does not expand
4. Rest of Malassez	15. Radiolucent
5. Enamel organ	16. 20–40 years
6. 1%	17. 40–60 years
7. 5%	18. Anterior mandible
8. 25%	19. Post mandible
9. 50%	20. Basal cell carcinoma
10. Round	21. Kallmann syndrome
11. Oval	22. Gorlin-Goltz syndrome

63. **Radiograph of dentigerous cyst (Fig. 9.2):**

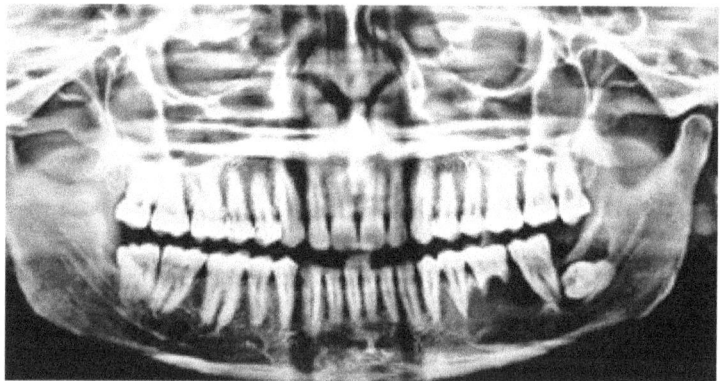

Fig. 9.2: Radiograph illustrating dentigerous cyst

    a. What is the likely diagnosis?
    b. Age range for this cyst
    c. Commonly affects which teeth?
    d. Next commonly affected teeth
    e. If cyst causes swelling in the gingival region it would be called

f. Where is it attached on tooth?
g. Appearance of cyst on radiograph
h. Best X-ray to diagnose this cyst
i. What are the effects of this cyst on adjacent teeth
j. Proportion of odontogenic cysts this can forms.

1. Idiopathic bone cyst	11. Gingival cyst	21. Displaced
2. Radicular cyst	12. Eruption cyst	22. Resorbed
3. Dentigerous cyst	13. Radiopaque	23. 5%
4. 0–15 years	14. Radiolucent	24. 60%
5. 18–40 years	15. Enamel	25. 25%
6. 40–60 years	16. Dentine	26. ADJ
7. Mandibular third molar	17. Amelo-dentinal junction (ADJ)	
8. Mandibular premolar	18. OPG	
9. Maxillary third molar	19. Periapical	
10. Maxillary canines	20. Postero-anterior mandible	

64. Radiograph of cementoma (Figs 9.3A to C):

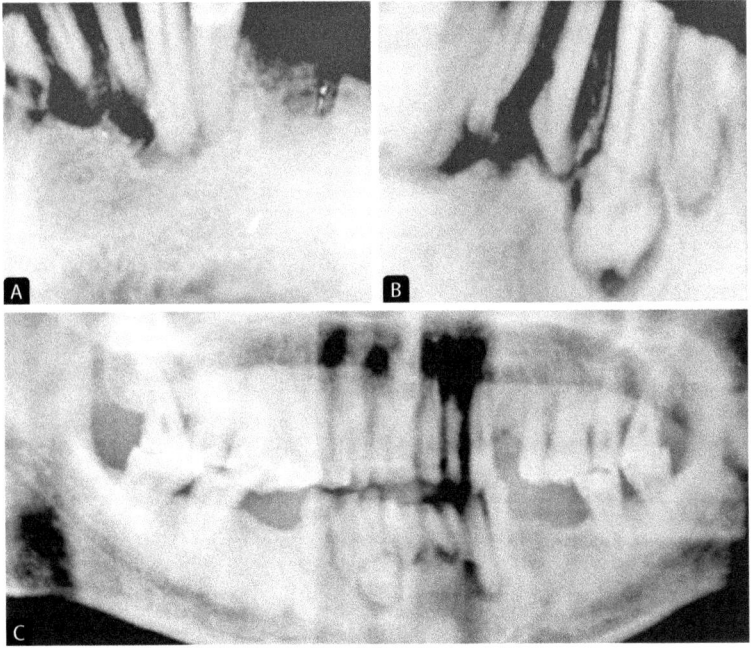

Figs 9.3A to C: Radiological appearance of cementoma

a. What is diagnosis?
b. Usually discovered at this age
c. The usual size of lesion is
d. Commonly affects
e. Pattern of definition of the the lesion

f. Radiographic appearance
g. Behaviour of the lesion
h. Shape of the lesion
i. Sex commonly affected

1. Cemento-ossifying fibroma	14. Maxillary anterior teeth
2. Calcifying epithelial odontogenic tumor (CEOT)	15. Well-defined
	16. Poorly defined
3. 0–18 years	17. Radiopaque
4. 18–40 years	18. Radiolucent
5. 60+ years	19. Malignant
6. 0–1 cm	20. Locally invasive
7. 1–3 cm	21. Benign
8. 71 cm	22. Golf ball
9. True cementoma	23. Rugby ball
10. Fibroma	24. Tennis ball
11. Maxillary molar	25. Male
12. Mandibular molar	26. Female
13. Mandibular anterior teeth	27. Equal in males and females

65. **Radiograph of zygoma or occipito-mental facial fracture OM0° & OM30° (Fig. 9.4):**

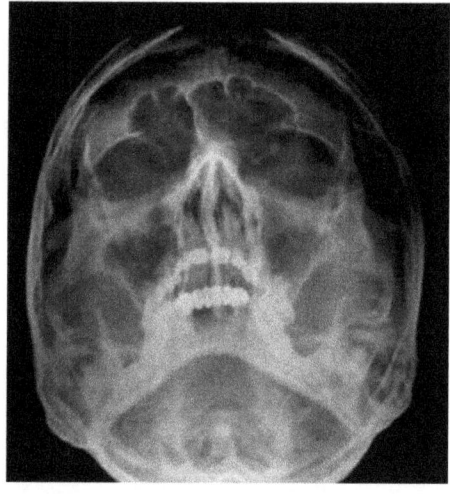

Fig. 9.4: Radiograph showing facial fracture OM30°

a. What is the diagnosis?
b. Which X-ray is used to diagnose this fracture?
c. On which side of the face, this usually occurs?
d. Common cause of this lesion
e. What lines should you follow while interpreting above X-ray?
f. Which eponymous instrument is used to correct this problem?
g. Which nerve is frequently involved in this fracture?
h. What is the common appearance of antrum in this condition?
i. What question should you be asking patient?

1. Fractured mandible	10. Sport	19. Inferior dental
2. Fractured maxilla	11. Interpersonal injury	20. Infra-orbital
3. Fractured zygoma	12. Car accident	21. Supra-tochlear
4. Lefort 1	13. Work related lying	22. Clear
5. Lefort 2	14. Winter	23. Narrowed
6. Lefort 3	15. Campbell	24. Cloudy
7. OM 0° and 30°	16. Joves	25. Have you lost consciousness
8. Left	17. Howarth elevator	26. Can you feel cheek?
9. Sport	18. Gillies Hook	27. Affected by paraesthesia

66. **Bone lesions—Radiograph of osteomyelitis (Fig. 9.5):**

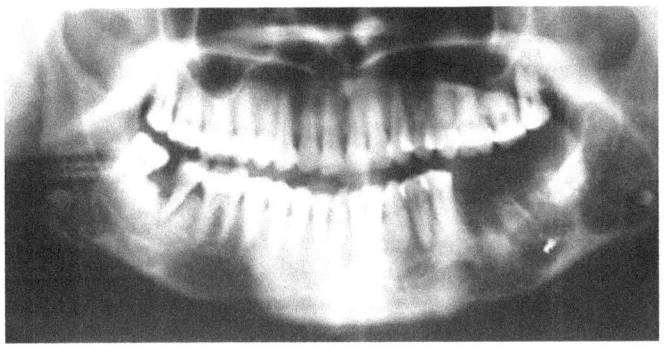

Fig. 9.5: Radiographic image of osteomyelitis.

a. What is the likely diagnosis?
b. What is dead bone called in this condition?
c. What is new formed boned called?
d. Appearance of radiographic lesion.
e. Where does it occur most commonly?

1. Paget's disease	6. Partition	11. Maxilla
2. Multiple myeloma	7. Occipital bone	12. Mandible
3. Osteomyelitis	8. Surgery	13. Temporal bone
4. Involucrum	9. Moth eaten	
5. Sequestrum	10. Burnt leaf	

67. **Non-odontogenic cyst—upper occlusal radiograph of nasopalatine cyst (Fig. 9.6):**

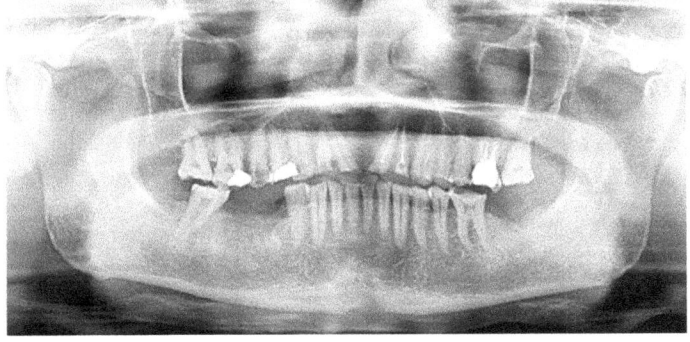

Fig. 9.6: Radiograph showing nasopalatine cyst

a. What is the diagnosis?
b. Age group commonly found is.
c. What percentage of total population gets affected by this cyst?
d. Site commonly involved
e. Outline of the lesion.

1. Radicular cyst	9. 10%
2. Nasopalatine duct cyst	10. 20%
3. Aneurysmal bone cyst	11. Anterior maxilla
4. Adenocystic carcinoma	12. Mid maxilla
5. 0–20 years	13. Oral maxilla
6. 20–40 years	14. Smooth and well-defined
7. 40–60 years	15. Smooth and partly-defined
8. 0.1%9.1%	16. Rough and partly-defined

68. **Radiograph of skull—multiple myeloma/malignant tumour:**
    a. What is the diagnosis?
    b. What is the sex predilection in patients with this tumour?
    c. Commonly found.
    d. Age group usually found in affected is.
    e. In which ethnic group this tumour is prevalent?
    f. Which cell causes this condition?
    g. Classic radiographic appearance is.
    h. Describe locularity of the lesion.
    i. Protein detected in urine in this condition.

1. Paget's	8. Skull vault	15. Caucasians
2. Thalassemia	9. Maxilla	16. Afro-Caribbean
3. Hyperparathyroidism	10. Mandibular	17. Plasma cells
4. Multiple myeloma	11. 0–20 years	18. Pepper pot
5. Male	12. 20-40 years	19. Moth eaten
6. Female	13. 40-60 years	20. Radiolucent/radiopaque
7. Bence-jones protein	14. Asian	21. Multilocular

69. **Photo of sialograph of parotid gland-Sialadenitis (Figs 9.7A and B):**

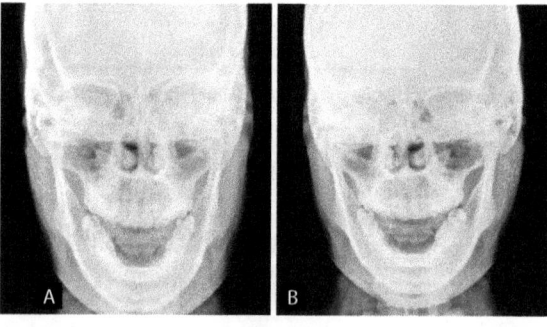

Figs 9.7A and B: Sialogram of a right and left parotid gland (A) Right side; (B) Left side

a. What is the likely diagnosis?
b. What type of radiograph is this?
c. Which site is shown in the X-ray?
d. Description of this condition.
e. What is the cause of this disorder?
f. Treatment of this condition.

Oral Radiology

1. Salivary calculi	9. Submandibular gland
2. Adenoid cystic carcinoma	10. Sublingual
3. Pleomorphic adenoma	11. Sunray
4. Sialadenitis	12. Sialectasis
5. Sialography	13. Tree in winter
6. CT scanning	14. Osteoarthritis
7. Positron emission tomography (PET) scanning	15. Rheumatoid arthritis
8. Parotid gland	16. Inflammation of glandular tissue

70. Ameloblastoma (Fig. 9.8):

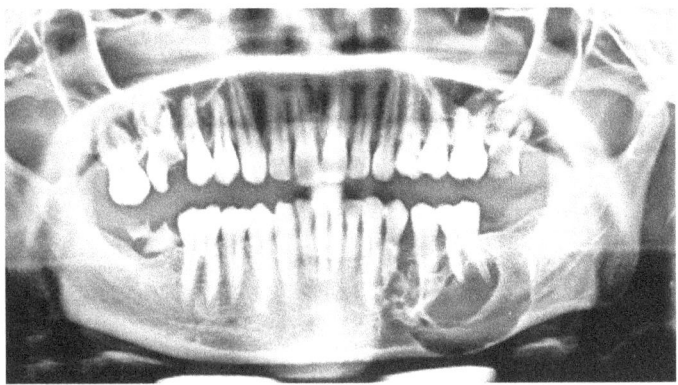

Fig. 9.8: Radiologic representation of ameloblastoma

a. What is the likely diagnosis?
b. In which a age group, it is likely to occur?
c. Site.
d. Locularity of lesion.
e. Radiographic description
f. Outline.

1. Ameloblastoma	10. Posterior maxilla
2. Fractured mandible	11. Anterior maxilla
3. 0–18, 18–35	12. Mononuclear
4. 35–50, 50+ years	13. Sunray
5. Posterior mandible	14. Stafne bone cyst
6. Smooth scalloped	15. Corticated
7. Soap-bubble	16. Orange peel
8. Smooth and rough	17. Non corticated
9. Stafne bone cyst	18. Multilocular

CASE DISCUSSIONS

Case 1: Osteomyelitis

A 47-year-old female with a chief complaint of pain and swelling following the extraction of a right mandibular second molar (LR7) by her general dental practitioner (GDP) a month ago. Discuss the steps you will take to reach diagnosis.

History of Presenting Complaint
- Pain in lower right second molar area; intense pain with a feeling of sensation of loose teeth
- Swelling present.

Medical History
Non-contributory.

Dental History
- One month ago extraction was performed of LR7 was performed with repeated injections of local anaesthesia
- Patient was prescribed four week course of clindamycin. There was a delay in presentation of symptoms initially. However, on cessation of the medication, symptoms recurred.

Social History
- Smoking habits: Approximately 20 cigarettes a day for the past five years
- No history of alcohol consumption.

Clinical Examination
- Extra-oral:
  - Swelling in lower right molar area
- Intra-oral:
  - Extraction socket was red and inflamed indicative of local osteitis. After four week course of clindamycin, there were no signs of infection at the extraction site.
- Investigations:
  - A full blood profile including erythrocyte sedimentation rate and c-reactive protein: Normal
  - MRI scan: There was a blush present in the bone marrow cavity suggested oedema but lacked evidence of extensive bone involvement
  - Bone scan: The report suggested the possibility of osteomyelitis but should be considered in conjunction with the MRI
  - After six months, patient was again back with pain
  - Following investigations were further carried out
    Cone beam computed tomography: This test demonstrated the presence of bony defects in the LR7/8 area. This finding is compatible with chronic/recurrent osteomyelitis. Further imaging of CBCT indicated bone involvement **(Figs 9.9 and 9.10)**
    Biopsy: Uninformative
    Microbiology: There is a presence of growth of mixed anaerobes, some Viridans streptococci and *Actinomyces naeslundii*.

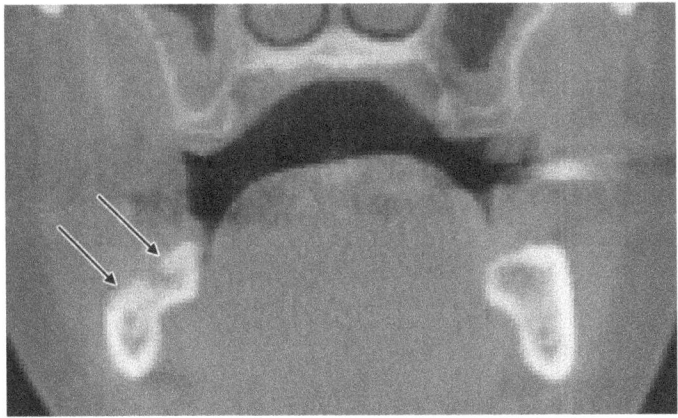

Fig. 9.9: Coronal slice of the CBCT scan: Irregular loss of the buccal and superior alveolar cortices (arrowed) evident

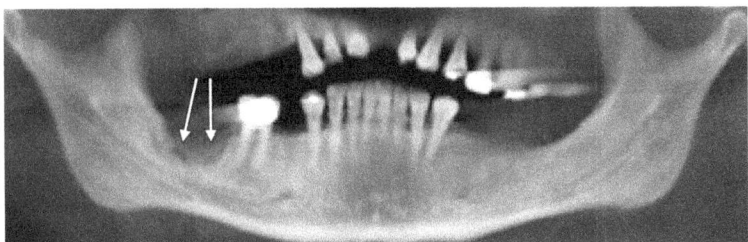

Fig. 9.10: Reconstructed panoramic image from the CBCT scan: Area of bone loss associated with the extracted lower right second molar tooth (arrowed) is illustrated

Treatment

- A second more intense course of anti-microbial therapy was commenced with a mixture of IV and oral antibiotics (azithromycin, teicoplanin, co-amoxiclav, clindamycin and metronidazole) continued over four weeks. The patient responded to the treatment and became symptom free for six months. She again complained of intense pain with general malaise
- Ceftriaxone IV and metronidazole postoperatively for a further four weeks

Follow-up

- Patient is symptom free and under long-term review

Differential Diagnosis

- Fibrous dysplasia
- Ewing-sarcoma
- Chondrosarcoma
- Osteosarcoma
- Carcinomatous metastases of other organs
- Cemento-ossifying fibroma
- Malignant non-Hodgkin-lymphoma.

Case 2: Periapical ameloblastoma

A male patient, aged 20 years complained of a small swelling in the vestibular area of the lower right second mandibular molar area. Discuss the steps to diagnose the pathology?

History of Presenting Complaint

The affected area was tender. The involved tooth was of grade two mobility. No noticeable nerve deficit or adenopathy in the head and neck region.

Medical history

- Not significant
- Patient had a good health.

Dental history

- The affected tooth was extracted by GDP
- Lesion was surgically removed. It was submitted for pathologic examination
- Round bur was used to ground away several millimetres of the bony socket before wound closure
- After 2 years, there was evidence of signs of recurrence.

Social history

Non-confirmatory.

Clinical Examination

On examination, facial asymmetry and firm swelling in right buccal vestibule of second mandibular molar region adjacent to the extraction site was evident.

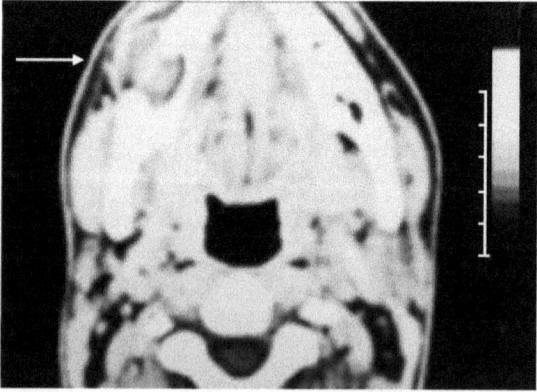

Fig. 9.11: Axial CT scan demonstrating perforation of the buccal cortex and extension of the lesion into the buccal soft tissues

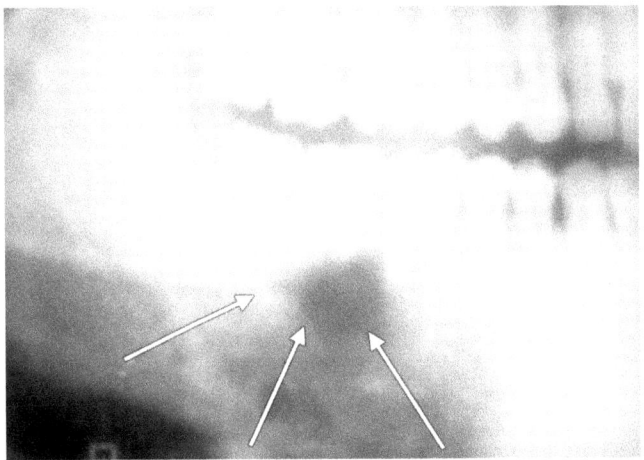

Fig. 9.12: Panoramic radiograph of periapical lesion of the second right mandibular molar with extensive root resorption

Investigations
- Vitality testing: Positive
- CT scans **(Fig. 9.11)**
- Intra-oral biopsy: It was performed under local anaesthesia.

Radiographic Examination
- Relatively defined radiolucent lesion evident in the periapex
- Mesial and distal root apices were resorbed **(Fig 9.12)**
- Expansion of buccal cortex along with the invasion of mandibular down to the dental canal was present in initial radiographs.

Histopathological Examination
The pathology report confirmed the diagnosis as plexiform ameloblastoma.

Treatment
- En bloc surgical resection of the involved mandible chemistry
- Under general anaesthesia, a routine intra-oral and extra-oral (Risdon) supra-periosteal approach for mandible was performed
- An anteroinferior 2.7 mm, reconstruction plate adapted at border of mandible. After unscrewing the plate, tumour was resected en bloc along with the overlying soft tissues and the alveolar nerve with 2 cm bony margins.

Follow-up
Six years post-operatively, patient has no signs of recurrence.

Differential Diagnosis
- Jaw lesions
- Infiltrating neoplasms of the maxillary sinus
- Odontogenic keratocyst
- Central giant cell granuloma
- Calcifying epithelial odontogenic tumour (CEOT)
- Odontogenic myxoma
- Calcifying odontogenic cyst.

Answers

1. a. T b. F c. F d. T e. F
2. a. F b. F c. F d. F e. T
   f. T
3. a. F b. T c. T d. T e. F
4. a. T b. T c. T d. T e. F
   f.
5. a. F b. F c. T d. T e. F
   f. F g. F h. T
6. a. T b. T c. T d. T e. T
   f. T g. F
7. a. T b. F c. T d. F e. T
   f. F
8. a. T b. T c. T d. T e. T
   f. F
9. a. F b. T c. F d. T e. F
10. a. T b. F c. T d. F e. T
11. a. T b. T c. F d. T e. F
    f. T
12. a. F b. F c. F d. F e. T
13. a. F b. F c. F d. F e. T
14. a. F b. F c. T d. T e. F
    f. F
15. a. F b. F c. T d. F e. F
16. a. T b. F c. T d. T e. T
    f. F g. F
17. a. T b. F c. F d. T e. T
    f. T
18. a. F b. T c. F d. T e. F
    f. T

19.	a.	F	b.	T	c.	F	d.	T	e.	F
20.	a.	T	b.	T	c.	T	d.	T	e.	T
21.	a.	T	b.	T	c.	T	d.	F	e.	F
	f.	??	g.	T						
22.	a.	T	b.	T	c.	T	d.	F	e.	F
23.	a.	T	b.	T	c.	T	d.	F	e.	T
24.	a.	F	b.	T	c.	T	d.	T	e.	F
25.	a.	T	b.	F	c.	T	d.	F	e.	T
26.	b	27.	b	28.	b	29.	d	30.	c	
31.	c	32.	a	33.	d	34.	a	35.	c	
36.	a	37.	a	38.	d	39.	c	40.	b	
41.	a	42.	d	43.	b	44.	b	45.	b	
46.	a	47.	a	48.	b	49.	b	50.	c	
51.	b	52.	b	53.	b	54.	a	55.	a	
56.	a	57.	d	58.	a	59.	a	60.	c	
61.	c									
62.	a.	3	b.	5	c.	8	d.	14	e.	16
	f.	17	g.	23	h.	21				
63.	a.	3	b.	4	c.	7	d.	10	e.	12
	f.	26	g.	14	h.	18	i.	21	j.	25
64.	a.	9	b.	3	c.	7	d.	13	e.	16
	f.	19	g.	22	h.	23	i.	27		
65.	a.	3	b.	7	c.	8	d.	11	e.	15
	f.	18	g.	27	h.	24	i.	25		
66.	a.	3	b.	5	c.	4	d.	9	e.	12
67.	a.	2	b.	7	c.	9	d.	14	e.	15
68.	a.	4	b.	19	c.	8	d.	13	e.	16
	f.	17	g.	18	h.	20	i.	21	j	7
69.	a.	4	b.	5	c.	8	d.	12	e.	16
70.	a.	1	b.	4	c.	5	d.	18	e.	7
	f.	6								

CORRECT ANSWER FOR FALSE STATEMENTS

1. b. X-ray, gamma and cosmic rays.
   c. Short wavelength.
2. e. Photoelectric interaction and Compton interaction.
   a. Genetic and somatic effects.
   c. Somatic effects
4. d. Also deterministic.
   e. <50/per million.
5. g. Intraoral radiographs are best for dental diagnosis.
7. f. UK Department of Health.
8. f. It is medical physicist.
12. b. Should be changed 10–14 days
    c. Film will become Dark
14. b. high temperature of developer.
    a. 1 msv.
15. a. Overdevelopment.
    b. Reduced temperature.
    d. Due to Patient movement.
    e. Fixer splashes.

Chapter 10
Oral Surgery

Identify the following Statements as True (T) or False (F)

1. According to the National Institute of Care and Excellence (NICE) guidelines, the following are the indication of removal of lower third molar:
   a. Treatment of facial pain
   b. Mesioangular impaction
   c. Crowding of lower anterior teeth
   d. Single episode of pericoronitis
   e. Plaque formation
   f. Prophylactic removal
   g. Pathology of follicle including cyst.

2. With regards to cranial nerves:
   a. Superior oblique muscle is supplied by the abducens nerve
   b. The lateral rectus muscle is supplied by oculomotor nerve
   c. The facial nerve is motor to muscles of mastication
   d. The trigeminal nerve is motor to muscles of facial expressions
   e. Palatoglossus is innervated by hypoglossal nerve
   f. The posterior third of the tongue is sensory supplied by glossopharyngeal nerve
   g. Upper face and lower face, both are bilaterally innervated by facial nerve
   h. Ptosis of the eyelid is caused due to palsy of optic nerve
   i. The intrinsic muscle of the tongue is supplied by glossopharyngeal nerve
   j. The incidence of permanent nerve injury after wisdom tooth removal is 5%
   k. The incidence of temporary inferior dental or alveolar nerve injury subsequent to third molar surgery is 10%.

3. The jaw elevator muscles are:
   a. Digastric muscles
   b. Inferior belly of lateral pterygoid muscles
   c. Mesial pterygoid muscles
   d. Temporalis
   e. Superior belly of lateral pterygoid muscles
   f. Geniohyoid muscles
   g. Mylohyoid muscles
   h. Masseter.

4. **With regards to extracting primary teeth:**
   a. Similar principles are applied as for permanent dentition
   b. May require general anaesthesia
   c. It is important to protect the airway during removal of teeth under general anaesthesia
   d. Small root fragments cannot be left in situ
   e. Submerged tooth is more common in maxilla
   f. A submerged tooth is associated with crowding.

5. **During extraction of lower third molar:**
   a. The patient should be warned of lingual nerve damage if extraction is done with forceps
   b. Bone removal should be done with chisel and mallet under local anaesthesia (LA)
   c. Horizontal impacted teeth are the most difficult teeth to extract surgically
   d. Relationship of inferior alveolar dental nerve with third molar can be determined using radiographs
   e. General anaesthesia is usually indicated.

6. **Radiological signs associated with increased risk of nerve injury during removal of third molar:**
   a. Presence of enlarged pericoronal space
   b. Interruption of lamina dura of inferior alveolar canal overlying the tooth
   c. Darkening of root due to crossing over of inferior alveolar canal
   d. Sclerotic bone around the roots of the tooth
   e. Diversion of inferior dental canal.

7. **With regards to surgical removal of tooth:**
   a. Is more traumatizing, depending upon the amount of bone removed and surgical complexity
   b. Patient should be prescribed antibiotics to reduce post-operative infections
   c. Radiographs are always required for surgical assessment
   d. In case of failed forcep extraction, dentist should immediately proceed with surgical removal of teeth
   e. Surgical removal of teeth may compromise implant placement
   f. Post-surgical pain, occurring after one week is likely to be related to surgical trauma.

8. **With regards to preprosthetic surgery:**
   a. Is less frequently required as dental implants are effective tooth replacement than dentures
   b. Sufficient non-keratinised mucosa around implants is essential to maintain health of surrounding soft tissues
   c. Can be carried out to increase the space between maxillary tuberosity and mandibular retromolar pad

d. Can be used to reduce mandibular tori
e. Can be used for sulcus deepening
f. Mental foramen can be surgically moved into inferior position
g. Muscles can be re-attached to more favourable positions that will prevent displacement of denture on contact.

9. **With regards to oro-antral fistula:**
   a. Maxillary permanent third molar is most susceptible to oro-antral fistula
   b. Patients are advised not to blow their nose
   c. Paraesthesia of upper lip is the most common complaints amongst patients with oro-antral fistula
   d. Closure should be done by buccal advancement flap
   e. Greater palatine nerve should be avoided in palatal rotation flap
   f. Oro-antral fistula is an endothelium lined tract between the mouth and maxillary sinus
   g. Saline nasal spray should be used in treatment
   h. Amoxicillin is the drug of choice in the treatment
   i. Buccal fat pad flap repair is the next surgical treatment of choice if initial treatment with buccal advancement flap has failed.

10. **With regards to parotid disease:**
    a. CoxA causes the most common childhood infection affecting bilateral parotid enlargement
    b. Adenoma is a salivary neoplasm common in parotid gland
    c. Adenocarcinoma presents with unilateral parotid swelling and facial palsy
    d. Meal time syndrome is caused by salivary retention cyst
    e. Polymorphous low-grade adenocarcinoma is a benign tumour of parotid gland
    f. Sarcoidosis is associated with Sjorgen disease
    g. Acute parotitis is associated with Haerd-Ford syndrome
    h. 'Cold abscesses' are associated with tuberculosis.

11. **Fractured mandible:**
    a. Angle of the mandible is the most common fracture site
    b. Condylar neck is the second most common fracture site
    c. Commonly affects both sides equally
    d. The most uncommon cause of fractured mandible is interpersonal trauma
    e. Open reduction and internal fixation are the most common treatment of fractured mandible
    f. Gunning splints are used for fractures in children <10 years
    g. Inter-maxillary fixation is treatment of choice for edentulous mandible fractures
    h. The most common nerve injured is lingual nerve.

12. Midface fractures:
a. Severe trauma can cause lengthening of face and obstruct the airway
b. The most common symptom of fractured orbital floor is subconjunctival haemorrhage
c. Inferior oblique muscle is commonly tethered in fractured orbital floor
d. Step deformity is the classic X-ray seen on occipitomental view in orbital floor fractures
e. Detached retina is a medical emergency associated with orbital floor fracture
f. Le Fort II fracture detaches the tooth bearing portions of the jaw via fracture line form the anterior margin of the anterior nasal aperture running laterally and back to lower third of pterygoid plate
g. Le Fort I can occur with other facial fractures
h. Le Fort II fracture can cause infra-orbital nerve paraesthesia
i. Le Fort III fracture can cause separation of fronto-zygomatic suture and deformity of zygomatic arches bilaterally
j. Internal fixation with range of plating techniques is fracture of choice for mid face fractures
k. Nasal fracture resembles four-pointed star on occipito-mental X-ray
l. Nasal fractures are frequently associated with deviation and crumpling of the septum
m. Naso-ethmoid fracture is diagnosed by bilateral black eye, nasal deformity, septal deviation, epistaxis and obstruction and possibility of cerebrospinal fluid (CSF) leak.

13. Osteoradionecrosis:
a. Is suppurative type of osteomyelitis
b. Affects maxilla more commonly
c. Can occur following hyperbaric oxygen treatment of squamous cell carcinoma
d. Is same as focal sclerosing osteomyelitis
e. Occurs due to reduction in vascularity secondary to endarteritis obliterans
f. Surgical management is similar to osteomyelitis
g. Can be prevented.

14. Orofacial infections are:
a. Common following contaminated facial lacerations
b. Common cause of lost working days
c. Usually of fungal or viral aetiology
d. Best managed by prescribing antibiotics
e. Commonly the result of endogenous commensal organism.

15. Apical surgery:
a. Can be carried out using semi-lunar incision when tooth is restored with crown
b. Is indicated when surgical repair of a root perforation is required

c. Can be undertaken on posterior teeth
   d. Can involve apicectomy of buccal roots of maxillary molar tooth
   e. May not require removal of all gutta percha from the wall of the cavity of root end
   f. Successful when no regeneration of periapical bone.

16. **To which spaces infection can spread directly from lower wisdom tooth:**
    a. Submasseteric space
    b. Pterygomaxillary space
    c. Submandibular space
    d. Cavernous sinus
    e. Maxillary sinus.

17. **Facial infection:**
    a. Infections from upper lateral incisors frequently spreads buccally
    b. Infections from maxillary canine may spread superficially to the side of the nose
    c. Second mandibular molar teeth can result in sublingual spread of infection
    d. Swelling due to cellulitis is mainly due to pus
    e. Cellulitis is an uncommon cause of Ludwig's angina
    f. Cavernous sinus thrombosis is more likely with lower face via facial vein.

18. **Oral surgery instruments:**
    a. 'Eagle beak' forceps are designed to penetrate oral bifurcation area and to split the roots
    b. Universal forceps are used to grip the roots of the teeth and to dilate sockets
    c. Elevators are always used to remove impacted teeth
    d. A Bard-Parker handle with No 11 Blade is usual scalpel
    e. Warwick James are periosteal elevators
    f. Chisels are particularly useful for disto-angular impacted third molars
    g. No. 8 round tungsten carbide bur is used for tooth division
    h. The commonly used suture size for intra-oral procedures is 4/0.

19. **Advantages of marsupialization of cysts over enucleation:**
    a. Cyst cavity open for inspection
    b. Whole cyst lining available for histological analysis
    c. Easier for patient to look after in terms of oral hygiene
    d. May be used to prevent damage to vital structure
    e. Less bone removal therefore less trauma
    f. Healing is faster than enucleation
    g. Does not allow tooth eruption through the cysts.

20. **Incisional biopsy is indicated in which of following lesions:**
    a. Squamous cell carcinoma of lateral border of tongue
    b. Fibroepithelial polyp on buccal mucosa

c. Capillary haemangioma on the lower lip
d. Sublingual keratosis
e. Palpable lump in the submandibular gland.

21. **Signs and symptoms of fractures of zygomatic arch:**
    a. Anosmia
    b. Limitation of mouth opening
    c. Deviation of mandible on opening to the ipsilateral side
    d. Deviation of mandible on opening to the contralateral side
    e. Diplopia
    f. Epistaxis.

22. **Regarding submandibular gland:**
    a. Damage to lingual nerve will cause loss of sensation to posterior-third of the tongue
    b. Submandibular gland wraps around posterior border of mylohyoid
    c. The buccal branch of facial nerve is at risk of trauma
    d. Hypoglossal nerve loop is under mandibular duct
    e. The safest site for an incision is on the lower border of the mandible to prevent damage to facial nerve.

23. **With regards to temporomandibular joint:**
    a. The articular surface of the joint is covered with fibrocartilage
    b. The articular surfaces is covered with hyaline cartilage
    c. The articular disc is composed of hyaline cartilage
    d. The middle part of the disc is vascular
    e. The disc attaches to the articular capsule anteriorly
    f. The temporomandibular ligament is related to the lateral aspect of the joint
    g. The stylomandibular ligament is remnant of deep cervical fascia as it passes medial to parotid gland
    h. The stylohyoid ligament extends from the tip of styloid process to the lingula
    i. The sphenomandibular ligament is remnant of Meckel's cartilage.

24. **Mandibular orthognathic surgery:**
    a. Is always undertaken via an intra-oral approach
    b. Is usually associated with nerve damage following sagittal split technique
    c. Require both pre-operative and post-operative orthodontics
    d. Causes facial swelling that can be reduced with systemic steroids
    e. Should be discussed with appropriate patients by their general dental practitioner.

25. **Patient with cleft lip and palate:**
    a. Dental abnormalities may include missing teeth
    b. Speech may be described hypernasal
    c. There may be eustachian tube dysfunction
    d. Osseointegrated implants are recommended
    e. Childhood surgery prevents the need for later orthognathic surgery.

26. Craniofacial anomaly of craniosynostosis:
   a. Includes the syndrome Crouzon and Apert
   b. Does not require surgical treatment until patient has reached adult age
   c. May require surgery on more than one occasion
   d. Results in disturbed growth of mandible
   e. Requires management by large multidisciplinary team
   f. Good age of surgery is between 5-7 years of age.

27. Suture materials:
   a. Polyglycolic acid sutures are easy to handle, less expensive and have minimal tissue reaction
   b. Catgut suture material is absorbable suture material
   c. Polyglycolic acid suture material is absorbable suture material
   d. Nylon is nonabsorbable suture material
   e. Polyesters and propylenes are absorbable suture materials.

28. Surgical procedures:
   a. Necropsy is histopathological study of tissue removed before death of an individual
   b. Autopsy is histopathological study of tissue removed after death of individual
   c. Incisional biopsy is performed by removing a wedge-shaped segment of pathological tissue along with surrounding adjacent normal tissue
   d. Biopsy is the study of tissues removed from living organism to confirm diagnosis through histopathological study
   e. Excisional biopsy is performed using a fine needle aspiration.

29. Extraction forceps:
   a. Ash forceps are used for extraction of all the teeth
   b. Forceps No.151 may be used for mandibular anterior teeth
   c. Allies forceps helps in grasping of tissues
   d. Mead forceps are used for maxillary anterior teeth.

30. Impaction:
   a. Impacted supernumerary teeth occur in mandibular anterior region
   b. In position C impaction, highest portion of tooth is above cervical line of second molar
   c. Distoangular is the most difficult impaction to remove due to its bulk present in vertical ramus
   d. Class IV impaction involves vertically impacted canine between lateral incisor and first premolar
   e. In class II impaction, space between distal surface of third molar while ramus is less than mesiodistal diameter of crown of second molar.

Identify the Single Best Answer for the following

31. **Agent used in gas sterilisation:**
    a. Chlorhexidine
    b. Sodium hypochlorite
    c. Cetrimide
    d. Ethylene oxide.

32. **The formation of dry socket usually occurs at:**
    a. 5th post-operative day
    b. 6th post-operative day
    c. 1st post-operative day
    d. 3rd or 4th post-operative day.

33. **The treatment approach for pericoronitis associated with impacted mandibular third molar is:**
    a. Antibiotics and analgesic therapy
    b. Operculectomy
    c. Extraction of impacted molar
    d. Irrigating under the operculum.

34. **Out of the following options, all are the objectives of alveolectomy, *except*:**
    a. To increase the inter-maxillary gap
    b. To decrease the inter-maxillary gap
    c. To correct the pre-maxillary excess
    d. To correct sharp knife-edged bony ridge.

35. **The treatment of choice for haemorrhagic bone cyst is:**
    a. Excision
    b. Incision
    c. Caldwell-Luc operation
    d. Surgical exploration followed by curettage.

36. **Osteoradionecrosis of the jaw bone is a complication of:**
    a. Physiotherapy
    b. Chemotherapy
    c. Surgery
    d. Radiotherapy.

37. **The most common site of mandible fracture is:**
    a. Symphysis of the mandible
    b. Body of the mandible
    c. Angle of the mandible
    d. Coronoid process.

38. **Dish face deformity is the characteristic feature of:**
    a. Le fort I
    b. Le fort II
    c. Le fort III
    d. None of the above.

39. The use of Gill's approach is to:
    a. Reduce the fractured zygoma
    b. A common approach for condylar surgery
    c. Block inferior alveolar nerve
    d. Managing angle fracture.

40. The splint most frequently used for fixation of the fractured mandible in children is:
    a. Acrylic cap splints
    b. Gunning splint
    c. Cast metal splint
    d. All of the above.

41. The direct structural and functional contact between bone and implant is called as:
    a. Fibrous integration
    b. Fibro-osseous integration
    c. Osseo-integration
    d. None of the above.

42. Which among the following causes parasthesia of lip?
    a. Fracture of the mandible
    b. A benign tumour of mandible
    c. Removal of mandibular 3rd molar
    d. Periapical abscess of first molar.

43. What causes mucoceles?
    a. Infection
    b. Tooth extraction
    c. Trauma
    d. Sialolithiasis.

44. Ruston bodies are absent in:
    a. Primordial cyst
    b. Gingival cyst of neonate
    c. Infected dentigerous cyst
    d. Apical periodontal cyst.

45. What is the other name for marsupialization?
    a. Waldron's operation
    b. Caldwell-Luc operation
    c. Partsch's operation
    d. None of above.

46. Bone blend consists of:
    a. Bone and sodium hypochlorite
    b. Bone and sterile saline
    c. Bone and blood
    d. Bone and sulfuric acid.

47. The following non-bone materials can be used as graft?
    a. Plaster of Paris
    b. Cartilage
    c. Sclera
    d. Calf bone.

48. White grafts:
    a. Behave in same manner as autogenous grafts
    b. Never rejected
    c. Are immunologically biocompatible
    d. Are rejected without evidence of vascularisation.

49. The material most commonly used as a dental implants:
    a. Polymers
    b. Titanium
    c. Steel
    d. Ceramics.

50. Determines stability of the dental implants:
    a. Quality of the bone
    b. Quantity of the bone
    c. All of the above
    d. None of the above.

51. The type of implant recommended when there is inadequate bone for the placement of implant:
    a. Endosteal implants
    b. Transosteal implants
    c. Subperiosteal implants
    d. Screw type of implants.

Identify the answers to the following Extended Matching Questions

52. With regards to oral infections:
    a. Pregnant women with soft, red, fluctuant swelling on the gingivae
    b. Purple swelling of the hard palate that does not blanch on applying pressure in a young man
    c. A pink swelling associated with multilocular radiolucency in the mandible
    d. Soft, well-circumscribed swelling on the midline of the palate
    e. A sensile fluctuant swelling on the lower lip, bluish in colour. Patient has history of trauma
    f. Multiple oral ulcers and fever in a child
    g. Multiple unilateral ulcers in elderly women
    h. A single sinus ulcer on buccal mucosa of 20-year-old
    i. Corrugated lesions bilaterally on tongue
    j. Irregular ulcers on the soft tissues in HIV positive patient.

1. Abscess	10. Herpes simplex virus (HSV)
2. Adenoma	11. Epstein-Barr virus (EBV)
3. Central giant cell granuloma	12. Coxsackie virus
4. Fibroepithelial polyps	13. Candida
5. Torus	14. Varicella zoster virus
6. Pyogenic granuloma	15. *Treponema pallidum*
7. Mucococle	16. *Staphylococcus aureus*
8. Haemangioma	17. Peripheral giant cell granuloma
9. Kaposi sarcoma	

53. **Anatomy:**
    a. Inserts on lateral surface of angle of lower ramus of mandible
    b. Inserts on pterygoid fossa below condylar process of mandible and intra-articular cartilage of TMJ
    c. Inserts on the medial and anterior aspect of coronoid process of mandible
    d. Elevates mandible and posterior fibres retracts
    e. Elevates, protracts and laterally displace mandible to opposite side for chewing
    f. This passes from sphenoid bone to the lingula next to inferior dental canal
    g. This arises from the styloid process and is attached to the angle of mandible
    h. The TMJ has fibrous capsule which is attached to articular margins. The lateral part of capsule is thickened to form
    i. The joint cavity is divided into two by dense fibrous connective tissue
    j. The upper cavity of the joint is long and includes both a concave surface of the temporal bone and convex bulge on the underside of the zygomatic arch. The lateral bulge is called.

1. Lateral pterygoid	7. Glenoid fossa
2. Masseter	8. Lateral ligament
3. Medial pterygoid	9. Meniscus
4. Temporalis	10. Sphenomandibular ligament
5. Articular eminence	11. Stylomandibular ligament
6. Condylar head	

54. **Non-tumour soft tissue lumps of mouth:**
    a. Bony lump found in the centre of palate
    b. Mucous extravasation cyst affecting lower lip
    c. Cyst from floor of mouth arising from sublingual gland tends to re-occur if marsupialized. It can pass deep into mylohyoid and can appear at neck and floor of mouth in the form of swelling
    d. A developmental cyst is commonly located at the lateral canthus of the eye and most often found in midline of the neck above mylohyoid.
    e. Giant cell lesion sometime found in soft tissues but commonly within the bone. It occur secondary to hyperparathyroidism. Diagnosis is usually suggested after enucleation and histopathological examination shows giant cells in fibrous stroma.

f. An over vigorous response to low grade recurrent trauma can be pedunculated and range from small lumps to lesions covering entire palate
g. Red fleshy nodular swelling in response to recurrent trauma and non-specific infection. Histology shows proliferation of vascular connective tissue results in bleeding readily
h. Present at birth, presents as pedunculated nodule histological examination reveal large granular cells
i. Increased inflammatory response to plaque during pregnancy causes lesion similar to pyogenic granuloma
j. A red, fleshy swelling often nodular occurring as response to chronic irritation. Histological examination reveals vascular lesions with multinucleated giant cells.

1. Basal cell carcinoma	9. Mucoceles
2. Brown's tumour	10. Stafne's bone cyst
3. Dermoid cyst	11. Torus mandibularis
4. Epidermoid cyst	12. Torus palatinus
5. Fibroepithelial polyp	13. Congenital epulis
6. Mucoepidermoid cyst	14. Epulis
7. Pyogenic granuloma	15. Giant cell granuloma
8. Ranula	

55. **Benign tumours of mouth:**
    a. Resembles white or pink cauliflower and caused by papilloma virus
    b. A smooth, soft slow growing yellowish lump present in cheek or neck
    c. A tumour comprises completely of Schwann cells
    d. A rare tumour histiocytic origin which usually arises as a nodule on the tongue. Always excised with margins
    e. Rare tumour of fibroblasts of peripheral nerve which usually affects tongue may be part of Von Recklinghausen disease. Can undergo sarcomatous change
    f. May be neoplasm or developmental anomaly. A well-demarcated fibro-osseous lesion of the jaws. It presents as painless, slow growing swelling expanding both buccal and lingual cortices. Similar histology as fibrous dysplasia

1. Lateral pterygoid	7. Glenoid fossa
2. Masseter	8. Lateral ligament
3. Medial pterygoid	9. Meniscus
4. Temporalis	10. Sphenomandibular ligament
5. Articular eminence	11. Stylomandibular ligament
6. Condylar head	

56. **Odontogenic tumours:**
    a. Not true neoplasm but malformation of dental hard tissue. They are either compound or complex in their classification
    b. Most common odontogenic tumour. Commonly found in men and Africans can be aggressive and invades surrounding tissue. Two types of histologically presentations are plexiform and follicular

c. Characteristically, it is seen as a radiolucency on X-ray with scattered radiopacities. Requires excision with margins
d. Can occur both in hard and soft tissues. These arising in jaws are tumour of odontogenic mesenchyme. It mostly occurs in young men and arises within bone having soap bubble appearance.
e. Rare tumour affecting young adults appears as unilocular radiolucency on X-ray causing painless expansion of jaws. Enucleation is curative.
f. Tends to occur in anterior maxilla in females. Conservative excision. Does not reoccur.

1. Adenoameloblastoma
2. Ameloblastoma
3. Ameloblastic fibroma
4. Calcifying epithelial odontogenic tumour
5. Myxoma
6. Odontoma.

57. Anaesthesia:
a. Loss of pain sensation without loss of consciousness
b. Contraindicated in cases of porphyria
c. Vasoconstrictor local anesthetic agent
d. Decreases the chances of toxicity
e. Causative agent in allergic reactions
f. Vasoconstrictor added in local anaesthetia solution
g. An amide derivative most commonly used local as well as topical agent
h. Natural local anesthetic drug
i. Fungicide in local anaesthesia
j. Preservative in local anesthesia
k. Prolongs the duration of LA
l. Most frequent complication associated with local anesthesia.

1. Anesthesia
2. Analgesia
3. Xylocaine
4. Benzocaine
5. Procaine
6. Cocaine
7. Centbucridine
8. Lidocaine
9. Paraffin
10. Methylparaben
11. Beeswax
12. Halothane
13. Adrenaline
14. Esters of PABA
15. Sodium chloride
16. Thiopentone sodium
17. Syncope
18. Shock
19. Swelling
20. Ludwig's angina
21. Hypersensitivity reaction
22. Malignant hyperthermia
23. Thymol

58. Post-operative extraction complications:
a. Post-operative complication of outpatient general anaesthesia
b. Circulatory complications
c. Patient with internal haemorrhage can suffer this with administration of local anaesthesia

d. Systemic complications of local anaesthesia
e. Local complication of local anaesthesia

1. Tachycardia	13. Toxicity
2. Hypertension	14. Delirium
3. Fainting/syncope	15. Airway obstruction
4. Vomiting	16. Hematoma
5. Nausea	17. Lipoma
6. Hyperventilation	18. Acanthosis
7. Laryngeal spasm	19. Swelling
8. Arrythmias	20. Chronic inflammation
9. Malignant hyperthermia	21. Eye infection
10. Hyperthyroidism	22. Neuroma
11. Acute inflammation	23. Neuritis
12. Cardiac disorder	

59. **Space infections:**
    a. Diffused inflammation of soft tissues
    b. Board like swelling of floor of mouth with elevation of tongue
    c. Common causative organism
    d. Firm, painful and diffuse swelling with paucity of pus
    e. Infection occurring around erupting or partially impacted third molars
    f. Acute, potentially life-threatening toxic cellulitis.

1. Ludwig's angina	9. *Prevotella*
2. Cellulitis	10. *Porphyromonas*
3. Neuritis	11. *Haemophilus influenzae*
4. Streptococci	12. *Moraxella catarrhalis*
5. Staphylococci	13. Focal infection
6. Pericoronitis	14. Arthritis
7. Otitis media	15. Subacute bacterial endocarditis
8. Phelgmon	16. Bacterial endocarditis

60. **Implants in dentistry:**
    a. Common material used for implants
    b. Time required for maxillary osseointegration
    c. Time required for mandibular osseointegration
    d. Endosseous implants
    e. Subperiosteal implants
    f. Most common type of implant
    g. Ceramic implants
    h. Minimum distance between two adjacent implants
    i. Implants used in atrophic mandible
    j. Minimum time required for healing of implant.

1. Mucosal inserts	13. 4 mm
2. Subperiostal implant dentures	14. 3 mm
3. Aluminium oxide	15. 5 mm
4. Titanium	16. 8 mm
5. 4 months	17. 1–2 months
6. Steel	18. 3–6 months
7. Two piece implant	19. 9–12 months
8. Blade vent implants	20. Single pin staples
9. Tricalcium phosphate	21. Endosteal implant
10. 1 mm	22. 6 months
11. Hydroxylapatite	23. Plymers
12. Screw	24. Ceramic

61. Neurological disorders:
   a. Sensory and motor nerve
   b. Definite trigger zones
   c. Fifth cranial nerve
   d. Tic douloureux
   e. Nerve that supplies muscles of mastication
   f. Cluster headache
   g. Herpes zoster is also called
   h. Loss of taste
   i. Treatment of choice for trigeminal neuralgia.

1. Trigeminal nerve	11. Periapical cyst
2. Trigeminal neuralgia	12. Phenytoin
3. Glosspharyngeal nerve	13. Alarm clock headache
4. Chorda tympani	14. Frey's syndrome
5. Hypoglossal	15. Sphenopalatine neuralgia
6. Histamine cephalgia	16. Carbamazepine
7. Neuritis	17. Amoxycilline
8. Shingles	18. Mandibular division
9. Periodic migranous neuralgia	19. Glossitis
10. Maxillary nerve	20. Analgesia

CASE DISCUSSION

Case 1: Complications of Extracting Teeth

Access

- Small mouths is always a complication but can be managed
- Crowded and malpositioned teeth will require transalveolar approach
- Trismus due to infection leading to patient's inability to open mouth
- Submasseteric abscess should be managed in hospital with external drainage and airway protection.

Pain

- Has local anaesthesia worked? Does it require further local anaesthesia may be regional block, infiltration and intraligamentary injection
- Whether it is Pain or pressure that patient is feeling? if pressure—reassure and proceed with extraction

- If pain persists and signs of LA are present → There is presence of acute infection
- Draining abscess should be considered.

Inability to Move Tooth
- Check radiographs
- If bulbous/diverging roots/long root/ankylosis or sclerotic bone
- Raise flap
- Use transalveolar procedure.

Breaking the Tooth
- Is common occurrence and assist extraction
- Most often crown fracture leaving roots in situ
- Small (< 3 mm) pieces of deeply buried apex can be left
- Provide patient with antibiotics, tell patient and review
- Large pieces of roots should be removed as they have high incidence of infective sequelae.

Fracture of Alveolar or Basal Bone
- Is common
- If fracture only involves the alveolus containing extracted tooth, remove dry pieces of bone which are not attached to periosteum and close the wound
- If alveolar carrying other teeth are involved, remove tooth by transalveolar approach and splint remaining teeth
- Basal bone fracture is rare, adequate analgesia (LA or systemic) and reduction and fixation.

Loss of Tooth
- Stop and look inside the mouth, is it under mucoperiosteum or in tissue spaces
- Look in suction apparatus
- Is it in the antrum or inferior dental canal
- Swallowed or inhaled
- Chest X-ray is mandatory, if tooth is not found.

Damage to Other Teeth/Tissues, and Extraction of Wrong Tooth
- Prevent by confirming with the patient the teeth to be removed and making careful notes. Plan the procedure
- If wrong tooth is extracted, replant if feasible and then remove correct tooth
- Make patient aware of the incident and document it.

Displaced Jaw
- Reduce—immediate reduction with LA around dislocated jaw joint
- Place thumbs over molar teeth and exert downward and backward pressure
- Advice jaw support when yawning, etc.

Pain, Swelling and Trismus
- Pain can be quite severe and respond best to non-steroidal anti-inflammatory drugs (NSAIDs)
- Pre-operatively LA works wells and leaves patient pain free and numb for the duration
- Trismus is due to pain and muscle spasms and can be reduced by adequate analgesia
- Swelling can be reduced by high dose peri-operative steroids
- Haemorrhage can be controlled by biting on pressure packs
- Antibiotic prophylaxis can be beneficial.

Bleeding
- Immediate: When true haemostasis not achieved
- Reactionary: Within 48 hours after surgery due to local and general increase in blood pressure resulting in opening up of small dividing vessels
- Secondary: Occurs ~7 day post-operatively due to infection destroying clot or ulcerating local vessels
- Treatment: Squeeze the socket, pack socket with collagen and place the suture, BIPP or whitehead varnish.

Case 2: Dento-Facial Infections

Vast majority of infections in this area requires surgical treatment. These infections are bacterial usually arising from necrotic pulps, periodontal pockets or pericoronitis. These can be life-threatening, if allowed to progress to fascial space in neck or cavernous sinus or as a focus for infective endocarditis.

Microbiology
- Mostly anaerobes—predominant bacteroides and streptococci (aerobe and anaerobe), usually sensitive of penicillins
- Bacteroides are always sensitive to metronidazole.

Diagnosis

Diagnosis is made clinically based on pain, swelling, temperature and discharge.

Apical Abscess
- Teeth are tender to percussion and non-vital
- Discoloured or crowned
- History of trauma or root canal treatment
- Intrabony pus tracks through soft tissue and discharge in buccal sulcus usually (upper lateral incisors discharge palatally)
- Associated with periostitis with severe thickening.
- Treatment:
  - Drainage of pus via root canal
  - Incision of any fluctuant abscess (Fig. 10.1)
  - Extraction under local anesthesia
  - Antibiotic coverage:
    Amoxicillin 500 mg TDS postoperatively for 5–7 days
    Metronidazole 400 mg TDS PO for 5–7 days or combination of both drugs.

Periodontal abscess
- Arise in pre-existing dental pockets
- Initial treatment is incision or drainage/elimination of pocket/extraction is considered.

Pericoronitis
- Inflammation and infection of a gum flap (operculum overlying partially erupted tooth usually over permanent lower third molar which gets traumatised by over erupted permanent upper third molar)
- Treatment removal of opposing upper third molar, irrigation under operculum with saline or chlorhexidine and antibiotics if required
- Molars associated with recurrent episodes of pericoronitis needs removal.

Dry socket
- Is osteitis of socket following extraction
- Common in mandible after removal of molars permanent lower third molar
- Predisposing factors—smoking, surgical trauma, LA history, bone disease, medications or immunodeficiency
- Diagnosis:
  - Pain onset after 2–4 days usually post-extraction
  - Worse than preceding toothache
  - Socket looks inflamed and exposed bone is visible.
- Treatment:
  - Clean socket by irrigation and dress the exposed bone by alvogyl, bismuth subnitrate and iodoform paste (BIPP) or zinc oxide eugenol (ZOE) pack
  - Topical metronidazole as an alternative
  - Chlorhexidine and hot salt mouth washes
  - Non-steroidal anti-inflammatory drugs are systemic analgesic of choice
  - Prophylactic anaerobicidal such as metronidazole.

Actinomycosis
- Persistent low grade infection, multiple sinuses (Fig. 10.2)
- Treatment:
  - Drainage
  - Amoxicillin 500 mg twice daily for 6 weeks
  - Doxycycline 100 mg once daily as an alternative.

Staphylococcal lymphadenitis
- Especially seen in children
- Small occult skin or mucosal breach allows ingress
- Mimic slapped face due to exotoxin
- Drain and give flucloxacillin 125–500 mg thrice daily (depending on age).

Atypical Mycobacteria
- Lymphadenitis with no obvious cause
- Cold nodes, non-febrile patients
- Drain and excise
- Culture up to 12 weeks
- Clarithromycin most useful conventional antibiotic
- Excision of nodes is definite treatment.

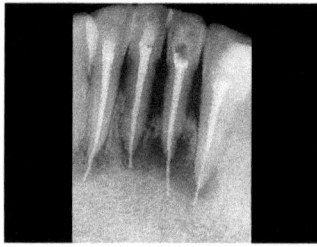

Fig. 10.1: Intra-oral periapical (IOPA) indicating periapical abscess

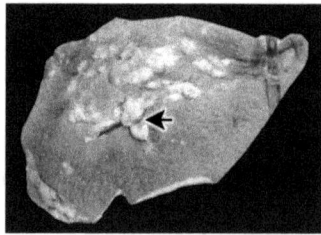

Fig. 10.2: Clinical presentation of *Actinomycosis*

Case 3: Cyst of the Jaws

Cysts are abnormal epithelium lined cavities often contain fluid but if they become too infected, they might contains pus. Jaw cysts predominantly arise from odontogenic epithelium, grows by epithelial proliferation, bone resorption by prostaglandins and variations in intra-cystic osmotic pressure.

Diagnosis
- Detected as asymptomatic radiolucencies on X-rays
- Painless swellings
- Always on buccal cortex (almost)
- Infected cysts presents with pain, swelling and discharge
- Vitality test associated teeth
- Orthopantomogram and intraoral periapical radiographs to screen for size and co-existing pathology
- Aspirations is useful
- Cysts can present with pathological fractures, especially mandible.

Treatment
- Enucleation with primary closure: Removing cyst lining from the bony walls of the cavity, repositioning the access flap. Any relevant dental pathology treatment can be carried out at same time, e.g. apicectomy
- Enucleation with packing and delayed closure in badly infected cysts, particularly large cysts unsuitable for primary closure. Pack with whitehead's varnish or BIPP
- Enucleation with primary bone grafting—rarely useful
- Marsupialization: This is opening of the cyst to allow continuity with oral mucosa, healing is slower than enucleation and cavity persists for some time. It is useful to allow tooth eruption through the cavity or where enucleation is contraindicated
- Always submit cyst lining for histopathology.

Classification
Epithelial Cysts
- Developmental odontogenic cysts:
  - Odontogenic keratocyst
  - Dentigerous cyst
  - Eruption cyst
  - Lateral periodontal cyst (Figs 10.3A and B)
  - Gingival cyst of adults
  - Glandular odontogenic cyst
- Inflammatory odontogenic cysts:
  - Radicular cysts
  - Residual cysts
  - Paradental cysts
- Non-odontogenic cysts:
  - Nasopalatine cyst
  - Nasolabial cyst.

Non-epithelial cysts
- Solitary bone cyst
- Aneurysmal bone cyst.

Clinical Features of Cysts

Cysts	Presentation	Characteristic features
Keratocysts	• Presents 2nd/3rd decade • Males population more prevalant than female • Angle of mandible	• Frequently symptomless, incidental finding on radiographs • Causes tooth displacement and occasional paraesthesia of lower lip • Treatment includes enucleation/cryotherapy and Carnoy solution
Dentigerous	• Presents 3rd–4th decade • Males population more prevalant than female • Mandibular 3rd molar followed by maxillary canine	• May grow large in size before treatment • Most discovered on radiographs take due to facture of took eruption
Eruption	• 1st and 2nd decade • Males population more prevalant than female • Deciduous/permanent teeth anterior to first permanent molar	• Smooth swelling of normal or blue-coloured mucosa over erupting-tooth
Radicular	• 3rd and 4th decade • Males population more prevalant than female • Tooth bearing areas of jaw • Anterior maxilla • Most common odontogenic cyst	• Slow enlarging swelling, symptomless, incidental finding on radiograph of non-vital teeth • Treatment includes enucleation and endodontic therapy or extraction
Residual	• 4th and 5th decade • Males population more prevalant than female • Mandibular premolar area	• Slow enlarging swelling • Frequently symptom less • Treatment—enucleation
Nasopalatine	• 4th, 5th and 6th decade • Males population more prevalant than female • Nasopalatine canal	• Swelling of anterior palate or floor of nose • Treatment—enucleation
Nasolabial	• 4th, and 5th decade • Female population more prevalent than male • Nasolabial fold	• Swelling in soft tissues • Treatment—enucleation.
Solitary	• 2nd decade • Female population more prevalent than male • Mandible	• Discovered on radiographs • Treatment—opening cysts, gentle curettage, closure heals cysts
Aneurysmal	• 2nd decade • Female population more prevalent than male • Posterior mandible	• Firm swelling • Expanding rapidly • Treatment include small cysts—enucleation • Long cysts—excision and reconstruction

Answers

1. a. F b. F c. F d. F e. F
   f. F g. T
2. a. F b. F c. F d. F e. F
   f. T g. F h. F i. F j. F
   k. F
3. a. F b. F c. T d. T e. T
   f. F g. F h. T
4. a. T b. T c. T d. F e. F
   f. F
5. a. T b. F c. F d. T e. F
6. a. F b. T c. T d. F e. T
7. a. T b. F c. T d. F e. T
   f. F
8. a. T b. F c. T d. F e. T
   f. T g. T
9. a. F b. T c. F d. T e. F
   f. F g. F h. F i. T
10. a. F b. F c. T d. F e. F
    f. F g. F h. F
11. a. F b. F c. F d. F e. ??
    f. F
12. a. T b. F c. F d. F e. F
    f. F g. T h. T i. T j. T
    k. F l. T m. T
13. a. F b. F c. F d. F e. T
    f. T g. T
14. a. F b. T c. T d. F e.

15.	a.	T	b.	T	c.	T	d.	T	e.	F
16.	a.	T	b.	F	c.	T	d.	F	e.	F
17.	a.	F	b.	T	c.	T	d.	F	e.	F
	f.	F								
18.	a.	F	b.	F	c.	T	d.	F	e.	F
	f.	T	g.	F	h.	F				
19.	a.	T	b.	F	c.	F	d.	T	e.	F
	f.	F	g.	F						
20.	a.	T	b.	F	c.	F	d.	T	e.	F
21.	a.	??	b.	T	c.	T	d.	F	e.	F
	f.	F								
22.	a.	F	b.	T	c.	F	d.	F	e.	F
23.	a.	T	b.	F	c.	F	d.	F	e.	F
	f.	T	g.	T	h.	F	i.	T		
24.	a.	F	b.	T	c.	T	d.	T	e.	T
25.	a.	T	b.	T	c.	T	d.	T	e.	F
26.	a.	T	b.	F	c.	T	d.	F	e.	T
	f.	T								
27.	a.	T	b.	T	c.	F	d.	T	e.	F
28.	a.	F	b.	T	c.	T	d.	T	e.	F
29.	a.	T	b.	T	c.	T	d.	F		
30.	a.	F	b.	F	c.	T	d.	T	e.	F
31.	d	32.	b	33.	c	34.	b	35.	d	
36.	d	37.	a	38.	c	39.	a	40.	a	
41.	c	42.	c	43.	c	44.	a	45.	d	
46.	b	47.	a	48.	d	49.	b	50.	d	
51.	c									
52.	a.	6	b.	9	c.	18	d.	5	e.	13
	f.	10	g.	15	h.	16	i.	11	j.	10

53.	a.	2	b.	1	c.	4	d.	??	e.	??
	f.	10	g.	11	h.	8	i.	9	j.	5
54.	a.	12	b.	9	c.	8	d.	3	e.	2
	f.	5	g.	7	h.	13	i.	14	j.	15
55.	a.	9	b.	3	c.	5	d.	10	e.	4
	f.	6								
56.	a.	6	b.	2	c.	4	d.	5	e.	3
	f.	1								
57.	a.	2	b.	16	c.	6	d.	13	e.	10
	f.	10	g.	8	h.	6	i.	23	j.	10
	k.	13	l.	17						
58.	a.	4,5	b.	1, 2, 8	c.	2	d.	3, 9, 6, 13	e.	16
59.	a.	2,8	b.	1	c.	4	d.	1	e.	6
	f.	1								
60.	a.	4	b.	21	c.	5	d.	7	e.	20
	f.	21	g.	3, 9, 11	h.	14	i.	2	j.	18
61.	a.	1	b.	2	c.	1	d.	2	e.	1
	f.	6	g.	8	h.	20	i.	16		

CORRECT ANSWER FOR FALSE STATEMENTS

1. d. Second and third episode of pericoronitis
   e. Plaque formation is a risk factor.
   f. Prophylactic removal does not confer additional health benefits
2. a. Trochlear nerve
   b. Abducens nerve
   c. Trigeminal nerve
   d Facial nerve
   e. All motor muscles of tongue except palatoglossus
   g. Lower face unilaterally and upper face bilaterally innervated
   h. Oculomotor nerve
   i. Hypoglossal nerve
   j. 0.5%
   k. 2%
4. e. Mandible
   f. Lack of permanent successor
5. b. Chisel & Mallet to be under GA → Removal of distolingual bone from disto-angularly impacted third molar
   c. Disto-angularly impacted are most difficult to extract surgically
   e. Conscious sedation is a likely option
7. f. Related to alveolar osteitis
8. b. Keratinised mucosa
   d. Only require surgery if interfering with lingual flange of the denture.
9. a. Maxillary first molars
   c. unable to drink fluid without bubbling through the nose
   e. Palatine artery should be avoided
   f. Epithelium lined
   g. Ephedrine should be used
   h. Cefuroxime is the drug of choice
10. a. Mumps
    b. Pleomorphic adenoma
    d. Salivary calculi
    e. Pleomorphic adenoma
    f. Recurrent obstructive sialadenitis
    g. Sarcoidosis
11. a. Condylar neck
    b. Angle of the mandible
    c. Left side
    d. Common cause

g. Gunning splints
  h. Inferior alveolar nerve
12. b. Diplopia
  a. Inferior rectus muscle
  b. Hang drop sign
  c. Retrobulbar haemorrhage
  d. Le fort I fracture
  k. Malar fracture
1. a. Spreads Palatally
  d. Oedema and is extensive when involve lax tissue.
  f. Cavernous sinus thrombosis is more likely with upper face via facial vein to cavernous sinus.
2. a. Cowhorn forceps
  a. Bard-Parker handle with No 15 blade
  b. Howarth
  g. No 8 round tungsten carbide is used for bone removal
1. a. loss of sensation to anterior 2/3rd of the tongue
  a. Lingual nerve loop under mandibular duct
  b. Incisions are placed two finger beneath below the lower border to avoid damage to marginal mandibular branch of facial nerve
2. b. Fibrocartilage
  a. Avascular
  b. The disc attaches to anterior margin of articular eminence, articular margin of the condyle and lateral pterygoid muscle
  h. Extends from the tip of styloid process to the angle of mandible
3. a. Mandibular orthognathic surgery is undertaken extraorally for vertical ramus
4. a. Adult patient may still require orthodontic expansion surgery followed by osteotomy to advance maxilla—as adult cleft, lip and palate patient has hypoplastic maxilla, class 3 skeletal base and dental occlusion with crossbite.

Chapter 11
Human Disease and Medical Emergencies

Identify the following Statements as True (T) or False (F)

1. **Anaemia:**
   a. Is said to be present in an adult male, if the haemoglobin (Hb) concentration is less than 13.5 g/dl and in an adult female of less than 11.5 g/dl
   b. Is associated with koilonychia
   c. Elective surgery in patients with an Hb <10 g/dl can be undertaken
   d. Microcytic anaemia is caused due to presence of chronic disease
   e. The total iron binding capacity (TIBC) is reduced/low in microcytic anaemia
   f. Macrocytic anaemia is caused due to low folate
   g. Pernicious anaemia is macrocytic anaemia
   h. Coeliac disease can be seen in patients with iron deficiency anaemia
   i. Chronic exposure to nitrous oxide can cause microcytic anaemia
   j. Lifelong intramuscular (IM) hydroxycobalamin 1mg injection is used to treat B_{12} deficiency
   k. Folinic acid is used to treat folate deficiency
   l. Sickle cell type contraindicates dental treatment under general anaesthesia
   m. The presence or absence of haemoglobin-s (sickle cell) should be determined before general anaesthesia in risk groups
   n. Haemolytic anaemia is the commonest anaemia
   o. TIBC is increased in normocytic anaemia.

2. **Haematological malignancy:**
   a. Acute myeloblastic leukaemia is the most common childhood leukaemia
   b. Acute lymphoblastic leukaemia has 90% cure rate in favourable cases
   c. All can present as gingival hypertrophy and bleeding
   d. Chronic lymphocytic leukaemia is uncommon
   e. Chronic lymphocytic leukaemia is characterised by the presence of Philadelphia chromosome
   f. Chronic myeloid leukaemia usually affects below 40 years
   g. Acute leukaemia have cells that retain most of the appearance of normal white cells
   h. Multiple myeloma is B-lymphocyte disorder
   i. Hodgkin's lymphoma has the poor diagnosis

j. Primary amyloidosis is a plasma cell dyscrasia
   k. Non-steroidal anti-inflammatory drugs (NSAIDs) can be safely prescribed in anaemia and haematological malignancy.
3. **Bleeding disorders:**
   a. Platelet disorders can present as purpura and nose bleeds
   b. Cannot be caused by Von Willebrand's disease
   c. Haemophilia A is factor XI deficiency
   d. Haemophilia A is a sex-linked recessive and it affects males predominantly
   e. Bleeding from mouth is uncommon in haemophilia A
   f. Factor IX deficiency is also known as Christmas disease
   g. In Von Willebrand disease, there is combined platelet and factor IX disorder affecting males and females
   h. Heparin effects can be reversed by protamine sulfate in an emergency
   i. Normal therapeutic range is an International Normalized Ratio of 2-4, simple extractions are safe at this level
   j. The activated partial thromboplastin time (APTT) is normal in haemophilia A.
4. **Cardiovascular system:**
   a. Hypertension is a risk factor for renal failure
   b. Local anaesthesia (LA) solution with adrenaline, if injected intravascularly can trigger angina in susceptible patients
   c. Breathlessness is a principal sign in right heart failure
   d. Dependent oedema and venous engorgement are prominent in left heart failure
   e. Arrhythmias can be diagnosed from history of palpitations and irregular pulse
   f. The death rate of myocardial infarction associated with GA is 50%
   g. Preoperative glyceryl trinitrate is recommended for patients with angina receiving treatment under LA
   h. Patients with history of rheumatic fever and congenital cardiac lesion are susceptible to infective endocarditis following dental treatment.
5. **An angina patient:**
   a. Can be safely treated under LA
   b. Is likely to be taking daily aspirin
   c. May not be at risk of postoperative haemorrhage
   d. Suffers from pressing chest pain that may radiate to the jaw and left arm and not relieved by nitrates
   e. May be taking drugs that cause oral signs
   f. During dental treatment should be treated in supine position.
6. **Features of bacterial endocarditis include:**
   a. Boutonniere's deformity
   b. Night sweats
   c. History of recent dental extractions

d. Splinter haemorrhages
   e. Finger clubbing
   f. Splenomegaly
   g. Roth's spots
   h. Osler nodes.

7. **The following conditions require long-term anticoagulation therapy:**
   a. Atrial fibrillation
   b. Previous deep vein thrombosis
   c. Cardiac pacemaker
   d. Prosthetic heart valves
   e. Ventricular fibrillation.

8. **The following procedures require antibiotic cover for patient with past medical history of rheumatic fever:**
   a. Inferior dental nerve block
   b. Impression of new denture
   c. Placing class I composite restoration
   d. Scaling and polishing
   e. Extraction of a tooth
   f. Subgingival periodontal therapy
   g. Basic dental examination.

9. **The following are non-water soluble vitamins:**
   a. Retinol
   b. Thiamine
   c. Tocopherol
   d. Riboflavin
   e. Vitamin D
   f. Niacin
   g. Vitamin K
   h. Biotin
   i. Vitamin C
   j. Folic acid.

10. **Regarding vitamin deficiency:**
    a. Vitamin A deficiency cause xerophthalmia
    b. Vitamin D deficiency can cause rechecking and flattening of back of skull in growing children
    c. In adults, vitamin D deficiency results in osteomalacia and osteoporosis
    d. Vitamin K deficiency can cause haemorrhaging to occur
    e. Vitamin C deficiency causes Beri-Beri
    f. Vitamin B deficiency causes Scurvy.

11. **Causes of hypertension are:**
    a. Conn's syndrome
    b. Crohn's disease

c. Phaeochromocytoma
d. Chronic glomerulonephritis
e. Unknown
f. Cushing syndrome
g. Acromegaly
h. Obstructive sleep apnoea
i. Thyroid problem.

12. **The modifiable risk factors for ischaemic heart disease are:**
    a. Smoking
    b. Hypotension
    c. Lack of exercise
    d. Hypercholesterolaemia
    e. Gender
    f. Hypertension
    g. Diabetes
    h. Obesity
    i. Age
    j. Family history.

13. **Respiratory disease:**
    a. Laryngotracheitis is an lower respiratory tract infection
    b. Chronic obstructive airway disease is defined as the presence of productive cough for at least three months in two successive years
    c. Intravenous (IV) conscious sedation can be used safely in chronic obstructive airway disease (COAD) patient
    d. Upper respiratory tract infection contraindicates elective GA
    e. Smoking is the primary cause of chronic obstructive pulmonary disease
    f. Asthmatic patients are unlikely to be allergic to penicillin
    g. GA drugs that release histamine should be avoided in asthmatic patients
    h. NSAIDs can be prescribed, if patients has taken drug before without hypersensitivity reaction
    i. Cystic fibrosis is an inherited autosomal dominant disorder
    j. Cystic fibrosis also affects pancreas, liver and kidneys
    k. Open pulmonary tuberculosis is highly infective and the dental treatment for the patient should be postponed.

14. **Cause of haemoptysis:**
    a. Bronchial carcinoma
    b. Asthma
    c. Pulmonary tuberculosis
    d. Pneumonia
    e. Bronchiectasis
    f. Mitral stenosis
    g. Bronchitis
    h. Pulmonary embolism.

15. **Gastrointestinal disease:**
    a. Peptic ulceration is unlikely to present with haematemesis
    b. Peptic ulceration is uncommonly due to infection with *Helicobacter Pylori*
    c. The treatment of peptic ulceration is combination of anaerobicidal with proton-pump inhibitor
    d. Alginates can provide symptomatic relief of dyspepsia
    e. Persistent epigastric pain should be investigated for gastric carcinoma
    f. Crohn's disease has preference for the colorectum area
    g. Ulcerative colitis presents as crohn's disease during initial stages
    h. Cobblestoning of mucosa is predominantly seen is coeliac disease
    i. Dermatitis herpetiformis can be seen in patients with coeliac disease
    j. Familial polyposis coli is associated with Frey's syndrome
    k. Pancreatitis is often a manifestation of alcohol abuse.

16. **Hepatic disease:**
    a. Hepatic disease can cause problems with production of clotting factors only
    b. Paracetamol and NSAIDs can be preserved safely in hepatic disease
    c. Intrahepatic cholestasis is reflected by decreased aspartate transaminase levels on liver function test
    d. Primary biliary cirrhosis causes intrahepatic cholestasis without hepatitis
    e. Gallstones cannot cause extrahepatic cholestasis
    f. Strict infection control should be employed.

17. **With regards to hepatitis:**
    a. Hepatitis B virus (HBV) is transmitted through punctured wounds or contact with infection body fluids
    b. Hepatitis C virus (HCV) is the most common blood-borne viral infection
    c. Hepatitis D occurs in conjunction with hepatitis B infection
    d. Hepatitis E is a water-borne disease
    e. Alcohol is an uncommon cause for hepatitis
    f. Autoimmune diseases can cause hepatitis
    g. Hepatitis A spreads via oro-faecal route
    h. HBV and HCV are leading causes of liver cancer
    i. HBV is unlikely to be transmitted from infected mother to the baby at the time of birth
    j. There is effective vaccine available to prevent HCV
    k. HBV can be transmitted from HBV positive family member who is in frequent contact with uninfected child
    l. Patient may require antibiotic cover for invasive procedure
    m. Increased bleeding following invasive procedure due to impaired synthesis of clotting factor
    n. Impaired drug metabolism.

18. **Renal disorders:**
    a. Facial oedema is prominent in nephrotic syndrome
    b. The severity of renal impairment is measured by creatinine clearance
    c. Chronic renal failure is commonly caused by glomerulonephritis
    d. Dialysis and renal transplants are mainstay of treatment
    e. Increased risk of infection and bleeding tendency
    f. Veins are sacrosanct
    g. Patient should receive dental treatment on the day of dialysis
    h. Renal transplant patient may require increased steroid dose prior to extensive dental treatment
    i. May not require antibiotic prophylaxis.

19. **Endocrine diseases:**
    a. Treatment should interfere with the mealtime of diabetic patient
    b. Have reduced resistance to dental infections
    c. May have accelerated periodontal disease
    d. Are prone to dental cysts
    e. Should not be given lidocaine with adrenaline as local analgesics
    f. Diabetes insipidus may occur temporarily after head injury
    g. In Addison's disease, secondary hypoadrenocorticism is common due to increased adrenocorticotropic hormone (ACTH)
    h. Cushing syndrome is primary condition due to therapeutic administration of synthetic steroid or adenoma
    i. Hyperthyroidism signs are bradycardia and hoarse voice
    j. Hypothyroidism is the most common cause of Graves' disease
    k. Hyperparathyroidism can be secondary to low plasma calcium levels
    l. In hypoparathyroidism, Chvostek's sign is positive
    m. Hypopituitarism does not lead to hypothyroidism
    n. Hypoparathyroidism does not cause delayed tooth eruption and enamel hypoplasia.

20. **Pregnancy:**
    a. A pregnant women should be placed in supine position
    b. Should be prescribed NSAIDs rather than paracetamol
    c. Can be safely treated using conscious sedation technique
    d. Rarely causes aggravation of gingivitis
    e. Can present with pyogenic granuloma at the gingival margins
    f. Can be given prilocaine and felypressin as LA.

21. **Addisonian crisis:**
    a. Patient's with secondary hypoadrenalism is at risk
    b. Patient's with Cushing's disease is at risk of an Addisonian crisis
    c. Patient's with secondary aldosteronism are at risk of an Addisonian crisis
    d. Patient's to be placed in horizontal position
    e. Patient's to be given glucagon
    f. Patient's to be give intravenous hydrocortisone
    g. Can present with vomiting, abdominal pain, weakness and hypovolemic shock.

22. Anaphylaxis:
a. Is mediated by immunoglobulin E (IgE) antibodies, which causes release of histamine and other vasoactive mediators
b. Is frequently caused by NSAIDs
c. Is caused by acute intravenous allergic response
d. Results in acute hypertension, bronchospasm and urticaria
e. Is managed by lying the patient flat and maintaining the airway
f. Is managed by giving 0-5 ml of 1:1000 adrenaline intravenously
g. In managed by giving oxygen
h. Is associated with antibiotics, blood products vaccines and NSAIDs, heparin and neuromuscular blocking agents.

23. Intramuscular injections:
a. Should not be given to patients with bleeding disorders
b. Is not appropriate for drug delivery in emergency due to slow absorption
c. Undergoes fast absorption when gluteal muscle is used
d. Intramuscular hydrocortisone can be used to mimic cortisol secretions in patients on long-term treatment with corticosteroids who suffer from adrenocortical suppression
e. Intramuscular vitamin K can be used for acute haemorrhage caused by liver disease
f. Vastus lateralis can be used for intramuscular injection.

24. Bone disease:
a. Marble bone disease is associated blue sclera and deafness
b. In osteogenesis imperfecta jaws are prone to fracture following extractions
c. In osteopetrosis there is increased bone density and brittleness with decreased blood supply
d. Achondroplasia is inherited autosomal recessive disorder
e. Cleidocranial dysostosis affects skull and clavicles
f. Fibrous dysplasia can be monostotic or polyostotic
g. Fibrous dysplasia is associated with Apert syndrome
h. Hands and feet are involved in Paget's disease of bone
i. In Paget's disease patient may suffer from symptoms of compression of cranial nerves.

25. With respect to fractures:
a. In simple fracture, there is no communication between the bone and the exterior
b. In greenstick fracture, the bone bends without actual separation of the fragments
c. In a comminuted fracture, there is communication between the bone and exterior
d. A complicated fracture occurs at the site of a disease process
e. In a impacted fracture the bone ends are driven together.

26. With regards to malignant disease:
    a. Hodgkin's is a type of leukaemia
    b. Acute leukaemia is a common childhood malignancy
    c. Patient with leukaemia presents with intra-oral bleeding
    d. Patient with multiple myeloma suffers from bone lesion and pain
    e. Oral squamous cell carcinomas are treated with chemotherapy.

Identify the Single Best Answer for the following

27. Type 1 diabetes is:
    a. Common in adults
    b. Involves scavenging of pancreas cells that secrete insulin
    c. Common in children and young adults known as juvenile diabetes
    d. Obesity is the only causative factor.

28. Which is the most common form of diabetes?
    a. Type 2 diabetes mellitus
    b. Type 1 diabetes mellitus
    c. Diabetes insipidus
    d. All of the above.

29. Estimated prevalence of epilepsy is:
    a. 1% of the population
    b. 4% of the population
    c. 8.5% of the population
    d. 20% of the population.

30. A specific investigation of diagnosing seizure disorder:
    a. Electrocardiogram
    b. Electroencephalogram
    c. Electroconvulsive therapy
    d. Event-related potentials.

31. Generalized tonic clonic epileptic seizure:
    a. Is also known as a grand mal
    b. Patient may have convulsions
    c. Patient may hallucinate
    d. Not associated with abnormal electrical activity.

32. If a patient has an epileptic seizure in the dental surgery:
    a. Should be given a muscle relaxant like midazolam
    b. Patient should have a mouth prop placed to prevent tongue biting
    c. Patient should be rolled onto their side
    d. If patient vomits, this should be wiped clear from their mouth.

33. Hypoglycaemia:
    a. Gets confused with other medical emergencies
    b. Occurs when the blood glucose drops below 4 mmol/litre
    c. Is treated by giving carbamazepine
    d. Is treated by giving adrenaline

34. **Sweating, clammy skin can be caused by:**
    a. Hypoglycaemia
    b. Low oxygen level (syncope)
    c. Myocardial infarction
    d. All the above.

35. **Vomiting can be caused by:**
    a. Myocardial ischaemia
    b. Adrenal insufficiency
    c. Post-epileptic seizure
    d. All the above.

36. **Low potassium levels are seen in:**
    a. Hyperaldosteronism
    b. Hyperthyroidism
    c. Hypothyroidism
    d. Hyperparathyroidism

Identify the answers to Extended Matching Questions

37. **Medical emergency drugs:**
    a. A 55-year-old patient develops chest pain during administration of local anesthesia. If the his pain does not improve despite returning patient to semi-supine position, oxygen and glyceryl nitrate spray
    b. A patient, non-diabetic losses consciousness. He does not regain consciousness despite receiving oxygen therapy and lies in supine position
    c. Prior to administration of nitrous oxide and oxygen inhalation sedation, a 8-year-old girl becomes irritable and develops shortness of breath
    d. A 65-year-old diabetic patient about to have extraction under local anesthesia becomes confused and sweaty. Patient did not have breakfast alongside her insulin injection. Patient did not lose consciousness.
    e. Just after receiving 3 gm amoxicillin orally, a 20-year-old man complains of feeling unwell, develops red skin rash and difficulty in breathing.

    | 1. Adrenaline (epinephrine)-1:1000 (1mg/mL) | 6. Aspirin |
    | 2. Adrenaline (epinephrine)- 1:1000 (1mg/10 mL) | 7. Atropine |
    | 3. Glucagon | 8. Glyceryl nitrate spray |
    | 4. Glucose | 9. Fresh frozen plasma |
    | 5. Hydrocortisone | 10. Salbutamol |

38. **Cardiorespiratory arrest:**
    a. A 25-year-old male suffers cardiorespiratory arrest shortly after arriving in accident and emergency (A and E) department with serious facial trauma
    b. A layperson is anxious about possibility of infection while performing basic life support.

c. A collapsed patient makes infrequent noisy gasps
d. A child's suffers cardiorespiratory system arrest
e. An appearance of asystole on electrocardiography rhythm strip during cardiopulmonary resuscitation.

1. Chest compression only (CPR) at the rate of 100/minute	6. Automated external defibrillator
2. Chest compression and rescue breaths in ratio of 30:2	7. Manual defibrillator
3. Jaw thrust	8. 1 mg epinephrine (adrenaline) IV
4. Head tilt and chin lift	9. 3 mg atropine IV
5. Five initial breaths before starting chest compression	

39. **Lymphadenopathy:**
    a. A 18-year-old female patient with history of sore throat, fever, malaise and enlarged lymph nodes
    b. A 45-year-old smoker with 15 kg weight loss and finger clubbing
    c. A 35-year-old Asian man with fever, night sweats and single cervical lymph nodes
    d. A 60-year-old male with large spleen and marked raised white cell count
    e. A 30-year-old female patient with bilateral facial road rash and joint pain

1. Carcinoma lung	6. Rheumatoid arthritis
2. Chronic lymphocytic leukaemia	7. Sarcoidosis
3. Epstein-Barr virus (EBV) infection	8. Systemic lupus erythematosus
4. Human immunodeficiency virus (HIV) infection	9. Toxoplasmosis
5. Hodgkin's lymphoma	10. Tuberculosis

40. **Endocrine disorders:**
    a. A 40-year-old woman hypertensive, obese with striae and has difficulty getting up from check
    b. A patient with bipolar affective disorder, polyuria and low urine osmolality
    c. A large patient with hyperhidrosis, headaches and carpal tunnel syndrome. Her condition was diagnosed following oral glucose tolerance test
    d. A 27-year-old woman with galactorrhoea.
    e. A 55-year-old woman with history of weight gain, dry hair and constipation.

1. Acromegaly	7. Hypothyroidism
2. Conn disease	8. Type and diabetes
3. Cushing disease	9. Thyroid stimulating hormone
4. Diabetes insipidus	10. Prolactinoma
5. Growth hormone deficiency	
6. Hypogonadism	

CASE DISCUSSIONS

Case 1: Managing Medical Emergencies in Dental Practice

Adrenal Crisis (Hypoadrenalism)

- Signs and symptoms:
  - Patient collapse
  - Rapid weak pulse
  - Pallor
  - Cold and clammy skin
  - Vomiting and diarrhoea.
- Causes:
  - Usually the patient is known to have Addison's disease or history of taking long-term steroids and has forgotten to take the tablets.
- Treatment:
  - Check airway, breathing, circulation, disability, exposure (ABCDE)
  - Call 999
  - Make the patients lie in supine position
  - Administer oxygen 15 litres/min
  - IV fluids and further IV hydrocortisone
  - Glucose may be needed, if hypoglycaemic.

Anaphylaxis

- Signs and symptoms:
  - Urticaria or angioedema
  - Flushing and pallor
  - Respiratory distress
  - Stridor, wheeze or hoarseness
  - Hypotension and tachycardia
  - May develop over 15–30 minutes after oral administration of a drug or rapidly over few minutes following intravenous drug administration.
- Treatment:
  - ABCDE, Call 999
  - Administer oxygen 15 litres/min
  - Position the patient flat with elevate legs
  - Give 0.5 ml epinephrine (adrenaline) 1 mg/ml (1:1000 IM)
      (0.25 ml for 6-12 years of age, 0.12 ml for 6 month–6 years of age)
  - Repeat adrenaline at ~10 minutes interval, if no improvement.
- Principles of treatment:
  - Requires prompt treatment of
      Laryngeal oedema
      Bronchospasm
      Hypotension.

- Further management:
  - Transfer to accident and emergency (A and E)
  - Administer chlorpheniramine 10 mg in 1ml IM or slow IV
  - Hydrocortisone sodium succinate 200 mg by slow IV injection
  - Infuse fluids intravenous, if not responding quickly to adrenaline
  - Basic and advanced life support, if cardiorespiratory symptoms
  - Endotracheal intubation or tracheostomy, if required.

Asthma

- Signs and symptoms:
  - Persistent shortness of breath poorly relieved by bronchodilators
  - Restlessness and exhaustion
  - Tachycardia greater than 110 beats/min and low peak expiratory flow
  - Respiration may be so shallow in severe cases that wheezing is absent.
- Life-threatening:
  - Cyanosis, poor respiratory efforts
  - Decreased heart rate, altered level of consciousness or confusion, exhaustion.
- Serve (child):
  - Too breathless to talk or feed
  - Inability to complete sentences in one breath
  - Respiratory rate (RR) > 40 (2 – 5 years), Heart rate (HR) > 140 (2-5 years)
  - RR > 30 (> 5 years), HR > 125 (> 5 years).
- Treatment:
  - ABCDE
  - Sit patient upright, administer oxygen
  - 2 puffs (100 µg/puff) of short acting beta-agonist inhaler (salbutamol), repeat dose may be required
  - Additional doses through spacer device
  - One puff every 30 seconds up to 10 puffs for a child
  - Reassure and allow home, if recovered.
- Causes:
  - Exposure to antigen but precipitated by many factors including anxiety.
- Principles of treatment:
  - Oxygenation
  - Bronchodilation.
- Further management:
  - If little response, call 999
  - Transfer patient to accident and emergency
  - Hydrocortisone sodium succinate IV adult 200 mg, child 100 mg
  - Add ipratropium 0.5 mg to nebulised salbutamol
  - Aminophylline slow IV injection of 250 mg in 10 ml over at least 20 minutes, monitor pulse during injection.

- Caution in epilepsy:
  - Rapid injection of aminophylline may cause arrhythmias and convulsions.

Syncope
- Signs and symptoms:
  - Nausea and closing of visual fields
  - Feels faint/dizzy/light headed
  - Collapse or loss of consciousness
  - Sweating, pallor, slow pulse, decreased blood pressure.
- Treatment:
  - ABCDE, lay flat, elevate legs, give oxygen, check pulse at carotid
  - Expect prompt recovery, offer glucose in water/sweet tea.
- Causes:
  - Pain or anxiety.
- Principles of treatment:
  - Need to encourage oxygenated blood flow to brain
  - May need to block vagal activity with atropine and allow increase in heart rate.
- Further management:
  - If patient is slow to recover, review the treatment given if not adequate give 0.3–1 mg atropine IV.

Cardiac Emergencies: Angina and Myocardial Infarction
- Signs and symptoms:
  - Sudden onset of severe crushing pain across front of chest, which may radiate towards the shoulder and down left arm into the jaw and neck
  - Pain from angina usually radiates down left arm
  - Skin pale and clammy
  - Breathlessness
  - Nausea/vomiting
  - Weak pulse and hypotension
  - If pain not relieved by glyceryl trinitrate, then cause is myocardial infarction.
- Treatment:
  - ABCDE (Fig. 11.1)
  - Comfortable position (usually sitting up) in presence of breathlessness
  - Angina:
    - Is relieved by rest and nitrates
    - Glyceryl trinitrate 400 mg metered dose – 2 activations sub-lingual
    - Give oxygen
    - Allow home, if attack is mild and patient recovers rapidly.
- Myocardial infarction:
  - If suspected—Give oxygen
  - Aspirin tablet 300 mg chewed

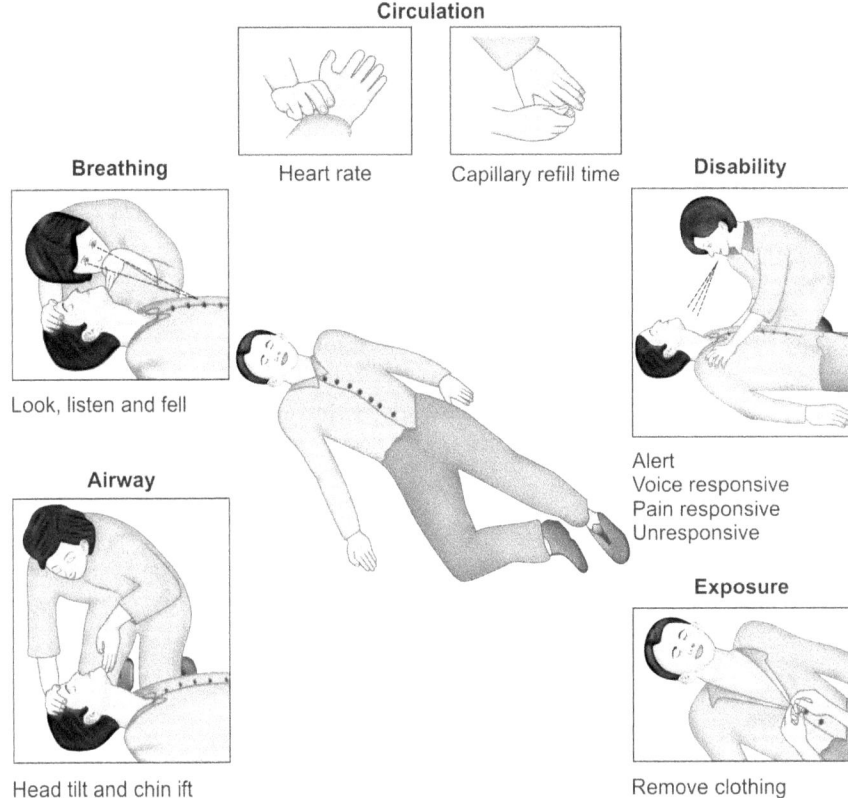

Figs 11.1: Treatment of Airway, breathing, circulation disability and exposure (ABCDE)

    Ensure automated external defibrillator is immediately accessible (should it be required).
- Causes:
  - Angina results from reduced coronary artery lumen diameter because of atheromatous plaques
  - Myocardial infarction is usually the result of thrombosis in a coronary artery.
- Principles of treatment:
  - Pain control and vasodilation of blood vessels to reduce load on heart.
- Further management:
  - Transfer to accidents and emergency
  - Treatment of myocardial infarction made on basis of two or three out of the history, ECG changes and enzymes changes suggestive of myocardial infarction
  - Diamorphine 5 mg (2.5 mg in older patient) by slow IV injection (1 mg/ml)
- Early thrombolytic therapy reduces mortality.

Epileptic Seizures
- Signs and symptoms:
  - Sudden collapse and loss of consciousness
  - Rigidity and cyanosis
  - Jerking movements of limbs
  - Noisy breathing
  - Tongue may be bitter
  - Frothing at mouth
  - Incontinence may occur
- Treatment:
  - ABCDE, safe environment: Prevent injury
  - Do not put anything in mouth
  - Do not attempt to restrain convulsive movements
  - Once jerking movements cease, recovery position and check the airway.
- Prolonged convulsive seizure (5 mins or more)/repeated seizure (> 3 in an hour).
  - Buccal midazolam—Oromucosal solution in single dose 10 mg
  - Paediatric dose of Buccal midazolam
    - 1–5 years: 5 mg
    - 5–10 years: 7 mg
    - – >10 years: 10 mg
- Causes:
  - Usually patient is known epileptic
  - Epilepsy may not be well-controlled
  - Seizure may be initiated by anxiety or by flickering light tube
- Principles of treatment:
  - Maintain oxygenated blood to brain
  - Protect from physical harm
  - Administer anticonvulsant.
- Further management:
  - Risk of brain damage increases with increased length of attack
  - If convulsive seizures continue for 15 minutes or longer or repeated rapidly (status epilepticus)
  - Transfer to accidents and emergency
  - Remove denture, insert Guedal or nasopharyngeal airway
  - Give oxygen
  - Give 10–20 mg IV diazepam (2.5 mg/30 s)
  - Check blood sugar to exclude hypoglycaemia as precipitant.

Diabetic Emergencies: Hypoglycaemia
- Signs and symptoms:
  - Shaking and trembling
  - Slurred speech
  - Vagueness
  - Sweating and pallor
  - Blurred vision

- - Tiredness and lethargy
    Confusion/aggression
    Stroppy/moody
  - Unconsciousness.
- Treatment:
  - ABCDE
  - Offer 15-20 g fast acting glucose, e.g. 3-4 glucose tablets, glass of orange juice or glucose gel
  - If patient is unconscious, inject 1 mg (1 unit) glucagon IM
  - Once consciousness return offer oral glucose
  - Call 999, if patient goes unconscious
  - Paediatric dose glucagon: <8 years of age or < 25 kg 0.5 mg IM.
- Causes:
  - Usually known diabetic
  - Patient may have taken medication as normal but not eaten before dental visit.
- Principle of treatment:
  - Return blood glucose level to normal by giving glucose or by converting patient's own glycogen to glucose by giving glucagon.
- Further management:
  - Transfer patient to accidents and emergency
  - Give up to 50 ml 20% glucose IV infusion followed by 0.9 % saline flush as glucose damages the vein
  - Expect prompt recovery and give sugary drink after gaining consciousness.

Stroke

- Signs and symptoms:
  - Confusion followed by signs and symptoms of focal brain damage
  - Facial weakness: Look for smile, Mouth or eye drooped—hemiplegia or quadriplegia
  - Arm weakness: Raise both arms?
  - Speech problem: Look for speak clearly and dysphagia
  - Locked in syndrome (aware but unable to respond)
  - Call 999.
- Treatment:
  - ABCDE
  - Call 999
  - Oxygen 15 litres/min
  - Nil by mouth.
- Causes:
  - Stroke results from either cerebral haemorrhage or cerebral ischaemia unrelated to dental treatment.
- Principle of treatment:
  - Maintain and transfer for further investigations.

Answers

1.	a. T	b. T	c. F	d. F	e. F
	f. T	g. T	h. F	i. F	j. T
	k. F	l. F	m. T	n. F	o. F
2.	a. F	b. T	c. T	d. F	e. F
	f. T	g. F	h. T	i. F	j. T
	k. F				
3.	a. T	b. F	c. F	d. F	e. F
	f.	g. F	h. F	i. T	j. F
4.	a. T	b. T	c. F	d. F	e. F
	f. T	g. T	h. T		
5.	a. T	b. T	c. F	d. F	e. T
	f. F				
6.	a. F	b. F	c. T	d. T	e. T
	f. T	g. T	h. T		
7.	a. T	b. T	c. F	d. T	e. F
8.	a. F	b. F	c. F	d. T	e. T
	f. T	g. F			
9.	a. T	b. F	c. T	d. F	e. T
	f. F	g. T	h. F	i. T	j. T
10.	a. T	b. T	c. T	d. T	e. F
	f. F				
11.	a. T	b. F	c. T	d. T	e. T
	f. T	g. T	h. T	i. T	
12.	a. T	b. F	c. T	d. T	e. T
	f. T	g. T	h. T	i. F	j. F
13.	a. F	b. T	c. F	d. T	e. T
	f. F	g. T	h. T	i. F	j. T
	k. T				

Human Disease and Medical Emergencies

14. a. T   b. F   c. T   d. T   e. T
    f. T   g. T   h. T
15. a. F   b. F   c. T   d. T   e. T
    f. F   g. T   h. F   i. T   j. F
    k. T
16. a. F   b. F   c. F   d. T   e. F
    f. T
17. a. T   b. T   c. T   d. T   e. F
    f. T   g. T   h. T   i. F   j. F
    k. T   l. F   m. T   n. T
18. a. T   b. T   c. T   d. T   e. T
    f. T   g. F   h. T   i. F
19. a. T   b. T   c. T   d. F   e. F
20. a. F   b. F   c. F   d. F   e. T
21. a. T   b. F   c. T   d. T   e. F
    f. T   g. T
22. a. T   b. F   c. F   d. F   e. T
    f. F   g. T   h. T
23. a. T   b. F   c. F   d. T   e. F
    f. T
24. a. F   b. F   c. T   d. F   e. T
    f. T   g. F   h. F   i. T
25. a. T   b. T   c. F   d. F   e. T
26. a. F   b. T   c. T   d. T   e. F
27. c   28. a   29. a   30. b   31. a
32. a   33. b   34. d   35. d   36. a
37. a. 6   b. 7   c. 10   d. 4   e. 1
38. a. 3   b. 1   c. 2   d. 5   e. 9
39. a. 3   b. 1   c. 10   d. 2   e. 8
40. a. 3   b. 4   c. 1   d. 10   e. 7

CORRECT ANSWERS FOR FALSE STATEMENTS

1. c. Would require elective surgery to be cancelled.
    a. Microcytic anaemia is caused due to Fe deficiency anaemia, chronic Blood loss (GI or menstrual), Diet
    b. Increasing TIBC in microcytic anaemia
    a. Decrease folate in Coeliac disease
    b. Macrocytic anaemia
    a. Folic acid 5 mg OD is used for treatment of Folate deficiency
    b. In homozygous patients have anaemia 6-10 g/dl—Red cell sickle when exposed, decreases oxygen tensions resulting in infarction of bone and brain. In heterozygous forms, cells are less fragile and sickle only in severe hypoxia.
    a. Iron-deficiency Anaemia is the most common type of anaemia.
    b. Decreased TIBC in Normocytic Anaemia
2. a. Lymphoblastic Leukaemia
    a. Chronic lymphocytic leukaemia is common
    b. Chronic myeloid leukaemia shows presence of philadelphia chromosome.
    g. Chronic leukaemia.
    i. Non-Hodgkin's lymphoma has poor diagnosis
    k. NSAIDs are not prescribed in anaemia and haematological malignancy
3. c. factor VIII deficiency
    g. Factor VIII
    j. Increased APTT in Haemophilia A
4. c. Left heart failure
    a. Right heart failure
    b. Only from ECG
5. f. Angina Patient are comfortable in upright or semi-reclined position than supine.
6. a. Rheumatoid arthriti.
7. e. Not compatible with life
10. e. B1 deficiency causes beri-beri
    f. Vitamin C deficiency causes scurvy
13. a. Laryngotracheitis is Upper respiratory tract infection
    c. Concious sedation in COAD patient compromise respiratory function and should be undertaken in hospital.
    f. Asthmatic patients are likely to be allergic to penicillins.
    i. Cystic fibrosis is inherited autosomal recessive disorder.

15. a. Peptic ulceration is likely to present haematemesis, epigastric pain, vomiting or Melaena.
    f. Crohn's disease has preference for Ileo-caecal area.
    h Cobblestoning to mucosa is seen in crohn's disease
    j. Gardner's syndrome.
16. a. Hepatic disease can cause problems with production of clotting factors, fibrinogen and drug metabolism.
    b. Also sedatives can be safely prescribed in Hepatic disease.
    c. Increased levels of aspartate transaminase on liver function test.
17. j. HBV
18. g. Day after dialysis.
19. g. Decreased ACTH
    i. Hypothyroidism
    j. Hyperthyroidism
20. a. Semi-reclined position because when in supine position pregnant uterus impedes venous return
    b. NSAIDS should be avoided in pregnancy
    f. Lidocaine with adrenaline
22. d. Results in acute Hypotension, bronchospasm and urticaria
    f. 0.5ml of 1:1000 Adrenaline IM
24. a. Brittle bone disease is associated with blue sclera and deafness
    d. Achondroplasia is Autosomal dominant disorder
    g. Fibrous dysplasia is associated with Albright syndrome.
    h Hands and feet are spared in Paget's disease of bone
25. c. In comminuted fracture there are multiple segments of Bone after high impact of trauma
    d. Pathological fracture occurs at the site of a disease process
26. a. Hodgkins is a type of Lymphoma
    e. Oral squamous cell carcinoma is treated with Surgery and radiotherapy

Chapter 12
Drugs and Therapeutics

Identify the following Statements as True (T) or False (F)
With regards to drugs used in general dental practice

1. **Aspirin:**
   a. Aspirin is not available directly to the public
   b. Aspirin is an anti-pyretic
   c. Aspirin can be used as an analgesic for children
   d. Aspirin may cause gastrointestinal ulceration
   e. Aspirin can be safely prescribed to asthmatic patients
   f. Aspirin prevents synthesis of prostaglandin E3
   g. Is a non-steroidal anti-inflammatory drug (NSAID)
   h. Aspirin does not interferes with warfarin
   i. Can be given in conjunction with selective inhibitor of cyclo-oxygenase-2 in patients with duodenal ulceration.

2. **Paracetamol:**
   a. Is a NSAID
   b. It acts as an analgesic but not as a anti-pyretic
   c. Can interfere with bleeding and coagulation time
   d. Hepatotoxic in large doses
   e. Dose is 500 mg–1000 mg QDS
   f. Is locally acting
   g. Can exacerbate asthma.

3. **Opioids analgesics:**
   a. Have anti-inflammatory properties
   b. Act locally to alter perception of pain
   c. They are recommended for mild-moderate pain of visceral origin
   d. Does not interfere with pupillary response
   e. Can be safely prescribed for head injury
   f. Can cause urinary retention
   g. Have risk of addiction
   h. Codeine cannot be used in combination with NSAID
   i. Morphine can be reversed by naloxone
   j. Buprenorphine can be given sublingually
   k. Papaveretum can be safely prescribed in women with child-bearing age
   l. Tramadol acts by two central methods.

4. **Steroids:**
   a. Are analgesic and causes pain relief
   b. Triamcinolone paste can be used in the management of lichen planus
   c. Topical steroids can cause adrenocortical suppression
   d. Benzydamine can be used in management of inflammatory mucosal conditions
   e. Betamethasone inhaler cannot be used on aphthae
   f. Triamcinolone acetonide cannot be injected into lesion
   g. Intralesional steroids can be used to treat granulomatous cheilitis
   h. Triamcinolone can be used intra-articularly
   i. Hydrocortisone can be used to induce arthroplasty in arthrosis of temporomandibular joint
   j. Long term steroid therapy does not cause hypertension and osteoporosis.

5. **Antidepressants:**
   a. Can be prescribed by general dental practitioner in dental practitioners formulary
   b. Can be used as co-analgesic
   c. Amitriptyline is monoamine oxidase inhibitors
   d. Amitriptyline can precipitate glaucoma
   e. Amitriptyline can be used safely in epilepsy
   f. Tricylics can cause xerostomia and difficulty with micturition
   g. Dothiepin cannot be used in patient with temporomandibular pain and dysfunction syndrome
   h. MAOIs are used for the management of atypical facial pain
   i. Selective serotonin reuptake inhibitor (SSRI) can cause hypertensive crisis induced by dietary and drug interaction
   j. Paroxetine and fluoxetine are monoamine oxidase inhibitors.

6. **Antiemetics:**
   a. Phenothiazine antiemetic is dopamine agonist
   b. Prochlorperazine can be safely prescribed in children
   c. Metoclopramide acts centrally only
   d. Metoclopramide reduces gut motility
   e. Domperidone can cause dystonia
   f. Domperidone can cross blood-brain barrier
   g. Cyclizine can aggravate heart failure
   h. Constipation does not cause nausea
   i. Common indication is to control postoperative nausea
   j. Ondansetron is selective 5-HT3 receptor agonist.

7. **Benzodiazepines:**
   a. Is commonly used anxiolytic drug
   b. Diazepam has short half-life
   c. Does not cause respiratory depression
   d. Can be used in management of temporomandibular pain and dysfunction syndrome

e. Midazolam is given intra-muscularly
f. Nitrazepam is short acting hypnotic
g. Temazepam can be used in rectal preparation
h. Lorazepam can be prescribed to epileptics
i. Chlormethiazole is used in the management of alcohol withdrawal
j. Zopiclone is benzodiazepine hypnotic
k. Chlormethiazole can control acute psychosis
l. Flumazenil is a benzodiazepine agonist
m. Carbamazepine is a benzodiazepine
n. Trimeprazine is used as a sedative to remove facial sutures
o. Chloral hydrate is useful as a sedative for children.

8. **Penicillins:**
   a. Penicillins are bacteriostatic
   b. Penicillins interferes with cell wall synthesis
   c. Penicillins has good tissue penetration including cerebrospinal fluid
   d. Are agonist to tetracycline
   e. Penicillins can cause hypersensitivity
   f. Penicillin is antibiotic of choice for anaerobic infection.

9. **Amoxicillin:**
   a. Is narrow-spectrum antibiotic
   b. Does not cause maculopapular rash
   c. Is a drug of choice in prophylaxis against infective endocarditis
   d. Does not interferes with action of oral contraceptive
   e. Can be prescribed during pregnancy.

10. **Tetracycline:**
    a. Is a broad spectrum antibiotics
    b. Unlikely to cause opportunistic infection
    c. Should be taken with milk due to better absorption
    d. Does not interferes with oral contraceptive
    e. May cause intrinsic staining of teeth
    f. May cause extrinsic staining of teeth
    g. May cause erythema multiforme
    h. Can be presented during pregnancy
    i. Can be used as a mouthwash in a dose of 25 mg dissolved in water
    j. Can be administered directly into periodontal pocket
    k. Is effective against protozoa.

11. **Erythromycin:**
    a. Is bactericidal
    b. Is a macrolide drug
    c. Active against penicillinase-producing organism
    d. Is active against chlamydia and mycoplasmas
    e. Not recommended during pregnancy
    f. Adult dose is 250–500 mg thrice daily for 5 days.

12. Clindamycin:
a. Risk of antibiotic induced colitis
b. Can be used as single dose prophylaxis for infective endocarditis
c. Cannot be used for cases of methicillin-resistant *Staphylococcus aureus*
d. Can be used in management of staphylococcal osteomyelitis
e. Has half-life of 6 hours
f. Is metabolised in liver.

13. Metronidazole:
a. Is bactericidal drugs
b. Effective against aerobic bacteria
c. Has half-life of four hours
d. Can cause disulfiram reaction when taken in conjunction with alcohol
e. Can be used during breast feeding/lactation
f. Should not be prescribed to chronic renal failure patient
g. Adult dosage is 200–400 mg four time daily.

14. Antifungals:
a. Acyclovir is an antifungal drug
b. Miconazole is a polyene anti-fungal drug
c. Nystatin is imidazole antifungal drug
d. Intraconazole is a triazole antifungal drug
e. Miconazole is used in the management of angular cheilitis
f. Fluconazole interacts with warfarin and potentiates its actions
g. Miconazole is used for oral thrush
h. Can be safely prescribed to liver disease patient
i. Are safe to be prescribed during pregnancy.

15. Antivirals:
a. Acyclovir is active against herpes simplex and zoster
b. Valacyclovir is active against Epstein–Barr virus
c. Famciclovir is active against cytomegalovirus
d. Zidovudine can prevent acquired immunodeficiency syndrome dementia complex
e. Zalcitabine and didanosine are nucleoside reverse transcriptase inhibitors
f. Interferon is an antiviral drug.

16. Decongestants:
a. Essential in management of oro-antral fistula
b. To be avoided in patient taking selective serotonin reuptake inhibitors
c. Prolonged use can lead to rebound vasodilation
d. Long-term use does not damage nasal cilia
e. Oxymetazoline is safe for long-term use
f. Systemic decongestants do cause rebound effect.

17. **Drugs relatively contraindicated in liver disease:**
    a. Aciclovir
    b. Terfenadine
    c. NSAIDs
    d. Sedatives
    e. Tetracycline
    f. Paracetamol
    g. Benzodiazepines
    h. Cefuroxime
    i. Carbamazepine
    j. Penicillin
    k. Co-trimoxazole
    l. Amphotericin
    m. Erythromycin.

18. **Drugs relatively contraindicated in renal failure:**
    a. Paracetamol
    b. Penicillin
    c. All opioids
    d. Amphotericin
    e. Tetracycline
    f. Antihistamine
    g. Acyclovir
    h. NSAIDs
    i. Benzodiazepine
    j. Metronidazole.

19. **Drugs contraindicated in pregnancy:**
    a. Antihistamine
    b. Co-trimoxazole
    c. NSAIDs
    d. Amphotericin
    e. Carbamazepine
    f. Benzodiazepine
    g. Tetracycline
    h. Aspirin
    i. Metronidazole
    j. Paracetamol.

20. **Drugs that cause xerostomia:**
    a. Antimalarial
    b. Antihistamine
    c. Atropine
    d. Antiemetics
    e. Tricyclic antidepressants
    f. Anti-Parkinson's agents.

21. **Drugs that cause lichenoid reactions:**
    a. Antimalarial
    b. Antiepileptic
    c. Antihypertensive drugs
    d. β-blockers
    e. Nifedipine
    f. Gold salts
    g. α-blockers
    h. Allopurinol
    i. Oral-hypoglycaemic drugs.

22. **Drugs causing gingival hyperplasia:**
    a. Phenytoin
    b. Rifampicin
    c. Diltiazem
    d. Carbamazepine
    e. Nifedipin
    f. Cyclosporin
    g. Verapamil.

23. **With regards to local anaesthesia:**
    a. Lidocaine 0.2% with 1:80000 epinephrine is commonly used local anaesthesia in dentistry
    b. Plain lidocaine provides more pronounced anaesthesia than local anaesthesia with epinephrine
    c. Prilocaine 3% with 0.03 IU/mL felypressin is commonly used dental local anaesthesia
    d. Lidocaine is long-lasting than bupivacaine

e. Prilocaine contains ester group
   f. A 1.8 mL cartridge of 2% lidocaine and 1:80,000 adrenaline contains
   g. 3.6 mg of lidocaine
   h. Amide local anesthesia is metabolised by liver
   i. Prilocaine has higher toxicity than lidocaine.

24. **With regards to action of local anaesthesia agents:**
   a. Local anaesthesia blocks hydrogen channel
   b. Local anaesthesia blocks calcium channels
   c. Local anaesthesia blocks potassium channels
   d. Local anaesthesia blocks sodium channels
   e. Local anaesthesia have membrane stabilising proteins
   f. Local anaesthesia prevents membrane depolarisation.

25. **Signs and symptoms of lidocaine overdose:**
   a. Tachycardia
   b. Hypertension
   c. Hyperventilation
   d. Convulsions
   e. Twitching
   f. Light headed.

26. **Antibiotic cover regime for adult patient with prosthetic heart valves requiring dental extraction:**
   a. Under general anaesthesia with 1 mg amoxicillin and 120 mg gentamiycin intravenously at induction with 500 mg amoxicillin orally 6 hours later
   b. Under general anaesthesia with 1g amoxicillin with 120 mg gentamicin IV at induction
   c. Under general anaesthesia vancomycin 1g by slow IV infusion and 120 mg gentamicin at induction
   d. Under local anaesthesia, 3 mg amoxicillin orally 1 hour before treatment
   e. Under local anaesthesia with 600 mg clindamycin orally, 1 hour before the procedure
   f. Under local anaesthesia, 600 mg clindamycin orally, 1 hour before the procedure and 600 mg clindamycin 6 hours later.

27. **Drugs commonly used in treatment of atypical facial pain:**
   a. Flumazenil   20 mg daily
   b. Amitriptyline   10–25 mg daily
   c. Protirelin   10–25 mg daily
   d. Nortriptyline   10–25 mg daily
   e. Fluoxetine   20 mg daily
   f. Dothiepin   25 mg daily.

Identify the Single Best Answer for the following

28. The mechanism of action of metronidazole is:
    a. Interferes with the synthesis of DNA
    b. Inhibits DNA gyrase
    c. Damages and interferes with DNA function
    d. Inhibits protein synthesis.

29. Inhalational anaesthetic agent with fastest onset of action is:
    a. Isoflurane
    b. Enflurane
    c. Nitrous dioxide
    d. Nitrous oxide.

30. The drug which can cause methaemoglobinaemia when used for larger doses for regional anaesthesia is:
    a. Bupivacaine
    b. Lidocaine
    c. Prilocaine
    d. Cocaine.

31. Patients with normal platelet counts and normal bleeding time may still bleed severely as a result of aspirin intake. The aspirin interferes with normal platelet function which may result in severe bleeding prior to a dental or surgical procedure, the aspirin function may last as long as:
    a. 4 hours
    b. 12 hours
    c. 2 days
    d. 7 days
    e. 5 days.

32. Aspirin is a non-opioid analgesic which is thought to work by inhibiting:
    a. Prostaglandin reductase and cyclooxygenase
    b. Cyclooxygenase
    c. Prostaglandin synthetase and cyclooxygenase
    d. Thromboxane synthetase.

33. Mediator that most likely to promote pain:
    a. Bradykinin
    b. Histamine
    c. Serotonin
    d. Prostaglandins
    e. Leukotrienes.

34. Mediator promoting greatest increase in vascular permeability, associated with acute inflammation:
    a. Serotonin
    b. Bradykinin

c. Prostaglandins
d. Leukotrienes.

35. A senior dental surgeon is concerned about the systemic effect of the tropically used drugs for plaque prevention, but the least preferred drug among the following options is:
   a. Vancomycin
   b. Polymyxin-B
   c. Kanamycin
   d. Clarithromycin.

36. The syndrome of acute salicylate overdose in children is characterized by:
   a. Marked hypothermia secondary to an antipyretic effect
   b. Vomiting
   c. Disturbance in acid-base and electrolyte balance
   d. Peripheral oedema.

37. The local anaesthetic agent which is primarily used for its good surface activity and low toxic potential is:
   a. Lidocaine
   b. Benzocaine
   c. Procaine
   d. Bupivacaine.

Identify the answers for Extended Matching Questions

38. Management of diabetes and hypoglycaemia:
   a. A 62-year-old man with poorly controlled diabetes despite maximum oral hypoglycaemic medicine.
   b. A 55-year-old patient with poorly controlled blood glucose, currently not taking any medication.
   c. A 45-year-old patient with hyperglycaemia and has chronic renal failure.
   d. A 67-year-old patient with type 2 diabetes to control pre-operative blood glucose levels
   e. A 37-year-old overweight, mild type 2 diabetes and mild hypertension, not taking any medication
   f. Drug that can be used in combination with metformin
   g. A 65-year-old male with type II diabetes and hypertension
   h. Case of severe hypoglycaemia, patient not able to take glucose orally.
   i. A 70-year-old patient with diabetic ketoacidosis
   j. A 60-year-old patients with increased blood glucose and increased HbA1C levels
   k. A 25-year-old male brought to accident and emergency department, unconscious, blood glucose 2 mmol/L.

1. Glucagon	9. Glibenclamide
2. Long acting insulin	10. Aspirin
3. Short acting insulin	11. Acarbose
4. Metformin	12. Heparin
5. Furosemide	13. Low calorie diabetic diet and exercise
6. Losartan	14. Gliclazide
7. Low dose aspirin	15. 50 mL of 50% glucose IV
8. Rosiglitazone	

39. **With regards to blood pressure and heart disease:**
    a. Antiplatelet therapy for atherosclerosis
    b. Immediate relief of angina
    c. Treatment of hypertension with angina
    d. Anticoagulation for unstable angina
    e. Thrombolysis medication in case of myocardial infarction
    f. Used in treatment of hypertension and asymptomatic left ventricular dysfunction
    g. Can be used in the absence of hypertension for its kidney protective effects
    h. Drug used for the treatment of fluid build-up due to heart failure
    i. Can be used along acetylsalicylic acid for prevention of thrombosis after placement of coronary stent
    j. Contraindicated in uncontrolled hypertension.

1. Furosemide	6. Low dose aspirin
2. Glyceryl trinitrate (GTN)	7. Low molecular weight heparin
3. Atenolol	8. Subcutaneous heparin
4. Enalapril	9. Streptokinase
5. Atropine	10. Clopidogrel

40. **Antibiotics**
    a. Used for the treatment of bacterial infections like pneumonia, *H. pylori*
    b. Used in prevention of bacterial endocarditis during dental treatment
    c. Contraindicated in patients with hypersensitivity to cephalosporins
    d. Second generation cephalosporins
    e. A macrolide antibiotic
    f. Initial drug treatment for community acquired lobar pneumonia
    g. Prophylaxis for recurrent urinary tract infection
    h. Initial treatment of meningitis in a teenager
    i. Used in treatment of mycobacterium infection
    j. Can cause intrinsic staining of teeth, if used in children below 12 years of age
    k. Treatment of osteomyelitis caused by *Staphylococcus aureus*.

1. Amoxicillin	7. Oral gentamicin
2. Clarithromycin	8. Rifampicin
3. Cefotaxime	9. Tetracycline
4. Erythromycin and amoxicillin	10. Oral nitrofurantoin
5. Erythromycin	11. Flucloxacillin
6. Cefuroxime	

CASE DISCUSSION

Case 1: Management of anaphylaxis.

Definition
- Anaphylaxis is life-threatening, systemic or generalised hypersensitivity reaction
- This is characterised by rapidly developing life-threatening airway, breathing and circulation problems usually associated with skin and mucosal changes.

Causes
Foods
- Protein in the food
- Allergic foods as peanuts, fish, shellfish, eggs and cow's milk
  - These reactions usually occur after swallowing. In few cases, reactions begin several hours after eating
  - Such allergies have been found to be associated with allergic conditions such as asthma, eczema and hay fever
- Insect stings reactions occur immediately in half hour, in particular stings of bees and wasps
- Natural rubber latex
  - Some common sources of latex:
    Contraceptives: Condoms, diaphragms
    Balloons and rubber bands
    Carpet backing and furniture filling
    Rubber gloves
    Medical/dental items such as catheters, gloves, disposable items.

Medicines
Anaphylactic reactions usually occur after the first dose of a course.

Idiopathic
Occasionally, especially in adults, the cause cannot be identified.

Symptoms and Signs
- Mild/moderate symptoms:
  - Burning, itching and tingling sensation in the mouth
  - Nasty taste in the mouth
  - Itching of skin, eyes and throat
  - Rapid development of nettle rash/wheals/hives (urticaria)
  - Swelling, particularly of the face and lips
  - Feeling hot or chilled
  - Rising anxiety
  - Flushed
  - Tummy, abdominal or stomach pain

- ➤ Nausea and/or vomiting
- ➤ Mild wheeziness.
- Severe symptoms:
  - ➤ Severe swelling of the tongue or throat associated with difficulty in breathing
  - ➤ Difficulty talking or hoarse voice
  - ➤ Severe wheeze or difficulty in breathing
  - ➤ Faintness or dizziness
  - ➤ Pale, blue colour and clammy skin
  - ➤ Unresponsive or any type of disorientation
  - ➤ Collapse.

Diagnosis

When patient is exposed to a trigger (allergen) he/she develops a sudden illness. It causes rapidly progressing skin changes, life-threatening airway, breathing circulation problems. Anaphylaxis is likely when all of the following 3 criteria are met:
- Skin or mucosal changes alone are not a sign of an anaphylactic reaction
- Skin and mucosal changes can be subtle or absent in up to 20% of reactions (Some patients can have only a decrease in blood pressure, i.e. a circulation problem)
- Patients can have either an A or B or C problem or any combination. Use the airway breathing circulation disability exposure (ABCDE) approach to recognise these. There can also be gastrointestinal symptoms (e.g. vomiting, abdominal pain, incontinence.

Airway problems

- Airway swelling, e.g. throat and tongue swelling (pharyngeal/laryngeal oedema). The patient has difficulty in breathing and swallowing and feels that the throat is closing up
- Hoarse voice
- Stridor: This is a high-pitched inspiratory noise caused by upper airway obstruction.

Breathing problems

- Shortness of breath: Increased respiratory rate
- Wheeze
- Patient becoming tired
- Confusion caused by hypoxia
- Cyanosis (appears blue): This is usually a late sign
- Respiratory arrest.

There is a range of presentation from anaphylaxis, through anaphylaxis with predominantly asthmatic features to a pure acute asthma attack with no other features of anaphylaxis. Life-threatening asthma with no features of anaphylaxis can be triggered by food allergy.

Circulation Problems
- Signs of shock: Pale, clammy
- Increased pulse rate (tachycardia)
- Low blood pressure (hypotension): Feeling faint (dizziness), collapse
- Decreased conscious level or loss of consciousness
- Anaphylaxis can cause myocardial ischaemia and electrocardiogram (ECG) changes even in individuals with normal coronary arteries
- Cardiac arrest.

Skin and/or mucosal changes
Cardiorespiratory arrest following an anaphylactic reaction.

Investigations
- Undertake the usual investigations appropriate for a medical emergency, e.g. 12-lead ECG, chest X-ray, urea and electrolytes, arterial blood gases, etc.
- Mast cell tryptase.

Drugs for Treatment
- Adrenaline (Epinephrine):
  - IM adrenaline dose in adults: 0.5 mg IM (500 micrograms = 0.5 mL of 1:1000) adrenaline.
- IM adrenaline dose in children:
  - \> 12 years:
    500 micrograms intramuscular (0.5 mL) i.e. same as adult dose
    300 micrograms (0.3 mL), if child is small or prepubertal.
  - \> 6 – 12 years:
    300 micrograms intramuscular (0.3 mL)
  - 6 months – 6 years:
    150 micrograms intramuscular (0.15 mL)
  - < 6 months:
    150 micrograms intramuscular (0.15 mL).
- Intravenous adrenaline (for specialist use only)
  - Ensure patient is monitored
  - Adrenaline intravenous bolus dose-adult:
    Do not give the undiluted 1:1000 adrenaline concentration intravenous.
  - Adrenaline intravenous bolus dose-children: 0.1-1mg/kg/min.
- IM adrenaline is the preferred route for children having an anaphylactic reaction.
- IV route is recommended only in specialist paediatric settings by those familiar with its use (e.g. paediatric anaesthetists, paediatric emergency physicians, paediatric intensivists and, if the patient is monitored and intravenous access is already available.
- A child may respond to a dose as small as 1 microgram/kg.

- Antihistamines (after initial resuscitation):
  - The dose of chlorpheniramine depends on age:
    - 12 years and adults: 10 mg intramuscular or intravenous slowly
    - 6 – 12 years: 5 mg intramuscular or intravenous slowly
- Steroids:
  - It is given after initial resuscitation
  - In asthma, early corticosteroid treatment is beneficial in adults and children
  - The dose of hydrocortisone for adults and children depends on age:
    - >12 years and adults: 200 mg intramuscular or intravenous slowly
    - > 6 – 12 years: 100 mg intramuscular or intravenous slowly
    - > 6 months – 6 years: 50 mg intramuscular or intravenous slowly
    - < 6 months: 25 mg intramuscular or intravenous slowly
- Other drugs:
  - Bronchodilators
  - Cardiac drugs.

Answers

1. a. F b. T c. F d. T e. F
   f. F g. T h. F i.
2. a. F b. F c. F d. T e. T
   f. F g. F
3. a. F b. F c. F d. F e. F
   f. T g. T h. F i. T j. T
   k. F l. T
4. a. F b. T c. F d. T e. F
   f. F g. F h. T i. T j. F
5. a. F b. T c. F d. T e. F
   f. T g. F h. T i. F j. F
6. a. F b. F c. F d. F e. T
   f. F g. T h. F i. T j. F
7. a. T b. F c. F d. T e. F
   f. F g. F h. T i. T j. F
   k. F l. F m. F n. F o. F
8. a. F b. T c. F d. F e. T
9. a. F b. T c. T d. F e. T
10. a. T b. F c. T d. F e. T
    f. F g. T h. F i. F j. T
    k. F
11. a. F b. T c. T d. T e. F
    f. F
12. a. T b. T c. F d. T e. F
    f. T

13.	a.	T	b.	F	c.	F	d.	T	e.	F
	f.	F	g.	F						
14.	a.	F	b.	F	c.		d.	T	e.	T
	f.	T	g.	T	h.	F	i.	F		
15.	a.	T	b.	F	c.	F	d.	T	e.	T
	f.	T								
16.	a.	F	b.	F	c.	F	d.	F	e.	T
15.	a.	F	b.	F	c.	T	d.	F	e.	F
16.	a.	F	b.	F	c.	T	d.	F	e.	F
	f.	F								
17.	a.	F	b.	T	c.	T	d.	T	e.	T
	f.	T	g.	T	h.	T	i.	F	j.	F
	k.	F	l.	F	m.	T				
18.	a.	F	b.	T	c.	T	d.	T	e.	T
	f.	F	g.	T	h.	T	i.	T	j.	F
19.	a.	F	b.	T	c.	T	d.	F	e.	T
	f.	T	g.	T	h.	T	i.	T	j.	F
20.	a.	F	b.	T	c.	T	d.	T	e.	T
	f.	T								
21.	a.	T	b.	F	c.	T	d.	F	e.	F
	f.	T	g.	T	h.	T	i.	T		
22.	a.	T	b.	F	c.	T	d.	F	e.	T
	f.	T	g.	T						
23.	a.	F	b.	F	c.	T	d.	F	e.	F
	f.	F	g.	T	h.	F				
24.	a.	F	b.	F	c.	T	d.	T	e.	T
	f.	T								
25.	a.	F	b.		c.	F	d.	T	e.	T
	f.	T								

26.	a.	F	b.	F	c.	T	d.	F	e.	T
	f.	F								
27.	a.	F	b.	T	c.	T	d.	T	e.	T
	f.	T								
28.	c	29.	d	30.	c	31.	d	32.	c	
33.	a	34.	d	35.	d	36.	c	37.	b	
38.	a.	2	b.	4	c.	9	d.	3	e.	13
	f.	8	g.	6	h.	1	i.	12	j.	14
	k.	18								
39.	a.	6	b.	2	c.	3	d.	8	e.	9
	f.	4	g.	4	h.	1	i.	10	j.	7
40.	a.	2	b.	1	c.	3	d.	6	e.	5
	f.	4	g.	20	h.	3	i.	8	j.	9
	k.	11								

CORRECT ANSWERS FOR FALSE STATEMENTS

2. a. Aspirin is directly available from pharmacies.
   c. Aspirin not be used in children as it causes Reye syndrome
   f. Prostaglandin E2.
   h. Aspirin interfere with Warfarin does
3. b. Paracetamol is both analgesic and anti-pyretic
   f. Paracetamol is centrally acting
4. b. Opiods analgesics acts centrally
   a. Used for severe pain
   b. Interferes with pupillary response
   c. Depresses respiratory function and interfere with pupil response
   h. Can be used at dosage of 8/15/30 mg
   k. Contraindicated due to presence of noscapine
5. a. Not analgesics but directly/indirectly aid in pain relief
   c. Topical steroids does not cause adrenocortical suppression as they are low potency steroid
   e. Can be used to spray apthae, spray = 100 μg.
6. c. amitriptyline is tricyclic
   e. Amitriptyline should be avoided in epileptic, diabetic and pregnant patient.
   a. MAOIs cause hypertensive crisis induced by dietary and drug interactions
   b. Paroxetine and Fluoxetine are SSRIs
7. a. Antagonist
   a. Prochlorperazine Can produce extrapyramidal symptoms
   b. Metoclopramide has both central and peripheral mode of action
   c. Metoclopramide increases gut motility
   j. Antagonist
8. b. Diazepam has long half life.
   a. Midazolam is administered IntraVenously.
   b. Nitrazepam long acting hypnotic.
   c. Diazepam can be used as rectal preparation. Temazepam is short acting hypnotic used as premedication
   a. Haloperidol controls acute psychosis
   b. Antagonist
   a. Chloral hydrate is used for removal of facial sutures
   b. Trimeprazine is useful sedative for children and also acts as anti-histamine
9. a. Penicillins are Bactericidal

a. Penicillins does not penetrate CSF
b. D: metronidazole is antibiotic of choice for anaerobic infections
c. Penicillins are antagonist to tetracycline

10. a. Amoxicillins are broad-spectrum antibiotics
    d. Amoxicillins interfere with action of oral contraceptives

11. b. Tetracyclines can cause opportunistic infections with Candida albicans
    c. tetracyclines absorption is inhibited by chelation with milk
    i. Can be used as mouthwash 250 mg dissolved in water to decrease secondary infection when patient has oral ulceration.
    k. Tetracyclines are effective against Spirochaetes

11. a. Erythromycins are Bacteriostatic
    f. Erythromycin adult Dosage 250-500mg QDS for 5 days

12. e. Clindamycin has half-life of 2-3 hours

13. c. Metronidazole has half-life of 8 hours
    g. Metronidazole adult dosage is 200-400mg TDS

14. a. Acyclovir is antiviral.
    b. Imidazole is an polyene anti-fungal drug

15. c. Ganciclovir is active against Epstein Barr Virus (EBV) and CytomegaloVirus (CMV)

16. b. Decongestants should be avoided in patient taking MAOIs.
    e. Oxymetazoline is safe for short-term use
    f. Systemic decongestants does not cause rebound effect.
    g Dose: Ephedrine nasal drops 1% 1-2 drops into nostrils 7-10 days QDS

23. a. Lidocaine 2% with 1:80000 with epinephrine
    e. Prilocaine contains amide group
    f. 1.8ml of 2% Lidocaine with 1:80000 adrenaline contains 36 mg of Lidocaine

27. a. Antibiotic Cover regime: Under GA with 1g amoxicillin and 120mg Gentamycin IV at induction with 500mg amoxicillin orally 6 hours later
    d. Under LA, 3g Amoxicillin orally 1 hour before treatment

Chapter 13

Dental Materials

Identify the following Statements as True (T) or False (F)

1. **Amalgams:**
   a. Lathe cut amalgams can be carved immediately
   b. Spheroidal amalgams are preferred for pinned restorations
   c. Are weakest in gamma 1 phase
   d. Increase proportion of copper in amalgam are least expensive
   e. High copper amalgams have less corrosion resistance, creep strength and durability
   f. A blended composition of alloy of silver tin AgSn and silver copper AgCu is the most resistant to tarnishing.

2. **Handling characteristics of amalgam:**
   a. The duration of trituration should be under 5 seconds
   b. Preparation cannot be overfilled
   c. Lathe cut amalgam can be carved immediately
   d. Preparations can be burnished
   e. Maximum strength can take up to 12 hours to develop
   f. Microleakage can be reduced by an anaerobic resin adhesive that bonds to set amalgam
   g. Waste amalgam should be stored in closed container under old radiograph fixing solution.

3. **Composites:**
   a. Most composite resins are based on urethane dimethacrylate
   b. Composites have high compressive strength, abrasion resistance but reduced modulus of elasticity
   c. Have reduced thermal expansion and setting contraction
   d. The interface between resin and filter is silane coupling agent
   e. Microfilled resins are suitable for load bearing situations and has good wear resistance
   f. Hybrid composites contains 30–60% filler by weight
   g. Sulfinic acid is used as an initiator to commence polymerisation
   h. Polymerisation shrinkage causes contraction forces of 4–7 MPa
   i. Mini-filled resin uses combination of 1–10 μm and 40 nm particle
   j. Modulus of hybrid resin composite is greater than amalgam
   k. Light emitting diode is preferred option for light activation
   l. Dual cure composites continue to cure chemically for polymerisation throughout the restoration even after removal of light

m. Composite resins can be used as fissure sealants
n. Flowable resin composites are preferred due to decreased contraction shrinkage
o. Lighter shades of composites resin cures better than darker shades
p. Beta-quartz inserts are used in composite resins to reduce polymerisation shrinkage
q. The resin component can absorb water and can cause hydrolytic breaking down of bonding agent.

4. **Acid–Etch:**
   a. Prophylaxis prior to etching is required
   b. Acid etching is required to allow resin composite retention in the cavity
   c. Bonding to enamel mainly occurs chemically
   d. 30–50% buffered phosphoric acid is used
   e. 'Macro-tags' contributes to the bond strength
   f. Etching time of 30 seconds is recommended for dentine
   g. Probe should be used to aid etchant penetration of pits and fissures
   h. The bond strength is greater, if an etchant solution is used instead of gel
   i. Composite resin tags can penetrate upto 50 µm in to enamel after acid etching
   j. Moisture control is important for the success
   k. Remineralisation of etched enamel can occur within 30 seconds, if in contact with saliva.

5. **Dentine bonding:**
   a. Oxalic acid cannot be used as dentine conditioner
   b. Bonding resins are mostly hydrophilic monomers
   c. Triethylene glycol dimethacrylate and hydroxyethyl methacrylate are examples of hydrophobic monomer
   d. Smear layer reduces sensitivity by occluding dentinal tubules
   e. Air-thinning of the material is preferred to prevent the air-inhibited layer permeating the resin
   f. Pre-curing adhesive bonding agent before placing composite increases bond strength
   g. If dentine bonding is done properly, the technique produces 'zero' microleakage
   h. Cannot be used for retention and seal of indirect porcelain and composite inlays.

6. **Glass ionomer cement:**
   a. Has increased solubility due to incorporation of phosphoric acid
   b. The glass has high level of fluoride, aluminium, calcium, sodium and silica
   c. Adhesion to enamel and dentine is only due to absorption of polyalkenoic acid onto collagen

d. Glass ionomer cement has reservoir effect for fluoride
e. Has similar coefficient of thermal expansion as of enamel and dentine
f. Tensile strength is 60% of resin composite
g. Is biocompatible
h. Can be used as luting cement for crown and bridges
i. Cannot be used as lining material in load bearing situation
j. Self-cure GIC has higher bond strength than light-cured glass ionomer cement
k. Can be used as a restorative cement
l. Glass ionomer cement has increased wear resistance compared to cermets
m. Glass ionomer cement and cermets have equivalent strength
n. Water balance during setting of glass ionomer cement is not critical.

7. **Resin-modified glass ionomer cements:**
   a. Can be polished immediately after setting
   b. Cannot be used in preparation below cemento-enamel junction
   c. Compomers have increased fracture toughness and wear resistance
   d. The resin in resin-modified glass-ionomer cements is tetraethylene glycol dimethacrylate
   e. The initial set of RMGIC is due to acid-base reaction
   f. Compomers can be used for restoration of deciduous teeth.

8. **Cements:**
   a. Zinc oxide is stronger than fluoro-aluminosilicate glass
   b. Zinc oxide eugenol has setting time of 6 hours
   c. ZOE can be used as a temporary dressing
   d. Addition of zinc acetate can accelerate setting time
   e. The strength can be increased with addition of hydrogenated resin to the powder
   f. Working time of zinc phosphate can increase, if mixed all at once
   g. Zinc polycarboxylate has liquid in 50% form of aqueous polyacrylic acid
   h. Calcium hydroxide is bacteriocidal
   i. Calcium hydroxide can induce mineralisation of adjacent pulp
   j. Heat increases setting time
   k. Can be used in stepwise excavation technique
   l. Resin bonded zinc oxide eugenol has increased strength than polycarboxylate cements
   m. Ortho-ethoxybenzoic acid cement can be used as a luting cement
   n. Can be used for pulp capping
   o. Can be used as a direct lining material with resin composite.

9. **Impression material:**
   a. Optosil is an additional cured silicone
   b. Additional cured silicone impressions should be casted immediately
   c. Condensation cured silicone are dimensionally stable

d. Polysulphides can be difficult to remove in cases with deep undercuts
e. Polyethers should not be stored with alginate impressions
f. Irreversible hydrocolloid can be used for crown and bridgework
g. Impression compound is useful in denture cases with severe resorption
h. Zinc oxide paste can be used in patient's existing denture or special tray to record edentulous ridges
i. Impression should be rinsed and immersed in a solution of sodium hypochlorite (1,000 ppm for 10 minutes)
j. Double mix technique uses combination of polyether and addition cured silicone
k. Special trays should be used for crown and bridgework impression.

10. **Casting alloys:**
    a. In dental casting gold alloys, 65% must have noble metal content
    b. Indium prevents oxidation of other metals during melting or casting
    c. Silver palladium alloys are less prone to porosity in comparison to gold alloys
    d. Nickle chromium has increased rigidity as compared to gold alloys
    e. Nickle chromium castings are more accurate than gold alloys
    f. Alloys for porcelain bonding should have lower melting than porcelain
    g. Cobalt-chromium alloys require phosphate bonded investment.

11. **Wrought alloys:**
    a. The stainless steel used in dentistry is austenitic steel
    b. Cobalt-chromium can be used for post fabrication in post and core crowns
    c. Pure titanium is used in implant systems
    d. Nitinol is easy to bend
    e. Titanium molybdenum alloy can be used for archwires.

12. **Ceramics:**
    a. Ceramics are compounds of non-metallic oxides only
    b. Quartz in dental porcelain is added for strength and colour
    c. Kaolin in dental porcelain is for strength and translucency
    d. Dental porcelain is reinforced with glass particles
    e. Firing shrinkage is 50%
    f. Empress crowns are built upon computer generated sintered core
    g. Are chemically inert.

13. **With regards to ceramic crowns:**
    a. Porcelain jacket crown requires porcelain thickness of 0.8 mm and 90° butt joint at margins
    b. Porcelain bonded crown have increased crack propagation
    c. Castable ceramics use lost wax technique to decrease firing shrinkage
    d. Glass ceramics crowns are least expensive
    e. 0.8 mm porcelain veneer has ability to hide tooth discolouration
    f. Porcelain crowns and veneer can be repaired.

14. **Denture Materials—Acrylic Resins:**
    a. The initiator in acrylic resin is hydroquinone
    b. The powder and liquid ratio should be mixed in 1:1 by weight
    c. The stringy stage is best for handling and packing
    d. Sodium alginate is used as a separator during denture fabrication
    e. Self-cure acrylics are resistant to abrasion
    f. The glass transition temperature for self-cure acrylic is 105°C
    g. They have low specific gravity
    h. Residual monomer can cause sensitivity reaction
    i. Strength of denture resins can be increased by using high performance fibres.

15. **Rebasing:**
    a. Self-cure polymethyl methacrylate is preferred for hard rebases
    b. Soft liners are based on silicon polymers
    c. Plasticised acrylic are more elastic
    d. Silicone polymer absorbs water
    e. Tissues conditioner comprises of powdered self-cure polymethyl methacrylate
    f. For tissue recovery lining should not be more than 1 mm.

Identify the Single Best Answer for the following

16. **Out of the following options, the elastic impression material is:**
    a. Zinc oxide-eugenol cement
    b. Polyether rubber base
    c. Low fusing compound
    d. Impression compound.

17. **Setting expansion of casting investment is:**
    a. 1.1–1.7%
    b. 0.8–1%
    c. 1.7–2%
    d. 0.1–0.5%.

18. **The dental amalgam alloys and mercury are mixed in the ratio of:**
    a. 1:1
    b. 2:1
    c. 1:3
    d. 1:4.

19. **Most common disadvantage of amalgam restoration is:**
    a. Porosity
    b. Marginal breakdown
    c. Contraction on setting
    d. Secondary expansion.

20. The maximum level of occupational exposure regarded safe to mercury vapours:
    a. 5 µg of mercury
    b. 35 µg of mercury
    c. 50 µg of mercury
    d. 1 µg of mercury.

21. The main resin constituent of composite resin is:
    a. Polycarbonate
    b. Urethane
    c. Dimethacrylate
    d. Polymethylmethacrylate.

22. The role of fillers in composite resin is:
    a. Increase coefficient of thermal expansion
    b. Increase working time
    c. Decrease working time
    d. Decrease setting time.

23. The firing temperature of high fusing porcelain is:
    a. 2350–2500°F
    b. 2500–3400°F
    c. 1000–1500°F
    d. 2000–4500°F.

24. The most dental resins are polymerised by:
    a. Chemical activation
    b. Light activation
    c. Heat activation
    d. None of the above.

25. Thickness of varnish should be:
    a. 0.01 mm
    b. 1.0 mm
    c. 0.1 mm
    d. 0.25 mm.

26. Stress is:
    a. An applied load or force
    b. An internal force opposing an applied load
    c. A deformation resulting from an applied load
    d. An external force opposing an applied load.

27. Proportional limit is:
    a. The minimum force required to cause a structure to break
    b. The maximum stress that can be induced without permanent deformation
    c. The maximum stress in a structure
    d. The maximum elongation under tension that can be measured before failure.

28. Modulus of elasticity of a dental material is:
    a. The strain at the proportional limit
    b. The stress at the proportional limit
    c. The stress/strain ratio within the proportional limit
    d. None of the above.

29. Hardness number which is not dependent on ductility of metal:
    a. VHN
    b. RHN
    c. KHN
    d. BHN.

30. The following has the highest modulus of elasticity:
    a. Enamel
    b. Amalgam
    c. Dentin
    d. Composite resin.

31. Which among the following hardness test is a micro hardness test?
    a. Shore-A
    b. Brinnel
    c. Knoop
    d. Rockwell.

32. The following refers to space lattice:
    a. Inter atomic imbalance
    b. Arrangement of atoms
    c. Inter atomic movement
    d. Arrangement of nucleus.

33. Name the time dependent properties of dental materials:
    a. Resilience
    b. Creep
    c. Elastic limit
    d. Ultimate strength.

34. The knoop hardness number for microfilled composite restorative material is
    a. 50–60 KHN
    b. 15–20 KHN
    c. 40–48 KHN
    d. 25–35 KHN.

35. The following conducts electricity
    a. Acrylic
    b. Porcelain
    c. Graphite
    d. Carbon.

36. The property among the following is present for adhesion between solid and liquid:
    a. Mechanical interlocking should be present
    b. Liquid should wet solid surface
    c. Should have high contact angle
    d. None of the above.

37. The flow of a material is:
    a. Continuous change of the material under a given load
    b. The homogenous of gypsum products
    c. Dimensional change of the material during setting
    d. The consistency of a material when mixing.

38. What type of conversion is sublimation?
    a. Solid to liquid and then to gas
    b. Solid directly to gas
    c. Gas to liquid and then to solid
    d. Gas directly to liquid.

39. The contact angle when solid gets wet completely:
    a. 0–90°
    b. 90°
    c. 0°
    d. >90°

40. What is ultimate tensile strength?
    a. Longitudinal compressive strength
    b. Stress before rupture
    c. Stress after rupture
    d. Horizontal compressive strength.

41. Which material among the following has KHN close to?
    a. Pure gold
    b. Amalgam
    c. Composite
    d. Porcelain.

42. The type of behaviour determined by Maxwell-voigt model is:
    a. Viscoelastic behaviour
    b. Elastic behaviour
    c. Plastic behaviour
    d. All the above.

43. The melting point of silver is:
    a. 960° Centigrade
    b. 1063° Centigrade
    c. 850° Centigrade
    d. 1123° Centigrade.

44. **The material for which Brazilian test is used to determine the ultimate tensile strength:**
    a. Ductile materials
    b. Brittle materials
    c. Flexible materials
    d. Malleable materials.

45. **Simplest alloy among the following:**
    a. Brittle materials
    b. Solid solution
    c. Eutectic alloy
    d. Malleable materials.

46. **KHN value of amalgam:**
    a. 67
    b. 450
    c. 90
    d. 343.

47. **4th state of matter:**
    a. Solid
    b. Colloid
    c. Liquid
    d. Gas.

48. **The hydrocolloid gel refers to:**
    a. Temperature lag between gelation and liquefaction temperature
    b. Moisture absorption
    c. Phenomenon of conversion of gel into sol
    d. All the above.

49. **The function of palladium when added to polyvinyl siloxane:**
    a. Helps as a surfactant
    b. Act as a scavenger
    c. Act as a plasticizer
    d. Acts as a catalyst.

50. **What is syneresis?**
    a. Shrinkage
    b. Gelation
    c. Seen as water loss in a hydrocolloid gel
    d. Water absorption.

51. **Syringe material has:**
    a. Medium viscosity elastomer
    b. High viscosity elastomer
    c. Medium viscosity elastomer
    d. Low viscosity elastomer.

Dental Materials

52. **Vulcanization is:**
    a. Zinc phosphate cement
    b. Reversible hydrocolloid
    c. Setting of Mercaptan impression material
    d. Zinc oxide-eugenol.

53. **The following materials undergoes hysteresis:**
    a. Irreversible hydrocolloid
    b. Impression plaster
    c. Reversible hydrocolloid
    d. Metallic oxide paste.

54. **The material used for preparing agar is:**
    a. Bullock meat
    b. Seaweed
    c. Chick cells
    d. Chemicals.

55. **Which among the following?**
    a. Alginate
    b. Impression compound
    c. Agar
    d. Polyethers.

56. **The following is an elastic impression material**
    a. Impression compound
    b. Wax
    c. Polyvinyl siloxane
    d. Zinc oxide eugenol (ZOE) paste.

57. **The function of trisodium phosphate in alginate**
    a. Reactor
    b. Retarder
    c. Accelerator
    d. Plasticizer.

58. **Name the best material for RPD impression:**
    a. Irreversible hydrocolloid
    b. Impression plaster
    c. Reversible hydrocolloid
    d. None of the above.

59. **This acts as a retarder in zinc oxide eugenol**
    a. $CaCl_2$
    b. Zinc acetate
    c. Glycerine
    d. Alcohol.

60. This acts as a accelerator in zinc oxide eugenol paste:
    a. Linseed oil
    b. Zinc acetate
    c. Olive oil
    d. All of these.

61. Which of the following statement is correct?
    a. Agar solidifies between 50–70°C
    b. Agar liquefies between 71–100°C
    c. Agar facilitates fabrication of metal dyes
    d. Agar cannot register fine surface details.

62. This dental material is most mucostatic
    a. ZOE paste
    b. Impression compound
    c. Alginate
    d. Elastomer.

63. What is a die?
    a. Impression of single tooth
    b. Replica of single tooth
    c. Impression of whole teeth
    d. Replica of whole teeth.

64. The function of gypsum is:
    a. Impressions
    b. Casts and dies
    c. Casts
    d. Die.

65. Plaster of Paris:
    a. Is wet calcined hemihydrate
    b. Is α- hemihydrate
    c. Is porous with irregular crystals
    d. Has a water powder ratio of 0.2.

66. ADA specification number for gypsum products is:
    a. 1
    b. 25
    c. 4
    d. 12.

67. This is a gypsum product:
    a. Stone
    b. Investment
    c. Plaster
    d. All of the above.

68. **Composite:**
    a. Resin
    b. Resin and Filler
    c. Filler
    d. None.

69. **The type of spatula is used to mix composite:**
    a. Stainless steel
    b. Brass
    c. Plastic
    d. None of the above.

70. **Trituration is:**
    a. Lysing amalgam alloy
    b. Removal of excess of mercury
    c. Mixing of amalgam alloy and mercury
    d. None of the above.

71. **Amalgam is:**
    a. A metallic powder composed of silver, tin, copper and zinc
    b. An alloy of two or more metals that have been dissolved in each other in the molten state
    c. An alloy of two or more metals, one of which is mercury
    d. A metallic substance in powder or tablet form that is mixed with mercury.

72. **The solid solution of silver and mercury is:**
    a. β_1
    b. γ
    c. γ_1
    d. γ_2.

73. **This method provides adequate mixing of mercury:**
    a. Dry mix
    b. Short mixing time
    c. Shiny mix
    d. None.

74. **The maximum percentage of carbon content of steel in dentistry:**
    a. 1.7%
    b. 19%
    c. 2%
    d. 4%.

75. **Cobalt-chromium alloys contains:**
    a. 30% cobalt and 60% chromium
    b. 1% palladium
    c. 60% cobalt and 30% chromium
    d. 20% gold.

76. **Pickling:**
    a. Process used to remove surface oxides from gold castings
    b. Is done by soaking the casting in baking soda
    c. Causes pores in gold
    d. Removes investment from gold casting.

77. **Passivating alloy:**
    a. Chromium, Gold, Titanium
    b. Chromium, Aluminium, Titanium
    c. Chromium, Molybdenum, Titanium
    d. Chromium, Iron, Titanium.

78. **The function of inlay wax is:**
    a. Invest inlay patterns
    b. Box models
    c. Temporarily cement inlays
    d. Make inlay wax patterns.

79. **The main ingredient of inlay wax is :**
    a. Candelilla wax
    b. Carnauba wax
    c. Paraffin wax
    d. Gum dammar.

80. **Nickel-titanium alloy:**
    a. Minimal spring back
    b. Unreliable spring back
    c. Low spring back
    d. None of the above.

81. **Annealing:**
    a. Soft hardening treatment
    b. Hard hardening treatment
    c. Stress relieving heat treatment
    d. Precipitating heat treatment.

82. **Average particle size of powdered gold is:**
    a. 10 um
    b. 30 um
    c. 15 um
    d. 0.1 mm.

83. **pH of polycarboxylate liquid:**
    a. 8
    b. 1.7
    c. 5
    d. 7.

84. **Torsional force is:**
    a. Compression
    b. Tensile force
    c. Transverse bending force
    d. Shear.

85. **Crocus cloth is:**
    a. Emery
    b. Rouge
    c. Garnet
    d. Pumice.

Identify the answers for Extended Matching questions

86. **Choose appropriate use for most appropriate material in clinical situations:**
    a. EDTA
    b. Non setting CaOH
    c. Setting CaOH
    d. Ledermix
    e. Sodium hypochlorite.

1. Direct pulp capping	4. Canal irrigant
2. Indirect pulp capping	5. Aid apexification
3. Steroid paste	6. Aid passage through canal narrowing

87. **Properties and characteristics of dental materials:**
    a. Internal force per unit cross-sectional area acting on the material
    b. Change in size of a material in response to a force
    c. The stress beyond which materials gets permanently deformed when a force is applied
    d. A measure of rigidity of material defined by stress: strain ratio
    e. An indication of how easy is to bend a piece of material without causing permanent deformation or fracture
    f. The amount of energy absorbed up to a point of fracture
    g. The energy absorbed by a material undergoing elastic deformation up to its elastic limit
    h. Resistance to penetration.
    i. Slow plastic deformation that occurs with application of static or dynamic forces over a time
    j. Abrasion of a substance
    k. When cyclic forces are applied a crack may nucleate and is increased by small increments each time the force is applied.

1. Elastic limit	7. Toughness
2. Elastic modulus	8. Hardness
3. Resistance	9. Creep
4. Stiffness	10. Wear
5. Strain	11. Fatigue
6. Stress	

88. Properties of dental materials:
a. Ability of a material to transmit heat
b. Rate at which temperature changes spread through material
c. The fraction increase in length for each degree of temperature increase
d. Ability of one material to flow across the surface of another.

1. Creep	5. Thermal conductivity
2. Wear	6. Thermal diffusivity
3. Hardness	7. Coefficient of thermal expansion
4. Fatigue	8. Wettability

89. Dental materials:
a. Increased tarnish resistance
b. Scavenger, prevents oxidation of other material during melting and casting
c. Increased strength and hardness
d. Decreased density and melting point
e. Increased density and melting point
f. Increased corrosion
g. Increased porosity
h. Decreased corrosion resistance
i. Increased tarnishing.

1. Copper	5. Zinc
2. Palladium	6. Gold
3. Platinum	7. Alumina oxide
4. Silver	8. Tin

90. Dental materials:
a. Accurate but liable to tear, requires purchase of water bath
b. Cheap elastomer, is prone to shrinkage and needs to be cast immediately.
c. Setting is a double decomposition reaction with calcium sulphate
d. Stable silicone elastomer, impression can be posted or stored prior to casting
e. Single mix, use stock strays. The material is stiff and removal can be stressful with deep undercuts, absorbs water and should not be stored with alginate impressions
f. Messy to handle but useful when long working time is required, used with special trays, stable but cast within 24 hours
g. Dispensed and mixed to give even colour. Used for recording edentulous ridges in special trays or in patient's existing dentures but contraindicated in undercuts.

1. Addition cured silicone	5. Polyether
2. Condensation cured silicone	6. Polysulphide
3. Impression compound	7. Reversible hydrocolloid
4. Irreversible hydrocolloid	8. Zinc oxide paste

91. Creep:
a. Time dependent plastic deformation.
b. At what temperature does amalgam undergoes creep?
c. Which type of restorations experience greater marginal breakdown?
d. Deformation of set amalgam during function is known as?

1. Stress	8. Low-creep alloys	15. Compressive strength
2. Strain	9. Static creep	16. Thermal expansion
3. Creep	10. Dynamic creep	17. Lathe-cut alloys
4. Boiling time	11. Medium-creep alloys	18. Corrosion
5. Melting point	12. Functional creep	19. Tarnish
6. Yield strength	13. Spherical alloys	20. High-copper amalgam
7. Higher-creep alloys	14. Trituration	21. Low-copper amalgam

92. Impression materials:
a. What is setting time of ZOE I paste?
b. What is the setting time of type II ZOE paste?
c. Name the materials used for duplicating casts or models
d. Which material undergoes addition type of polymerisation
e. Name the material which is most dimensionally stable of all dental materials
f. Which material is also known as mercaptan materials?
g. What are four types of elastomers?
h. Name one rigid material.

1. 10 minutes	11. Amalgam
2. Addition silicones	12. Zinc-oxide eugenol
3. 15 minutes	13. Polysulphide impression material
4. Condensation silicones	14. Rubber base
5. 1 minutes	15. Impression plaster
6. Agar	16. Ethyl alcohol
7. 17 minutes	17. 35 minutes
8. Alginate	18. Polyether
9. 20 minutes	19. Ethyl alcohol
10. Impression compound	

93. Gypsum products:
a. Dental stone of high strength and high expansion
b. If excess water than that required for hydration of hemihydrate is left in the specimen, what type of strength is obtained?
c. When plaster is mixed with silica, what is it called?
d. Beta-hemihydrate obtained by dry calcination of gypsum
e. When the specimen is dried of the excess water, strength obtained is called as?
f. Replica of entire arch
g. Water powder ratio of plaster of Paris ranges from
h. Investment containing die stone.

1. Type V	13. Dental plaster
2. Green strength	14. 0.4-0.5
3. Type III	15. Dental stone
4. Wet strength	16. Class I stone
5. Dry strength	17. Class II stone
6. Divestment	18. Dry calcination
7. Investment	19. 0.3–0.6
8. Casting shrinkage	20. Wet calcination
9. Type II	21. 0.1–0.2
10. Type I	22. Hygroscopic setting
11. Plaster of Paris	23. 0.2–0.5
12. Impression compound	24. Cast

94. **Dental cements:**
    a. What is an ion leachable glass?
    b. What is used as a pulp-capping agent?
    c. Name the universal luting cement.
    d. Which cement show chemical bonding with enamel?
    e. Which cement has severe effect on pulp?
    f. Name two biocompatible cements.
    g. Which cement are used as both cementing and temporary restorations?
    h. Name a substitute for eugenol.
    i. Name the cement that is least soluble in oral cavity.

1. Calcium-fluoro-alumino- silicate glass	14. Glass ionomer cement
2. Silicate cement	15. Alumina
3. Zinc phosphate	16. Silicophosphate
4. Zinc polycarboxylate	17. Glycerine
5. Zinc oxide eugenol	18. Olive oil
6. Zinc silicophosphate	19. Glacial acetic acid
7. Eugenol	20. Zinc acetate
8. Orthoethoxy benzoic acid	21. Fluorapatite
9. Varnish	22. Calcium phosphate
10. Carboxylic	23. Phosphoric acid
11. Resin cement	24. Acetic acid
12. Calcium hydroxide	25. Polyacrylic cement
13. Zinc oxide	

95. **Ceramics:**
    a. When and by whom was the first ceramic crown introduced?
    b. Which additive is used in porcelain for shade matching?
    c. What is used for polishing hard metal parts?
    d. What is the process of firing of ceramic is known as?
    e. What is clogging with debris of abrasive instrument called as?
    f. Which electrolyte is preferred for electroplating of copper dies?
    g. What process is used to remove clogged debris from abrasive instrument?
    h. Which is the most toxic form of mercury?
    i. Which two properties of porcelain bind it to metal ceramic restorations?

1. Copper sulphate acidified with sulfuric acid	14. Metallic oxides
2. Methyl mercury	15. Firing
3. Chemical bonding	16. Fonzi
4. Hydrostatic force	17. 1817
5. 1903	18. 1789
6. Mechanical interlocking	19. 1808
7. Chemical etching	20. Detachment
8. Dr Charles Land	21. Led lamp
9. Pfaff	22. Vacuum firing
10. Crocus cloth	23. Porcelain
11. Sintering	24. Feldspar
12. Abrasive dressing	25. Truing
13. Abrasive binding	

96. **Casting alloys:**
    a. Name the common dental casting alloys.
    b. Which metals are preferred to alloy with gold to improve its properties?
    c. Name one principal hardener
    d. Which metal acts as a grain refiner and scavenger?
    e. What acts as scavenger for oxygen
    f. Wet strength of gypsum product
    g. Which metal exhibits shape, memory and super elasticity?
    h. Which process is used to reverse the effect of cold working with help of heat?
    i. What is the process of formation of protective oxide film by reactive substance called as?
    j. Which metal decreases tarnish and corrosion?
    k. Which metal can be heat hardened but not cold worked?
    l. Greenish discoloration of porcelain is due to.
    m. Which alloys can be cold worked?
    n. In which material is greening shrinkage observed?

1. Nickel-titanium alloys	14. Passivation
2. Noble metal alloys	15. Gold
3. Annealing	16. Platinum
4. Zinc	17. Type 1
5. Copper	18. Ductility
6. Iron	19. Corrosion
7. Chromium	20. Cobalt chrome alloys
8. Indium	21. Greening
9. Casting shrinkage	22. Shrinkage molybdenum
10. Base metal alloys	23. Silica bonded investments
11. Silver palladium	24. Type 11
12. Green strength	25. Higher melting alloys
13. Nickel	

97. **Casting procedures:**
    a. Die material of choice with hydrocolloid impressions
    b. Material with high resistance to abrasion
    c. Process of elimination of wax from mould cavity
    d. Channel to provide molten alloy to mold after wax is removed.

e. Gypsum with least resistance to abrasion
f. Die material with lethal potential
g. Ring liners for mold expansion
h. Most commonly used die material in laboratory
i. To prepare pattern for metallic framework of RPD
j. To record under-cut edentulous portion of mouth.

1. Die stone	10. Ceramic liner	19. Tempering
2. Epoxy resin	11. Electroplated silver	20. Cold working
3. Gold	12. Asbestos	21. Work hardening
4. Nickel	13. Sprue former	22. Strain hardening
5. Distortion	14. Base plate	23. Corrosion resistance
6. Employ type I	15. Ceramic	24. Paraffin
7. Boxing	16. Phosphate investments	25. Ferrite
8. Casting	17. Impression	
9. Burn out	18. Cellulose	

98. Tarnish and corrosion:
   a. Surface discoloration or alteration of surface finish
   b. Forerunner of corrosion
   c. Deterioration of metal by reaction with its environment
   d. Type of corrosion that occurs between dissimilar metals in contact
   e. Metal when at maximum stress shows more reactivity than unstressed metal.
   f. What happens if metal reacts to form oxides, chlorides and sulphides in absence of electrolytes
   g. Which type of alloys resist corrosion?
   h. Type of corrosion that requires water or any other fluid as electrolyte.

1. Corrosion	10. Stress corrosion	19. Phosphate bonded investments
2. Tarnish	11. Crevice corrosion	20. Opaque
3. Galvanic corrosion	12. Electro corrosion	21. procelains
4. Metallurgy	13. Concentration cell corrosion	22. Titanium
5. Ceramics	14. Passivation	23. Aluminium
6. Noble metal alloys	15. Sulfides	24. Dry corrosion
7. Chemical corrosion	16. Chlorides	
8. Wet corrosion	17. Glazing	
9. Chromium	18. Composite	

99. Bonding:
   a. What is used for acid etching?
   b. Time of application of an etchant.
   c. Name the acid used for etching both enamel and dentine simultaneously
   d. Which is used to help in removal of smear layer?
   e. What aids in easy flow of bonding agents?
   f. What material helps in formation and stabilization of hybrid layer?
   g. Name the fluoride releasing bonding agents
   h. Which type of dentin bonding agent uses glycerol-phosphoric acid dimethacrylate?
   i. What are self-etching primers?
   j. Three step procedures are involved in which type of dentin bonding agent?

1. 37% phosphoric acid	14. 5th generation DBA
2. 60 second	15. 6th generation DBA
3. Maleic acid	16. 7th generation DBA
4. Citric acid	17. 10 second
5. Ist generation dentin bonding agents (DBA)	18. Dentin bonding agents
6. 45 second	19. Bisphenol A glycidyl dimethacrylate (BisGMA) resins
7. Oxalic acid	20. 10% phosphoric acids
8. 2nd generation DBA	21. HEMA
9. Conditioners	22. Fluoride
10. 3rd generation DBA	23. 65% phosphoric acid
11. 4th generation DBA	24. Composites
12. 30 second	25. Phenol
13. Primer	

100. Casting defects—Which among the following are the causes for the below mentioned errors in casting?
   a. Casting too large
   b. Distorted casting
   c. Rough surface
   d. Small casting
   e. Suck back porosity
   f. Back pressure
   g. Microporosity
   h. Incomplete casting
   i. Subsurface
   j. Pinhole porosity
   k. Fins on casting
   l. Gaseous inclusions

1. Too little expansion	13. Casting has rounded margins
2. Breakdown of investment	14. Due to bulk of investment, air is unable to escape
3. Air bubbles on wax	15. If the alloy enters rapidly, spherical voids appear in casting
4. Cracks in investment	
5. Wax elimination is not done completely	16. Shrinkage caused by rapid solidification
6. Molten alloy is highly viscous	
7. Molten alloy shrinks on cooling	17. Poor venting
8. Excessive expansion	18. Proper burnout
9. Investment has weak surface	19. Thick sprue is used
10. Investment has strong surface	20. No repeat heating of investment
11. Irregular voids in casting	21. Improper vacuum investing
12. Due to premature termination of flow of molten metal during solidification	22. Wax pattern gets distorted

CASE DISCUSSION

Case 1: Discuss Biocompatibility of Dental Materials.

Before any new material can be marketed, it must pass both laboratory and clinical trials to evaluate its biocompatibility. However, some adverse effects can become apparent after materials have been in clinical use. Material should be used with care or else it may prove hazardous to the patient or the dentist or the staff.

Hazards to Patient

- Allergic reactions.
  - Systemic effects:
    - Amalgam—Amalgam toxicity (use composite cast restoration)
    - Nickle—Nickle sensitivity, eczema
    - Acrylic monomer—Allergic reaction (decrease concentration of monomer, cobalt-chromium and stainless steel denture)
    - Burning mouth
    - Epimine—Polyether impression material
  - Directly toxic:
    - Beryllium present in nickel alloys is known as carcinogen
    - Fluoride in excess can be toxic
    - Ingestion and inhalation of air-borne dust must be avoided
  - Local damage:
    - Eye damage caused by curing lamp (use shield or ask patient to close eyes)
    - Thermal injury to pulpis caused by exothermic setting reaction
    - Damage to mucosa is caused by dentures which are thermal insulators
    - Damage to soft tissue caused by use of hot instruments
- Chemical injury: Noxious chemicals (etchant, hydrogen peroxide), if in direct contact with tissues.
- Hypersensitivity reactions: Can be caused by materials that cause systemic allergy.

Hazards to Staff

In the surgery.
- Allergic reactions:
  - Alginate dust
  - Mercury vapour
  - Nitrous oxide
  - Topical anaesthesia
  - Latex gloves
  - Methyl methacrylate (MMA) monomer
  - Dental adhesive system
  - Eye damage from light sources.

Hazard in the Laboratory

- Cyanide solution for electroplating vapours from low fusing metal dies
- Siliceous particles in investment materials
- Fluxes containing fluoride
- Hydrofluoric acid used for etching porcelain veneers
- Beryllium in some alloys
- PMMA powders
- MMA monomers
- Casting machines

Dental Materials

Answers

1. a. F b. T c. F d. F e. F
   f. F
2. a. F b. F c. F d. T e. F
   f. T g. T
3. a. T b. F c. T d. T e. F
   f. F g. T h. T i. F j. T
   k. F l. T m. T n. F o. T
   p. T q. T
4. a. F b. F c. F d. T e. F
   f. F g. F h. F i. T j. T
   k. F
5. a. F b. F c. F d. T e. F
   f. T g. F h. F
6. a. F b. T c. F d. T e. T
   f. F g. T h. T i. F j. F
   k. T l. F m. T n. F
7. a. T b. F c. T d. F e. F
   f. T
8. a. F b. F c. T d. T e. T
   f. F g. F h. F i. T j. F
   k. T l. F m. F n. T o. F
9. a. F b. F c. F d. F e. T
   f. F g. T h. T i. ?? j. F
   k. F
10. a. F b. T c. F d. T e. F
    f. F g. T
11. a. T b. F c. T d. F e. T

12.	a.	F	b.	F	c.	F	d.	F	e.	F
	f.	F	g.	T						
13.	a.	T	b.	F	c.	T	d.	F	e.	F
	f.	F								
14.	a.	F	b.	F	c.	F	d.	T	e.	F
	f.	F	g.	T	h.	T	i.	F		
15.	a.	F	b.	T	c.	F	d.	T	e.	F
	f.	F								
16.	b	17.	d	18.	a	19.	b	20.	c	
21.	b	22.	a	23.	a	24.	c	25.	b	
26.	b	27.	b	28.	c	29.	c	30.	a	
31.	c	32.	b	33.	b	34.	d			
35.	c	36.	b	37.	a	38.	b	39.	c	
40.	b	41.	d	42.	a	43.	a	44.	b	
45.	a	46.	c	47.	b	48.	a	49.	b	
50.	c	51.	d	52.	c	53.	c	54.	b	
55.	d	56.	c	57.	b	58.	a	59.	c	
60.	b	61.	b	62.	a	63.	b	64.	b	
65.	c	66.	b	67.	d	68.	b	69.	c	
70.	c	71.	c	72.	c	73.	c	74.	a	
75.	c	76.	a	77.	b	78.	d	79.	c	
80.	d	81.	c	82.	c	83.	b	84.	d	
85.	b									
86.	a.	6	b.	5	c.	1	d.	3	e.	4
87.	a.	6	b.	5	c.	1	d.	2	e.	4
	f.	7	g.	3	h.	8	i.	9	j.	10
	k.	11								
88.	a.	5	b.	6	c.	7	d.	8		

89.	a.	2	b.	5	c.	1	d.	1	e. 4
	f.	3	g.	4	h.	1	i.	4	
90.	a.	7	b.	2	c.	4	d.	1	e. 5
	f.	??	g.	8					
91.	a.	3	b.	5	c.	7	d.	10	
92.	a.	1	b.	3	c.	6, 8	d.	2	e. 2
	f.	13	g.	2, 4, 13, 18	h.	15			
93.	a.	1	b.	2, 4	c.	7	d.	11	e. 8
	f.	24	g.	14	h.	6			
94.	a.	1	b.	12	c.	3	d.	4, 14	e. 2
	f.	4, 5	g.	4, 11	h.	8	i.	11	
95.	a.	5, 8	b.	14	c.	10	d.	11	e. 13
	f.	1	g.	12	h.	2	i.	3, 6	
96.	a.	2, 10	b.	4, 5, 8, 13	c.	5	d.	8	e. 4
	f.	12	g.	1	h.	3	i.	14	j. 16
	k.	15	l.	21	m.	20	n.	23	
97.	a.	1	b.	2	c.	9	d.	13	e. 1
	f.	11	g.	10, 12, 18	h.	2	i.	8	j. 17
98.	a.	2	b.	2	c.	1	d.	3	e. 10
	f.	7, 23	g.	6	h.	8, 12			
99.	a.	1	b.	2	c.	3, 4, 7	d.	9	e. 13
	f.	18	g.	16	h.	5	i.	11	j. 10
100.	a.	8	b.	22	c.	2, 3, 9	d.	1	e. 11
	f.	13, 14	g.	16	h.	5	i.	15	j. 14
	k.	4	l.	15					

CORRECT ANSWERS FOR FALSE STATEMENTS

1. a. Spheroidal amalgams
   a. Gamma 2 phase Sn–Hg
   b. Increase in copper contents results in increased expense
   c. Increased strength, durability, creep and corrosion resistance
   d. Single composition of Cu-Ag-Sn alloy
2. a. Varies from 5–20 seconds
   a. Should be overfilled so Hg rich surface larger can be removed later
   b. Spheroidal
   a. 24 hours
3. b. Increase modulus
   b. 75–85% weight of fillers.
   i. 0.6–1μm
   k. Quartz tungsten halogen
   n. Increased shrinkage on curing
4. b. Cavity design
   c. Micromechanical
   a. Micro-tags formed at the core of prism in the individual crypt of dissolved hydroxyapatite crystals
   b. 15 seconds
   c. Probing is contraindicated
   d. No difference in bond strength
   k. Remineralisation after 24 hours indistinguishable from untreated enamel
5. b. Hydrophobic monomer based on BIS-GMA
   c. Hydrophilic
   e. Brush thinning is preferred to maintain sufficient film thickness
   g. No technique produces zero microleakage
6. a. Decreased solubility due to carboxylic and phosphoric acid
   c. Also due to ionic displacement of calcium and phosphate with polyacrylate ions
   f. 40%
   n. Absorption of water will result in dissolution and dehydration will lead to crazing
7. d. HEMA BISGMA
   a. Due to formation of polymerisation matrix which is strengthened by acid-base reaction
8. b. 24 hours
   b. Incremental mixing
   c. 40% PAA

Dental Materials

   d. Bacteriostatic
   j. Decreased setting time
   a. Phosphate > polycarboxylate resin bonded ZOE > accelerated ZOE >
28 Clinical Guide for Overseas Dental Examination
   b. calcium hydroxide.
   c. EBA cement should not be used as luting due to increased solubility
   o. Can be used with dentine adhesive system with direct/indirect pulp capping
9. d. Polyethers
   a. Polysulphides
   b. Stock trays
10. a. >75%
    f. Higher melting point
1. b. Cobalt-chromium-nickel
    d. Nitinol not easy to bend without fracture
2. a. Metallic and nonmetallic oxides
    a. Kaolin
    b. Quartz
    c. Alumina particles for increased strength e.30–40%
    f. Procera crown
3. d. Least expensive than Porcelain Jacket Crown
4. a. Benzoyl peroxide.
    b. ~2.5:1
    c. Dough stage
    a. Least resistance to abrasion
    b. 105 degree for Heat cure acrylic.
5. a. Heat cure preferred for hard rebases
    b. Silicone polymer are more elastic
    a. Polyethyl methacrylate (PEMA) to which mix of alcohol and ester is added
    b. Minimum 2 mm

Chapter
14 Law and Ethics of General Dental Council

Identify the following Statements as True (T) or False (F)

1. **The General Dental Council:**
   a. Was established in 1921
   b. The Dentist's Act 1984 consolidated the 1957 and 1983 Acts into one legislation
   c. The 2003 order also allowed registration of Dental Care Professionals
   d. It is optional for dentist to have dental indemnity
   e. The council is now made up of 15 members
   f. The membership now includes 8 members from dental profession
   g. The lay members are appointed by the Queen on the recommendation by her Privy council.

2. **The following are eligible for full registration with the General Dental Council:**
   a. Dentist qualified in Canada
   b. Dentist qualified in USA
   c. Dentist qualified in Sweden
   d. Dentist who have not completed Vocational Dental Training
   e. Dentist who have a Licentiate of Dental Surgery from a Royal College
   f. Icelandic and Norwegian graduates.

3. **Dentist with temporary registration:**
   a. Can practise under the supervision of General Dental Council
   b. It is granted for work in the community dental services
   c. Temporary registration is granted for the maximum period of 4 years
   d. Can work in oral and maxillofacial surgery unit in a UK hospital
   e. Completion of maximum period of temporary registration leads to full registration to practice dentistry in UK
   f. Are permitted to take 'on call' duties in a UK hospital.

4. **The Overseas Registration Exam:**
   a. Is in 3 parts
   b. Candidates are allowed 2 attempt for each part of overseas registration exam
   c. Candidates have to pass part-2 within 2 years of sitting part-1 exams
   d. Has to be passed by Iranian dentist for full registration
   e. Has to be passed by Greek dentists for full registration.

5. **A dentist can use following titles:**
   a. Dental practitioner
   b. Dental surgeon
   c. Doctor
   d. Dentist
   e. Orthodontist
   f. Surgical dentist.

6. **The specialities recognised by General Dental Council are:**
   a. Dental and maxillofacial radiography
   b. Dental public health
   c. Oral and maxillofacial pathology
   d. Special care dentistry
   e. Oral microbiology
   f. Oral surgery
   g. Maxillo-facial surgery
   h. Crown and Bridge
   i. Implants.

7. **Registered dental hygienist:**
   a. Can take radiographs and interpret them
   b. Can give inferior dental block analgesia
   c. Cannot take impression
   d. Cannot place rubber dam
   e. Cannot administer inhalation sedation
   f. Can restores teeth
   g. Can adjust unrestored surfaces
   h. Can diagnose disease.

8. **Registered dental therapists:**
   a. Can extract permanent teeth
   b. Can carry out direct restoration on primary teeth only
   c. Can carry out pulp treatments
   d. Can carry out pulpotomies in primary teeth
   e. Can plan patient's treatment
   f. Can prescribe tooth whitening independently
   g. Can replace crowns
   h. Can scale, clean and polish teeth
   i. Cannot refer patients to other health care professionals.

9. **Dental technicians:**
   a. Can fit removable partial dentures
   b. Can fit complete dentures
   c. Can fit immediate dentures
   d. Can carry out implant frame assessment
   e. Can do occlusal registration
   f. Can trace cephalographs

g. Can work independently in the clinic
h. Can carry out independent clinical examination
i. Can take tooth shade in the construction of prosthesis
j. Cannot repair dentures directly for public
k. Are to be registered with general dental council.

10. **Clinical dental technicians:**
    a. Can perform clinical procedure related to providing removable partial dentures (RPDs)
    b. Cannot carry out clinical examination
    c. Can provide complete dentures direct to patients
    d. Cannot fit removable appliances
    e. Can provide anti-snoring device
    f. Can re-cement crown
    g. Can remove sutures
    h. Cannot provide sports mouth guard.

11. **Orthodontic therapists:**
    a. Cannot fit headgears
    b. Can take orthognathic facebow readings
    c. Can fit orthodontic facebow
    d. Can insert active removable appliances
    e. Can prepare, insert, adjust and remove archwires
    f. Cannot measures and record plaque indices
    g. Can remove subgingival deposits
    h. Can also place active medicaments
    i. Can give or administer local anaesthesia
    j. Can activate orthodontic wires.

12. **The GDC can remove dentist from dentist's registration if:**
    a. Dentist is addicted to prescribed drugs or alcohol
    b. Dentist has not paid annual registration fees
    c. If dentist has been found guilty of serious professional misconduct
    d. Has committed/convicted of a criminal offence prior to qualifying as a dentist
    e. Has been removed from the equivalent register in another country
    f. Convicted of drunk driving offences
    g. Conviction of fraud relating to personal finances
    h. Convicted of anti-social behaviour.

13. **GDC disciplinary procedures can be initiated if:**
    a. A formal complaint has been filed by a patient
    b. Complaint by member of public, not your patient
    c. Complaint from a person acting in a public capacity
    d. GDC's solicitors
    e. Notification by the police
    f. Notification by the criminal court.

14. **GDC disciplinary procedures:**
    a. Are all screened by Chief Dental Officer
    b. Dentist's name can be erased for maximum period of 12 months
    c. The investigating committee can suspend registrants
    d. The professional conduct committee can suspend registrant for maximum up to 6 month
    e. The professional conduct committee can issues a reprimand
    f. Lay person cannot sit on disciplinary committees
    g. The professional performance committee cannot suspend registrants
    h. Health committee can impose conditions on individuals registrations
    i. Registrars can appeal to Privy Council against general dental councils decision of fitness to practice committee.

15. **Professional Conduct Committee:**
    a. Reprimand a dental professional
    b. Impose condition on registrants for maximum period of 2 years
    c. Can suspend dental professional
    d. Can have name erased from dentist's register
    e. Can be referred to Health Committee
    f. Can be referred to Professional Performance Committee.

16. **Restoration following erasure:**
    a. A dental professional can apply restoration to the register after 3 years
    b. A dentist can re-register at end of a period of suspension
    c. Suspension or erasure takes into effect immediately
    d. Continuing professional development will not be a requirement
    e. No fee is payable for restoration to the dentist's register.

17. **With regards to dental professional's health:**
    a. Preliminary screening is undertaken by chief investigation officer
    b. Medical examination is mandatory
    c. The dentist has 1 month to respond to an enquiry on health matters
    d. A dentist can submit report by his own medical examiner
    e. Investing committee decides if a dentist should be referred to health committee.

18. **Health Committee of the General Dental Council:**
    a. Can impose conditions on Dental professional registration
    b. Can suspend dentist/DCP from the register
    c. Can keep dental professional under review for indefinite period
    d. Can issue reprimand
    e. Impose conditions for up to 3 years
    f. Can refer all cases of suspension to Professional Performance Committee
    g. Can erase from Dentist register, if impairment is solely on health grounds.

19. **Professional performance committee can:**
    a. Suspend from dentist's register
    b. Erasure from dentist's register
    c. Impose conditions to continuing registration
    d. Appoint assessors, who are General Dental Council members
    e. Professional performance committee can commission National Clinical Assessment Service report.

20. **GDC will investigate professional misconduct, if referred by:**
    a. A professional colleague
    b. A health authority
    c. A member of public
    d. GDC solicitors
    e. A court of law officer.

21. **To practice dentistry in UK:**
    a. Dental professional should be citizen of the European Economic Area/the European Union country
    b. Registered with general dental council
    c. Should have complete Vocational Dental Training
    d. Sound mind and character
    e. Holds a Dental Degree.

22. **Dentists in UK are strongly advised to:**
    a. Undertake vocational or General Professional Training after qualifying from Dental school
    b. Continue training and education until retirement from profession
    c. Should be aware of scope of their practice and limitations
    d. Join Dental Professional Organizations
    e. Always be chaperoned when with a patient.

23. **Patients records:**
    a. Must be clearly handwritten
    b. Should be kept minimum of 5 years from the completion of last course of treatment
    c. Records of treatment of children should be kept until they are above 18 years plus
    d. Parents can take action in a court on behalf of the minor concerned
    e. Trustees and beneficiaries can take action on behalf of deceased
    f. Must include medical history
    g. Can be destroyed if patient dies
    h. Can be written up at the end of the week.

24. **Confidentiality and disclosures:**
    a. The records cannot be disclosed to third party
    b. The records can be shown to patient's spouse
    c. The records can be shown to police officers
    d. Can be shown to court of law

e. Can be shown to a specialist to whom patient is referred
f. The dentist must register as a data user with the data protection register under the Data Protection Act of 1984.

25. **Consent to treatment:**
    a. Can be written
    b. Can be verbal
    c. Can be implied
    d. Is not required for children under the age of 18 years
    e. Can be withdrawn by the patient
    f. Can be obtained by auxiliary staff.

26. **Written consent:**
    a. Must be obtained, if patient is having treatment under sedation
    b. Must be obtained, if patient is having treatment under General Anaesthesia
    c. Advisable for complicated or expensive treatment
    d. Obtained prior to the removal of impacted lower wisdom tooth
    e. Should contain details of procedure, type of anaesthetic agent and any risk of complications
    f. Patient should be aware if they are consenting for National Health Service (NHS) or private treatment.

27. **Consent for special cases:**
    a. Minimum age for valid consent is 18 years
    b. Child less than 16 years of age can consent for treatment, if they fully understands the treatment
    c. In case of GA for 17 years old, consent of parent or guardian is only required
    d. For mentally impaired patient, consent of patient carer should be obtained
    e. Non-life saving treatment should be delayed until consent is obtained
    f. Written consent should be obtained for patient's photographs
    g. In case of advance refusal by incompetent adult, General Dental Council must abide by that refusal
    h. Treatment of unconscious patient is valid.

28. **At present, general anaesthesia for dental treatment can be administered by:**
    a. A doctor
    b. A suitability trained dentist
    c. Consultant anaesthetist
    d. Trainee anaesthetist
    e. A staff-grade anaesthetist.

29. **Dental surgeon referring patient for treatment under general anaesthesia:**
    a. Should give full justification for the use of general anaesthesia
    b. Should include full medical history

c. Should explain patient about the risk involved
d. Should offer alternative methods of pain control to complete the treatment
e. Should obtain consent
f. It is their responsibility to ensure that protocols for general anaesthesia should be adhered.

30. **When carrying out treatment under general anaesthesia:**
    a. Dentist is responsible for recovery of patient
    b. Dentist is responsible for discharge of patient
    c. There must be protocol for providing advanced life support
    d. There must be arrangement in place to transfer patient to critical care facility
    e. There must be a presence of three appropriately trained staff present.

31. **Sedation for dental treatment:**
    a. Depresses central nervous system
    b. Communication with patient can be stopped once patient is sedated
    c. Suitably experienced and trained dental nurse can administer sedation
    d. Only one sedative drug should be administered
    e. Requires presence of four trained personnels
    f. Should be administered intravenously in children.

32. **Before undertaking dental treatment under sedation, Dental surgeon should:**
    a. Take full medical history
    b. Advise on appropriate method of pain and anxiety control
    c. Obtain written informed consent for sedation only
    d. Ensure proper equipment is available to administer sedation
    e. Appropriate drugs for resuscitation are readily available
    f. Dentist and staff should be trained in resuscitation techniques.

33. **While treating patient under sedation:**
    a. A chaperone must be present
    b. Patient should be monitored during sedation only
    c. Patient recovering must be supervised and protected
    d. Patient must be accompanied by responsible adult
    e. Monitoring of the patient should be undertaken by trained nurse responsible to sedationist
    f. Drugs must be available for resuscitation.

34. **Patient complaints:**
    a. Every dental practice should have complaint procedure
    b. Every dental hospitals should have complaint procedure
    c. Every department in the hospital or clinic should have their own complaint procedure

    d. Complaints from patients should be dealt with doctors and dentists only
    e. Should be answered in writing
    f. Complaints procedure should be available.
35. **Dealing with complaints:**
    a. Complaints cannot be made verbally
    b. Complaints should be acknowledged within a week of their receipt
    c. Dental practice should send written reply to complainant within three weeks
    d. National heart service trust should respond within 3 week of receiving complaint
    e. Chief medical officer of the national heart service trust should respond via written reply.
36. **Making a complaint:**
    a. Can only be made by patient
    b. Must be made within 3 month of the occurrence of the incident
    c. Complainant can request for independent review panel
    d. Review panel comprises convener and 2 independent lay members.
37. **Negligence, the following would not be negligent:**
    a. While treating a friend out of hour and something goes wrong
    b. Not treating patient to the standard of care that would be expected of a specialist
    c. If the patient did not suffer damage from dentist error
    d. If the dentist had duty of care at that time
    e. If dentist did not exercise reasonable skill and care
    f. Failure to refer to specialist.
38. **A claim of compensation for negligence against dentist is not likely to succeed:**
    a. If patient pleads 'Res ipsa Loquitur'
    b. If dentist exercised reasonable skill and care
    c. If damage occurs as the result of patient grabbing dentist working arm
    d. If negligent act was carried out by an employee
    e. If patient 'talked' Dentist to undertake treatment that dentist was unsure would be successful.
39. **The dentist (defendant) can use following in his defence:**
    a. The Bolam principle test
    b. The Bolitho judgement test
    c. The parent was under 18 years
    d. The incident occurred 10 years ago
    e. Dentist was carrying out a 'Good Samaritan act'.
40. **Employment:**
    a. All employees should have written contract of employment
    b. Contract must include termination procedures from employment

c. It is the duty of the employer to ensure the health, safety and welfare at work of all employees
d. Employer should provide instruction, training and supervision necessary to ensure health and safety
e. Provide working environment with no risk to employee's health.

41. The following law affects practice of dentistry:
    a. Control of Substances Hazardous to Health
    b. Ionising Radiation (Medical Exposure) Regulations (IRMER)
    c. The Dental Act
    d. Health and safety at work Act
    e. Data Protection Act
    f. Notification of Accidents and Dangerous Occurrences Regulations
    g. Financial Services Act.

Identify the Single Best Answer for the following

42. The GDC is governed and enabled by:
    a. The Dentists Act 1984, amended 2005 ("the Act")
    b. The Dentists Act 1981, amended 2004 ("the Act")
    c. The Dentists Act 1982, amended 2005 ("the Act")
    d. The Dentists Act 1985, amended 2006 ("the Act").

43. Dental care professionals regulated by General Dental Council are:
    a. Dental nurses, dental technicians, dental therapists and orthodontic therapists
    b. Dental hygienists, dental nurses, dental technicians, dental therapists, orthodontic therapists
    c. Clinical dental technicians, dental technicians, dental and orthodontic therapists
    d. Clinical dental technicians, dental hygienists, dental nurses, dental technicians, dental therapists, orthodontic therapists.

44. The purpose of General Dental Council is:
    a. Registering qualified professionals
    b. Setting standards of dental practice and conduct
    c. Helping patients with complaints about dental professionals
    d. All of the above.

45. The following sanctions is not within the power of the general dental council?
    a. Erasure from the dentists register
    b. Imposition of a suspended sentence of less than six months
    c. Reprimand a registrant
    d. Suspension of a registrant's registration for a maximum of 12 months.

46. After how long can a dental professional who has been erased may apply for restoration to the register
    a. After five years
    b. After three years

c. After two years
d. After seven years.

47. **The patient records to be kept after completion of last course of treatment for the period of:**
   a. 5 years
   b. 7 years
   c. 10 years
   d. 2 years.

48. **Written consent mandatory for:**
   a. Treatment under sedation
   b. Prior to removal of impacted lower wisdom tooth
   c. Complicated or expensive procedures
   d. All of above.

49. **What is Gillick competence?**
   a. Child patient can consent for himself or herself, if she or he understands treatment
   b. Consent from parents or legal guardians
   c. Ask for consent from parents/guardians on telephone
   d. None of the above.

50. **How many members constitute the general dental council**
   a. 12
   b. 15
   c. 17
   d. 10.

Identify the answers to Extended Matching questions

51. **The General Dental Council:**
   a. Who constitutes the Council?
   b. How the lay members are appointed?
   c. When was General Dental Council established?
   d. Who has the authority to appoint of lay members?

1. 1921	5. Lay members recommended by Privy Council of queen
2. The council is made up of 12 members	
3. 6 members of dental profession	6. 1956
4. Queen	

CASE DISCUSSION

Case 1: Consent

You are a senior house officer in an oral and maxillofacial surgery department. The patient is 24-year-old man with learning difficulties attends clinic for examination under anaesthetic and extractions. He attends the clinic with his carer. Discuss the consent procedure you would follow and law applied.

Treatment without consent is equivalent to assault. Treatment with consent but without any explanation of what entails is called negligence. Consent must be obtained before starting any treatment, physical examination or providing any care for the patient. Consent should be 'informed' consent which means that patient should understand treatment, aftercare and precautions if necessary. The clinician should discuss commonly occurring risks or side-effects from the treatment proposed. Patient should also be made aware of any alternative forms of treatment.

Adult

- No one can give consent on behalf of an adult, even if adult is incompetent
- Consent has to be obtained from patient
- Severity of his learning difficulty will determine whether he understands the treatment or not
- If patient has some difficulty in understanding, explain the procedure in the way that he can understand
- If patient cannot understand: Treatment can be given in patient's best interest
- Inability to consent should not prevent the treatment
- People close to patient can give some information
- Information should be sought from relative/carer of patient
- Agreement with those close to patient to carry out treatment, even if not consented
- Consent can be given in written, verbal or implied forms, consent should always be obtained by the clinician after explaining risks and benefits of the treatment.

Written Consent

- Extensive treatment
- Treatment under sedation or general anaesthesia
- Complicated and expensive treatment
- Carrying out procedure with specific risk (extraction of lower impacted wisdom tooth)
- Consent should be written in simple language that patient understands (without use of abbreviation and jargons) to describe procedure
- Signature on form does not prove that consent is valid. Patient should actually understand the risk and benefits of treatment.

Verbal Consent

- Should minimum be obtained for treatment
- Dentist—"would you like local anaesthesia for this filling?" Patient verbally agreeing or opening mouth to allow dentist to proceed would be valid consent
- Dentist to be confident that patient understands treatment
- No treatment if in doubt regarding patient's mental abilities

- Patient can withdraw consent anytime, if requested treatment should be stopped.

Implied Consent
- If patient has been presented with treatment plan and arranges further appointment for treatment plans to be carried out
- By attending an appointment
- Sitting in dental chair gives implied consent to dental examination (but not treatment)
- If patient requests local anaesthesia for filling and opens mouth for local anaesthesia to be administered.

Case 2: Complaints
You are general dental practitioner in new dental practice. Explain national heart service complaint system in your practice.
- Vast majority of complaints should be dealt in house
- Each practice must have complaint protocol to follow
- There should be a designated person in-charge of its administration
- Practice complaints procedures must be available to patient
- If patient makes verbal complaint, the designated person should discuss nature of problem with patient, relative or carer
- Discussion should take place in private office to protect patient's confidentiality
- All records relating to complaint must be kept separately
- Written complaint should be acknowledged within 2 working days
- Following investigation of the complaint, a written response should be sent out to patient within 10 working days of the original complaint
- Complaints can be made within 6 months of the event or 6 months from the time they noticed problem, provided it is less than 12 months after the incident
- A courteous and efficient system for dealing with complaints leads to their resolution without recourse to formal procedures
- If complaint cannot be resolved in-house, it will pass on to local health authority to look into it.

Outcomes of Complaint
- Complaint referred back to practice
- Conciliation
- Independent review panel of conveyor and 2 independent member
- Health care commission
- No further action
- Advising patient to contact health services ombudsman

Case 3: Consent for Minor

Discuss consent in relation to 14-years-old girl who is visiting group camp and requires treatment for dental abscess.
- Patient is minor and under 16 years
- Consent from parent or legal guardian is required
- Patient is away from home
- One of the following may be used to obtain consent which should be in writing:
  - a. Contact patient's parent/guardian by telephone
    b. Explain treatment and ask for consent
    c. Have second person to listen to phone call
    d. Write notes of the call on patient's records
  - Check if patient's parents or guardians have signed a letter giving group leader 'in loco parentis' right. In that case, this person can consent treatment. A copy of the 'in loco parentis' should be taken
  - Patient can consent herself, if she understand the treatment. This is called Gillick competence. Get another colleague to approve your treatment plan and patient's understanding of the treatment
  - Treatment should be limited to relief of pain; treatment should be reversible i.e. treat rather than extraction. Further treatment can only be given after obtaining parental consent. Any non-urgent matters to be referred back to patient's own dentist.

Answers

1.	a.	F	b.	T	c.	F	d.	F	e.	F	
	f.	F	g.	T							
2.	a.	F	b.	F	c.	T	d.	T	e.	T	
	f.	T									
3.	a.	F	b.	F	c.	F	d.	T	e.	F	
	f.	T									
4.	a.	F	b.	F	c.	F	d.	T	e.	F	
5.	a.	T	b.	T	c.	T	d.	T	e.	F	
	f.	F									
6.	a.	T	b.	T	c.	T	d.	T	e.	T	
	f.	??	g.	F	h.	??	i.	F			
7.	a.	T	b.	T	c.	T	d.	F	e.	F	
	f.	F	g.	F	h.	F					
8.	a.	F	b.	F	c.	F	d.	T	e.	F	
	f.	F	g.	T	h.	T	i.	F			
9.	a.	F	b.	F	c.	F	d.	T	e.	T	
	f.	T	g.	F	h.	F	i.	T	j.	F	
	k.	T									
10.	a.	T	b.	F	c.	T	d.	T	e.	T	
	f.	T	g.	T	h.	F					
11.	a.	F	b.	T	c.	T	d.	T	e.	T	
	f.	F	g.	F	h.	T	i.	F	j.	F	
12.	a.	T	b.	T	c.	T	d.	T	e.	T	
	f.	T	g.	T	h.	F					
13.	a.	T	b.	T	c.	T	d.	T	e.	T	
	f.	T									

14.	a.	F	b.	F	c.	F	d.	F	e.	T
	f.	F	g.	F	h.	T	i.	T		
15.	a.	T	b.	F	c.	T	d.	T	e.	T
	f.	T								
16.	a.	F	b.	T	c.	F	d.	F	e.	F
17.	a.	F	b.	F	c.	F	d.	T	e.	??
18.	a.	T	b.	T	c.	T	d.	T	e.	T
	f.	T	g.	F						
19.	a.	T	b.	T	c.	T	d.	F	e.	F
20.	a.	T	b.	T	c.	T	d.	T	e.	T
21.	a.	F	b.	T	c.	F	d.	T	e.	F
22.	a.	T	b.	T	c.	T	d.	T	e.	T
23.	a.	F	b.	F	c.	F	d.	T	e.	T
	f.	T	g.	F	h.	F				
24.	a.	T	b.	F	c.	F	d.	F	e.	T
	f.	T								
25.	a.	T	b.	T	c.	T	d.	F	e.	T
	f.	F								
26.	a.	T	b.	T	c.	T	d.	T	e.	T
	f.	T								
27.	a.	F	b.	T	c.	F	d.	T	e.	T
	f.	T	g.	T	h.	T				
28.	a.	F	b.	F	c.	T	d.	T	e.	T
29.	a.	T	b.	T	c.	T	d.	T	e.	T
	f.	F								
30.	a.	F	b.	F	c.	T	d.	T	e.	F
31.	a.	T	b.	F	c.	F	d.	F	e.	F
	f.	F								
32.	a.	T	b.	T	c.	F	d.	T	e.	T
	f.	T								

33.	a.	T	b.	F	c.	T	d.	T	e.	T
	f.	T								
34.	a.	T	b.	T	c.	F	d.	F	e.	T
	f.	T								
35.	a.	F	b.	F	c.	F	d.	F	e.	F
36.	a.	F	b.	F	c.	T	d.	T		
37.	a.	F	b.	F	c.	T	d.	F	e.	F
	f.	F								
38.	a.	F	b.	T	c.	T	d.	F	e.	F
39.	a.	T	b.	T	c.	F	d.	T	e.	F
40.	a.	T	b.	T	c.	T	d.	T	e.	T
41.	a.	T	b.	T	c.	T	d.	T	e.	T
	f.	T	g.	F						
42.	a	43.	d	44.	d	45.	b	46.	a	
47.	b	48.	d	49.	a	50.	a			
51.	a.	2, 3	b.	4, 5	c.	6	d.	4		

CORRECT ANSWERS FOR FALSE STATEMENTS

1. a. 1956
   a. Order 2005
   b. It is compulsory to have indemnity to remain on Dentist's Register
   c. 12 members
   d. 6 members
1. a. GDC registered consultant
   a. Only granted for NHS hospitals, dental schools and other approved institution
   b. 5 years
2. a. 2 parts
   a. Upto 4 attempts
   b. Within 5 years
3. e. Has to be on specialist register
6. g. Maxillo-Facial Surgery is medical speciality
1. e. Dental Hygienist can administer inhalation sedation if undergone proper training
2. a. Dental therapist can extract Primary teeth.
   b. Dental therapist can carry out direct restoration on both permanent and primary teeth
   f. Requires prescription of Dentist
1. a. GDC disciplinary procedures are all screened y fitness to practice case officer
   a. Erasure is permanent unless Dentist applies for restoration
   b. Interim orders committee can suspend Registrants.
   c. 12 months
   g. Professional performance committee can suspend registrants
2. b. 3 years
3. a. 5 years
   a. Only if interim order committee considers Dental professional as a risk to public or themselves
   b. CPD should be up to date and essential for re-admission to the register
4. a. Preliminary screening is undertaken by fitness to practice case officer
   a. But will stop investigation proceedings
   b. 28 days
5. g. No practice committee can erase based solely on health grounds
6. d. Performance is assessed by NCAS
   e. Investigating committee can commission NCAS report

Law and Ethics of General Dental Council

21. a. Can be citizen of any country and UK qualifications
    c. Only required for providing NHS dental care
    e. Dental Degree from EU or EEA or Licentiate of Royal College
1. a. Records can be typed/computerised
    a. 7 years
       18 + 7 =25 years.
    h. Records should be updated during or immediately after treatment
2. d. Unless there is a specific court order
3. f. Consent should always be obtained by clinician
27. a. 16 years
    c. Both parents and child should consent
1. f. It is treating Dentist's responsibility to ensure GA protocols are adhered not referring Dentist
2. e. Four people; Dentist, Dental Assistant, Anaesthetist, Anaesthetic assistant.
3. b. Communication with patient should be maintained throughout the procedure under sedation
    a. Dental surgeon can administer sedation
    b. If more than one drug is utilised, the provision of advance life support must be available immediately
    c. Three people; Dentist, Dental assistant, Dental/general nurse for patient monitoring
    d. IV unsuitable for children, relative analgesia is preferred.
4. c. written informed consent should be obtained for both sedation and treatment proposed.
5. c. NHS Trust have their own complaint procedure
6. d. Complaints should be dealt with designated personnel for handling complain;doesn't have to be Doctor or Dentist
7. b. Two working days
    a. 10 working days
    b. 4 weeks
    c. Chief Executive of the NHS trust should respond via written reply.
8. a. Complaint can be made by parent, guardian, friend or spouse
    b. Within 6 month to maximum 12 months
9. a. Liability is present everywhere
10. d. Dentist is responsible for acts of his employees
    e. Dentist should have refused treatment
11. c. Parents can sue if patient is under 18 years

Annexures

ANNEXURE 1

STANDARDS FOR DENTAL TEAM

The standards for dental team apply to the following people:

- Dentists
- Dental Nurses
- Dental Hygienists
- Dental Therapists
- Orthodontic Therapists
- Dental Technicians
- Clinical Dental Technicians.

The core nine ethical principles practiced by General dental practitioner are as follows:

1. Put patients' interests first
2. Communicate effectively with patients
3. Obtain valid consent
4. Maintain and protect patients' information
5. Have a clear and effective complaints procedure
6. Work with colleagues in a way that is in patients' best interests
7. Maintain, develop and work within your professional knowledge and skills
8. Raise concerns if patient is at risk
9. Make sure your personal behaviour maintains patients' confidence in you and the dental profession.

ANNEXURE 2

ELIGIBILITY CRITERIA FOR REGISTRATION

The following individuals are eligible for full registration without assessment of qualifications:

- Those people exhibiting a UK dental qualification
- Those who have successfully passed the Overseas Registration Exam or Licence in Dental Surgery
- Those who have acquired a qualification before 01/01/01 from Hong Kong, Singapore, Malaysia, South Africa, New Zealand and Australia with the exception of BChD MEDUNSA, BDS awarded between 01/01/97 to 31/12/00 and BChD Western Cape awarded before 31/12/97
- Exempt persons with a scheduled dental qualification from the European Economic Area.

ELIGIBILITY TO APPLY FOR INDIVIDUAL ASSESSMENT OF KNOWLEDGE AND SKILL

If you do not Meet the Criteria Above for full Registration

> You may be eligible for an individual assessment of your dental training, knowledge and skill
>
> This application route is only presented to exempt persons who have qualified overseas and is not a guaranteed route to registration.

If an Individual Fails to Meet any of the Above Criteria

- ORE is an exam which assesses clinical skills and knowledge of dentists who are not eligible for registration. Applicants are eligible to apply for full registration once they have passed overseas registration exam
- Temporary registration permits dentists who are not eligible for registration or assessment to practise dentistry, if they have had the offer of a supervised post for training, teaching or research purposes, for a limited time.

OVERSEAS REGISTRATION EXAM

- The ORE is a two part exam that overseas qualified dentists have to pass so as to get registered with the general dental council which in turn allows dentists to practice dentistry unsupervised in the UK
- It assesses clinical skills and knowledge of dentists from outside the EEA whose qualifications are not eligible for full registration with the general dental council in UK

- Candidates are anticipated to meet or surpass the standard of a freshly passed UK BDS graduate
- The exam is based on the UK dental curriculum and uses modern evaluation methods to ensure a toughness and consistency
- It has two parts and candidates are permitted up to four attempts at each Part of the ORE and a percentage mark out of 100 for Paper 1 and for Paper 2 will be given to the candidate along with an overall pass or fail award.
    - Part 1 exam:
        It is aimed to test candidates' application of knowledge to clinical practice
        It involves two computer-based exam papers:
        - Paper A covers clinically applied dental science and clinically applied human disease
        - Paper B covers aspects of clinical dentistry, including law and ethics and health and safety.
    - Each paper lasts 3 hours and consists of multiple short answer questions (extended matching questions and single best answer questions)
    - A candidate must pass both papers in order to progress to Part 2
    - The result will be sent to the candidate by email within 20 working days of the examination
    - The ORE candidates will have to pass Part 2 within 5 years of first sitting Part 1
    - Part 2 exam:
        It is aimed to demonstrate practical clinical skills of the candidate
        It consists of 4 components
        An operative test on a dental manikin: The test involves three procedures over a period of three hours which include preparation and restoration of teeth, etc. to evaluate operative skills
        An objective structured clinical examination: In this test, the candidate visits a series of maximum 20 stations for a period of 2 hours which test their clinical skills. It comprises of history-taking and assessment, communication skills, judgment and decision making, ethics and attitudes, and clinical examination
        A diagnostic and treatment planning exercise: This encompasses an actor who will provide an appropriate history with relevant information such as photographs, radiographs, study models or results of other special tests. The exercise does not include examination and may involve any of the above aspects of clinical dentistry
        A practical examination in medical emergencies (ME): The candidate is evaluated on two parameters namely, a structured scenario-based oral and demonstration of single handed cardiopulmonary resuscitation
        The exam results will be sent to the candidate by email within 20 working days of the exam.

ANNEXURE 3

CONTACT INFORMATION

Address: General Dental Council
                37 Wimpole Street
                London WIG 8DQ
                Phone No.: 02078873800
                Fax: 02072243294
Minicom: 1800102078873800 (via Type Talk)
Email: information@gdc-uk.org
Web: www.gdc-uk.org

ANNEXURE 4

APPLICATION FORM FOR REGISTERING AS A DENTIST WITH THE GENERAL DENTAL COUNCIL (OVERSEAS QUALIFIED)

Section 1: Registration Details (Please complete in BLOCK letters)

The details that you enter in this section will be your registered details. Your name and your qualification(s) will appear in the register and will be available to the public on our website or on request. We will not disclose to the public any other personal details you provide. Please note that the general dental council may choose to publish your full registered address in the future.

Registration number: *(office use only)*

Title: ☐ Mr ☐ Mrs ☐ Ms ☐ Miss

Last name:

First name:

Address:

Postcode:

Gender: ☐ M ☐ F

Date of birth: D D M M Y Y

Nationality: *(please see guidance)*

Other contact detail

To ensure we are able to process your application promptly, please provide contact telephone numbers and an email address. These details will not be made available to

Home phone:

Work phone:

Mobile phone:

Email address:

Dental Qualification/s	Awarded by	Awarded on

The above details are correct and my name has not been entered in the dentists' register before.

Signed: .... **Date:**

☐ **Return of documents**
Please tick if you would you like your documents returned. There is a £10 fee, payable by debit/credit card online through eGDC at the time the registration fee is paid.

☐ **Amendments countersigned**
Any amendments made on the application form or supporting documents must be countersigned. Do not use correction fluid.

Section 2: Character Reference *(See guidance notes)*

The character reference must be completed by someone who has known the applicant for at least a year and must not be signed by a member of the applicant's family.

The character referee must also sign the back of the passport photograph. By doing so, they are certifying that the image is a true likeness of the applicant.

Full name of applicant:

I (full name of referee):

Professional position:

Address of referee:

Postcode:

Declaration

I certify that I am not a relative of the applicant. I have known the applicant for at least 1 year and that they are the person they declare themselves to be, and: (please tick an option)

☐ **(a)** Am satisfied that, to the best of my knowledge that they are of good character and fit for registration

OR

☐ **(b)** The GDC should be aware of the following details of character which might affect their suitability for registration (please use a separate sheet if required).

Signed: .... Date: ☐☐☐☐☐☐☐☐

This certificate is only valid for three months from the date on which it was signed

Section 3: English language *(See guidance notes)*

The Dentists Act 1984 requires the general dental council to be satisfied that all applicants have the necessary knowledge of English prior to entry to our registers.

As an applicant who qualified from outside the European Economic Area (EEA) you must provide evidence of your language competence when you submit your application. We will assess your English language evidence in conjunction with our assessment of your qualifications, knowledge and skill.

Please refer to our guidance on how you can demonstrate the necessary knowledge of English language and the types of evidence we are likely to accept.

You must provide recent, objective evidence that you can read, write and interact effectively in English with patients, relatives and other healthcare professionals in relation to your role as a dental professional.

I confirm that I have read and understood the English language requirements

Please tick: ☐ Yes

Please tick as appropriate the evidence that you are submitting:

☐ International English Language Testing System certificate

☐ A recent primary dental qualification that has been taught and examined in English

☐ A recent pass in a language test for registration with a regulatory authority in a country where the first and native language is English

☐ Recent experience of practising in a country where the first and native language is English

☐ Other (please provide details in the box below)

Section 4: Health and Self-Declaration *(See guidance notes)*

Before answering the first two questions, please read the general dental councils health self-certification guidance.

1. Are you a carrier of any infectious disease, blood-borne virus or other transmissible disease or do you have any reason to believe that any such infectious or transmissible disease may be present?

   ☐ Yes ☐ No

   If yes, please give details of the infectious or transmissible disease or blood-borne virus on a separate sheet.

2. Do you have any health condition which may affect or has affected the safety of patients you treat and/or those you work with, and/or your ability to do your job safely?

   ☐ Yes ☐ No

   If yes, please give details of the medical condition on a separate sheet. If the GDC has any concerns about your health, we may need to obtain further information from any medical practitioner who is treating you. If you have answered yes to any of the statements above, please provide the full name and contact details for your occupational health practitioner and/or any other medical practitioner who is treating you.

3. Have you been convicted of a criminal offence and/or cautioned (other than a protected conviction or caution) and/or are you currently the subject of any police investigations which might lead to a conviction or a caution in the UK or any other country?

   Note: Dentists are exempt from The Rehabilitation of Offenders Act 1974. You must therefore tell us about prosecutions or convictions, including those that might otherwise be considered 'spent' under this act (other than a protected conviction or caution). Protected convictions and cautions are defined in the Rehabilitation of Offenders Act 1974 (Exceptions) Order 1975 (Amendment) (England and Wales) Order 2013.

   ☐ Yes ☐ No

If yes, please give details on a separate sheet, including the approximate date, offence, authority which dealt with the offence and any circumstances that you would want the Council to be aware of in consideration of your application.

4. To the best of your knowledge, have you been or are you currently subject to any proceedings by a regulatory or licensing body in the UK or any other country?

☐ Yes ☐ No

If yes, please give details on a separate sheet of the nature of the proceedings undertaken, or contemplated, including approximate date of proceedings, country where proceedings were undertaken and the name and address of the licensing or regulatory body concerned.

5. **Declaration by all applicants**

I consent to you contacting my character referee and give consent to contact any of the health practitioners whose names have been provided.

The Dentist Act 1984 includes a requirement for registrants to hold insurance or indemnity cover.

I have in place, or will have in place at the point at which I practise in the UK, insurance or indemnity arrangements appropriate to the areas of my practice. (please tick) ☐ **Yes**

I acknowledge that my professional registration will be at risk if I knowingly make a false statement in this declaration and undertaking, or if I act in any way which is incompatible with it. I further acknowledge and accept that should a question as to whether or not I have acted in accordance with this declaration and undertaking arise, it may be used by the GDC in fitness to practise proceedings against me.

I will advise the GDC of any future criminal proceedings/police investigations, convictions or cautions and any future health conditions which arise which affect the safety of patients I treat and/or those they work with, and/or my ability to do my job safely.

I have read and understand the General Dental Council's standards and health self-certification guidance and I will adhere to this guidance.

The information I have given here is true.

Signed: .... Date: ☐☐☐☐☐☐☐☐

Section 5: Payment for this Application Only

I wish to pay by: (please tick)

☐ **Credit/Debit Card**

Credit/debit card payments can only be made on our e-payment portal.

We will notify you by email when you can make the payment. This will normally be when your application has been processed and we can proceed with your registration.

In order to pay by credit or debit card you must have access to the internet and an email account.

Please provide the following details so that we can contact you. Please ensure that you check your email account regularly and contact us should your email address or phone number change.

Please make payment within 14 days of receiving your payment request form, otherwise your application may be delayed or returned to you.

Email address:

☐☐☐☐☐☐☐☐☐☐☐☐☐☐☐☐☐☐☐☐☐☐☐☐☐

Preferred contact telephone number:

☐☐☐☐☐☐☐☐☐☐☐☐☐☐☐☐☐☐☐☐☐☐☐☐☐

Payment for Future Annual Retention Fees

Bank/Building Society to pay by Direct Debit

Please complete this form if you wish to pay your future annual retention fees by Direct Debit. The completed form must be received by 30th September of the year prior to the year you are paying for.

Please complete form in BLOCK CAPITALS using a ball point pen

Name(s) of Account Holder(s) to be debited

☐☐☐☐☐☐☐☐☐☐☐☐☐☐☐☐☐☐☐☐☐☐☐☐

☐☐☐☐☐☐☐☐☐☐☐☐☐☐☐☐☐☐☐☐☐☐☐☐

Bank or Building Society Account No

☐☐☐☐☐☐☐☐☐☐☐☐☐☐☐☐☐☐☐☐☐☐☐☐

Branch Sort Code

☐☐☐☐☐☐

Name and full postal address of your United Kingdom Bank or Building Society

[   ]

Direct Debit Originators No

| 7 | 5 | 8 | 5 | 7 | 8 |

Your GDC registration number *(for office use only)*

☐☐☐☐☐☐☐☐

Instruction to your Bank or Building Society: Please pay the General Dental Council Direct Debits from the account detailed on this instruction subject to the safeguards assured by the Direct Debit Guarantee. I understand that this instruction may remain with the General Dental Council and if so, details will be passed electronically to my Bank/Building Society.

Signature of account holder(s): .... Date: ☐☐☐☐☐☐☐☐

Signature of account holder(s): .... Date: ☐☐☐☐☐☐☐☐

Banks and Building Societies may not accept Direct Debit instructions for some types of account.

The Direct Debit Guarantee

- This Guarantee is offered by all banks and building societies that accept instructions to pay Direct Debits
- If there are any changes to the amount, date or frequency of your Direct Debit the General Dental Council will notify you 10 working days in advance of your account being debited or as otherwise agreed. If you request the General Dental Council to collect a payment, confirmation of the amount and date will be given to you at the time of the request
- If an error is made in the payment of your Direct Debit by the General Dental Council or your bank or building society you are entitled to a full and immediate refund of the amount paid from your bank or building society
- If you receive a refund you are not entitled to, you must pay it back when the General Dental Council asks you to
- You can cancel a Direct Debit at any time by simply contacting your bank or building society. Written confirmation may be required. Please also notify us.

Guidance Notes for Completing This Form

(Advice for applicants and those signing the Character Section)
Please note we cannot accept any documents or application forms by fax or email. The documents and forms must be posted and addressed to the Registration Team, (New Registrations), General Dental Council, 43-45 Portman Square, London, W1H 6HN.

The Registrar must be satisfied that applicants for registration are fit to practise dentistry before registering them. We need:

- a signed character reference; and
- a declaration about health and character filled in by the applicant

Publication of your personal details

The general dental council's register rules and regulations require us to keep a register of the names of everyone who is registered with us. The registers are public documents and are published on our website. The dentists and dental care professionals registers contain the names and other information about a registrant the general dental council is legally obliged to make public.

Registered addresses are not public information. Please note that the general dental council may choose to publish your full registered address in the future, therefore the general dental council recommends that your registered address is either a business or a practice address. Using your business or practice address will assist, if necessary, with local resolution of complaints.
It is important to note that any formal notices issued by the general dental council will be sent to your registered address, therefore you must have access to correspondence at this address.

Change of Address

Please tell us if you change your address. If you do not do so, this could lead to important communications and notices, including those relating to the annual fee, going astray. To tell us of a change of address please call the Registration Team on 0845 222 4141 or email registration@gdc-uk.org.

Keeping Your Name on The Register

To keep your name on the Register you must pay your annual fee each year. We will notify you when your fee is due. You must pay this fee by law whether or not you have received the reminder.

Return of Documents

An administration charge of £10 should be added to the registration fee if you wish us to return any documents you have submitted.

Character Reference

If you are applying for registration within one year of graduation, the character reference must be provided by the head of your dental training school. If you are applying for registration more than one year after graduation, the character reference can be provided by another professional such as a doctor, a dentist or a lawyer who has known you for over one year. The character reference cannot be provided by a member of your family.
The general dental council will only use the information provided by the referee to assess fitness for registration. The person writing the character reference should include any information about your character or health which might raise a question about your suitability for registration. The Registrar will decide whether or not the information is relevant and whether any further inquiries need to be made.

Evidence of English language

The Dentists Act 1984 requires the general dental council to be satisfied that all applicants have the necessary knowledge of English prior to entry to our registers.

If the general dental council is satisfied about your knowledge of English from your initial application for registration we will not request further evidence or information.

If the general dental council is not satisfied that you have produced sufficient evidence that you have the necessary knowledge of English we will request further evidence and/or information. Please refer to "Evidence of English language competence: guidance for applicants" document, which can be found on the general dental council website (www.gdc-uk.org) for types of evidence we are likely to accept as demonstrating that a dental professional has the necessary knowledge of English.

If this further evidence still does not satisfy us, we will direct you to undertake a test before we register you. The test that we will direct you to undertake is the International English Language Testing System exam. You must achieve the pass scores relevant to your profession.

Health and Character Self-Declaration

Please read the general dental council's health self-certification guidance before completing the questions relating to your health within the self-declaration.

You must inform the general dental council if you have any condition present which might impair your fitness to practise. Having such a condition will not necessarily mean we will refuse registration.

If the registrar is satisfied that you are correctly managing any relevant health condition, by taking steps which will avoid any risk to patients and will ensure you have the ability to perform your job safely, you will not be refused registration on health grounds.

The registrar may refuse to register someone with a serious impairment (for example, substance abuse or serious mental illness) who cannot be trusted to self-regulate, although they can reapply if their condition improves.

You should tell us about any relevant condition on a separate sheet. While not a definitive list, examples of conditions we would expect to know about are:

- Uncorrected visual impairment
- The presence of any infectious disease, blood-borne virus (tuberculosis, hepatitis B) or other transmissible disease
- Prescribed medication which substantially impairs the immune response
- Psychiatric disease or problems
- Alcohol or drug related problems.

Because dentists are exempt from the UK Rehabilitation of Offenders Act 1974, you must tell us about any previous or pending prosecutions or convictions, including those considered "spent" under this Act (other than a protected conviction or caution). Protected convictions and cautions are defined in the Rehabilitation of Offenders Act 1974 (Exceptions) Order 1975 (Amendment) (England and Wales) Order 2013. We also need to know if you have been the subject of any professional proceedings in the past, or if any are being contemplated, by a regulatory or licensing body in the UK or any other country.

You will also need to advise the general dental council of any future criminal proceedings/police investigations, convictions or cautions.

We will treat the information you provide in confidence. We will only use it to assess your fitness for registration now and in the future and will only refuse registration on the basis of this information if we are not satisfied about your fitness to practise and or/good character. If you make a false statement, we may refuse your application for registration and/or prosecute you and/or charge you with professional misconduct.

A copy of the general dental council's Standards for the Dental Team is available on our website. It is important that you read and become familiar with the principles it includes. You will be responsible for applying these principles to your daily work and maintaining appropriate standards of personal behaviour.

Making a false declaration to the general dental council is a serious issue. If you declare that you have or will have appropriate indemnity in place and this is found to be false, there is a risk that you may be removed from the general dental council register or be subject to fitness to practise proceedings.

Indemnity

The Dentist Act 1984 includes a requirement for registrants to hold insurance or indemnity cover; it is a condition of registration for all dental professionals to have insurance or indemnity cover.

We understand that those who are not/have not yet registered with the general dental council will not yet have insurance or indemnity cover in place. The declaration on our application form is that you will have indemnity cover in place by the time you start to practise in the UK.

The only types of cover recognised by the general dental council are:
- Dental defence organisation membership – either your own membership or cover provided by your employer's membership;
- Professional indemnity insurance held by you or your employer; or
- NHS/Crown indemnity.

Your insurance or indemnity cover must be appropriate to the areas of your practice. If you are relying on arrangements made by your employer, you must check the indemnity position with them. All registrants must know the details of their indemnity cover when they start practising, and be able to provide these to the general dental council if asked to do so.

The general dental council will undertake audits of compliance with these requirements on a regular basis. You will need to make sure you have, or can access, the details of the policy should you need to provide them.

For more information on insurance or indemnity cover please see:
www.gdc-uk.org/dentalprofessionals/standards/pages/indemnity.aspx

Identity Document

The identity document that you submit with your application must be a colour photocopy correctly certified. This document should be an A4 size page.
The image of your identity document should be clear with the certification statement not overlapping any part of the identity document.

If you are submitting a certified photocopy of your passport it is important that the machine readable zone is clear.

Only one type of identity document should be provided on a single page. If you are submitting two types of identity documents, these should appear on two separate pages.

Passport Photo

You must supply us with a recent passport sized photo that has been certified by your character referee on the back of the photo.
The requirement for individuals applying for registration or restoration with the general dental council to submit a passport photo is aligned with the **UK Government requirements.***

You must make sure that your passport photo meets these requirements otherwise there may be delays to your application.

Your photo must be professionally printed and be 45 millimetres (mm) high by 35 mm wide—the standard size used in photo booths in the UK.
Your photo must be:
- In colour on plain white photographic paper
- Taken against a plain cream or light grey background
- Taken within the last month
- Clear and in focus
- Without any tears or creases
- Unaltered by computer software.

The image of you - from the crown of your head to your chin - must be between 29 mm and 34 mm high (see example below).

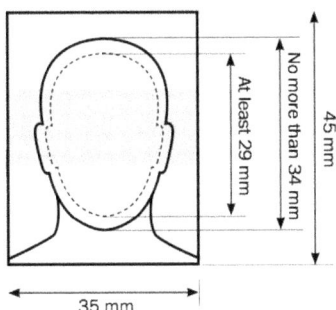

*Contains public sector information licensed under the Open Government Licence v3.0.

Other Documents Required

Please refer to the accompanying guidance information for documentation required to be submitted.

Important note: Any amendments, corrections or alterations made on the application form or supporting documents must be countersigned. Do not use correction fluid on any part of the application. Applications with amendments which have not been countersigned or where correction fluid has been used may not be accepted and your application may be returned to you as a result.

Continuing Professional Development

You must also undertake continuing professional development in 5 yearly cycles, as a condition of continued registration. Further information is available on our website www.gdc-uk.org

Registration fees

Please check our website or call the Registration Team on +44 (0)20 7167 6000 for current registration fees.

General

Please return your completed form, and your documents to the Registration Team (New Registrations), General Dental Council, 43-45 Portman Square, London, W1H 6HN. Please refer to section 4 of the form for payment by credit/debit card. When you have been registered you will receive a certificate of registration.

It is a criminal offence for anyone, other than a registered medical practitioner, to practise dentistry without being registered with the General Dental Council.

If the registrar is in any doubt about an application for reasons other than failure to comply with the continuing professional development requirements, they reserve the right to require you to attend an interview in person at the Council's offices.

Equality Monitoring Form

The GDC is committed to promoting and developing equality and diversity in all our work. We want to be sure that our policies and ways of working are fair and do not discriminate against individuals or groups. To help us to monitor the effectiveness of our policies and practices we ask you to complete the monitoring form. This information will be treated in the strictest confidence under the Data Protection Act 1998 and will be used to produce statistics to enable the GDC to look at the diversity profile of our staff, registrants and others with whom we work. Through this we can check a variety of processes to ensure equality and address issues as they arise.

AGE

☐ 16-21 ☐ 22-30 ☐ 31-40 ☐ 41-50 ☐ 51-60 ☐ 61-65 ☐ Over 65 ☐ Prefer not to say

DISABILITY Do you consider yourself to have a disability?

☐ Yes ☐ No ☐ Prefer not to say

(The Equality Act 2010 defines disability as a physical or mental impairment which has substantial long-term effect on a person's ability to carry out normal day to day activities).

RACE

White
☐ British
☐ Irish
☐ Any other White background (please specify)

Black or Black British
☐ African
☐ Caribbean
☐ Any other Black background (please specify)

Asian or Asian British
☐ Bangladeshi
☐ Indian
☐ Pakistani
☐ Any other Asian background (please specify)

Mixed Ethnic Background
☐ White and Asian
☐ White and Black African
☐ White and Black Caribbean
☐ White and Chinese
☐ Any other mixed ethnic background (please specify)

Chinese or any other ethnic group
☐ Chinese
☐ Any other ethnic background (please specify)

☐ Prefer not to say

SEX

☐ Female ☐ Male ☐ Prefer not to say

GENDER IDENTITY – is your gender identity the same as the gender you were assigned at birth?

☐ Yes ☐ No ☐ Prefer not to say

RELIGION/BELIEF

☐ Buddhist ☐ Christian ☐ Hindu ☐ None
☐ Jewish ☐ Muslim ☐ Sikh ☐ Prefer not to say
☐ Other religion/faith (please specify)

SEXUAL ORIENTATION

☐ Bisexual ☐ Gay man ☐ Gay woman ☐ Heterosexual ☐ Prefer not to say

MARITAL STATUS

☐ Civil partnership ☐ Divorced ☐ Married

☐ Separated ☐ Single ☐ Widowed ☐ Prefer not to say

Advice for Applicants who have Completed the Overseas Registration Examination

This advice sheet is intended to assist your application for full registration after successful completion of overseas registration examination and have received notification from the general dental council for the same.

APPLICATION PROCESS

Complete Application

- The application is considered complete when all of the necessary documents have been provided according to the Council's standards
- Any document having a 3 month time limit must be in date when the application is complete and the registration is being issued
- This application form, accompanying documents and registration fee should be posted to:

  Registration Team (New Registrations)
  General Dental Council
  43-45 Portman Square
  London W1H 6HN

Documents Required for Application to be Processed

- Completed application form
- The fee
- If applicable, you may need to provide the following supporting evidence
  - An original certificate of good standing
  - Original or certified evidence of the applicant's current passport
  - Original or certified evidence of the primary dental qualification
  - Translations
  - Evidence of name change
  - English language evidence.

Completed Application Form

- All sections of the application form must be completed
- Section 1:
  - Registered details of the candidate will be entered among which name and qualifications will appear in the register which will be available

to the public on the general dental council website whereas all other details provided in this section will not be available to the public.
- Section 2:
  - The Character Reference must not be more than three months old and should be provided by another professional such as dentist, lawyer, or doctor who has known you for over one year and who is not a member of your family.
- Section 3:
  - The Dentists Act 1984 necessitates the general dental council to be satisfied that all applicants have the necessary knowledge of English prior to entry to our registers
  - Submission of evidence of passing the International English Language Testing System exam at the relevant level within two years of a complete application for registration is satisfactory.
- Section 4:
  - The Health and Character Self-Declaration must be completed and signed by the applicant.

The Fee

- It is important to consider that the amount to be paid depends when the application is received by the Council instead of the issuing of the registration
- The relevant fees are shown on the website www.gdc-uk.org
- The registration fee can be made by debit or credit card and once registered; the payment is made by the end of December of each year to remain registered in the following year.

Certificate of Good Standing

- The certificate of good standing must be issued by the competent dental authority in the country in which the dentist has last worked
- The original certificate of good standing must be current and less than three months old.

Passport and Primary Dental Qualification

- The Council will only accept the original or certified copies of the current passport for evidence of nationality and identity
- The Council will only accept the original or certified copies of the primary dental qualification
- Full name must correspond on all documents. In case of change of name, documentary evidence, e.g. a certified copy of the marriage certificate should be included.

Translations for any Document not in English Must Follow the Guidelines

- The certified translation must be produced by a qualified translator which must be bonded to a photocopy of the specific document
- The Council will not accept a translation of a translation and translator should provide his contact details.

Certified Copies Must Meet All of the Following Criteria

- The document must be a first generation photocopy
- The person certifying the copy should provide the contact details of the person certifying, including the name, signature and address and confirmation in English writing that he has inspected the original documents
- The person certifying the documents cannot be the applicant himself, or his spouse.

PROCESSING TIMES

- Please refer to the Council's website www.gdc-uk.org for current processing times
- An Original Registration Certificate will be sent to the address of candidate upon successful inclusion to the Register to practise dentistry in UK
- Once registered, candidate must have professional indemnity to practise in UK.

CONTACT DETAILS

- In case of query
- Please contact the general dental council Registration Department on Tel: +44 (0) 20 7167 6100; Fax: +44 (0)20 7167 6100; Email: registration@gdc-uk.org.

REGISTRATION FOR OVERSEAS QUALIFIED PRACTITIONERS IN AUSTRALIA

General Registration

There are several pathways to General Registration for dentists with overseas qualifications:
1. Dentists who are registered to practise in New Zealand under Trans-Tasman mutual recognition
2. Dentists with eligible bachelor degrees from the United Kingdom, Republic of Ireland or New Zealand
3. Dentists with eligible degrees from Canada and compliant with the 'additional requirements'
4. Dentists with other qualifications: (a) Complete an Australian approved program of study; or (b) undertake the examination procedure conducted by the Australian Dental Council (ADC).

Pathway of Registration for Overseas Qualified Dental Practitioner

1. Initial assessments for dental practitioner

The dentist assessment process assesses the knowledge, judgement, clinical skills, and professional competencies of overseas-trained dentists seeking eligibility to apply for registration with the Dental Board of Australia (DBA), and whose qualifications are not otherwise approved for registration. The format of the assessment and examination process has been approved for the purposes of registration in Australia. It consists of three stages: an initial assessment, a written examination, and a practical examination.

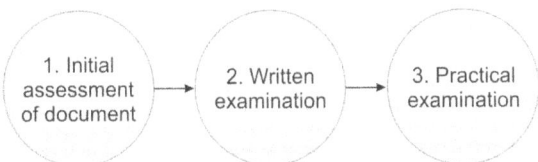

An initial assessment can be completed at any time of year by submitting an initial assessment of professional qualification application form for the relevant profession.

Once the application form and supporting documents have been received, applicants will be assigned an ADC candidate reference number. This number should always be used when you contact the ADC.

Timeframe: Approximately 8 weeks, not including time taken to submit any additional documents.

Cost: AUD $610

Process

- Download and complete an application form
- Submit application form as well as a completed application form, you are required to submit a clear, certified copy of your:
  - current passport (high quality color copy)
  - evidence of change of name (if applicable)
  - dental qualification, official certificate or testamur
  - academic transcript
  - internship certificate
  - evidence of registration or license to practise dentistry
  - two written professional references
  - evidence of practise or work history as a registered or licensed dentist.
- Receive an initial assessment outcome from the ADC: There are three possible outcomes—
  1. Your application was successful and you are now eligible to proceed to the written examination. A successful initial assessment does not expire.
  2. Your application is incomplete and you are required to submit additional information for further assessment.
  3. Your application was unsuccessful and you are ineligible to proceed with the ADC process.

2. Dentist written examination

The written examination is the second stage of the ADC assessment process. The Australian Dental Council (ADC) written examination for dentists is a computer delivered examination designed to test a candidate's knowledge of the science and practise of the dentistry. The examination also assesses the application of clinical judgement and reasoning skills relevant to dental practice in Australia.

The two-day examination is delivered by Pearson VUE on behalf of the ADC. Each computer-based examination consists of four papers each containing 80 scenario-based and single-best answer multiple choice questions. The examination is held in multiple locations in Australia and overseas. You should carefully read the written examination handbook for a comprehensive description of the format and requirements of the written examination. The handbook can be downloaded here.

Timeframe: Approximately five months

Cost: AUD $2,000

Time frames

Activity	Time frame
Written examination application period	Approximately 3 to 4 months before the examination
Authorisation to test emails sent	8 weeks before examination
Pearson VUE bookings open	8 weeks before examination
Pearson VUE bookings close	5 weeks before examination
Notification of examination results	6 weeks after examination
Application for verifications and appeals close	28 days from notification of results

To apply for a written examination, you must complete and submit a written examination application form, along with the relevant supporting documentation and full payment. The application should be downloaded and printed as a hard copy prior to completion. The application form contains detailed guidelines to assist you in completing the form. All supporting documentation must adhere to the ADC certification of document guidelines. Incorrectly certified documents will result in delays, or in the application being declined. Post your application and supporting documents to the address specified on the application form. You will receive an email notification when your application has been received.

Book a written examination

If your application is successful, the Australian Dental Council (ADC) will issue you with a Written examination authorisation letter. This letter contains information on the opening of your booking period and instructions on how to book your examination venue through the Pearson VUE booking system.

Written examination results will be released via the ADC candidate portal. Results are released approximately 6 weeks after the examination date. To be awarded a pass in the written examination, candidates must pass all four papers in one examination session. Your results profile will provide a grade for each paper attempted. Grades A, B, and C are pass grades and D and E are fail grades. A pass in the written examination is valid for 3 years and there are no limits on the number of times you can attempt the examination.

3. Dentist practical examination

The practical examination is the third and final stage of the ADC assessment process. ADC practical examination is the platform for candidates to demonstrate that they are competent to practise safely as a dentist in Australia. The practical examination assesses candidates across the range of the entry level competencies of the newly qualified dentist. The competencies can be viewed here.

The examination is held over 2 days; a technical skills day and a clinical skills day. Examinations are held most weeks of the year at the ADC examination center. Upon successful completion of the practical examination, candidates are eligible to apply for registration with the Dental Board of Australia (DBA).

You should carefully read the practical examination handbook for dentists for a comprehensive description of the format and requirements of the practical examination. The handbook can be downloaded here.

Timeframe: Approximately 6 to 9 months

Cost: AUD $4,500

Time frames

Activity	Time frame
Practical examination application period	At least 3 months prior to examination
Notification of application receipt	Within 2 weeks of receipt of application
Notification of allocated practical examination date	Within 6 weeks of practical examination application period
Notification of examination results	6 weeks after examination

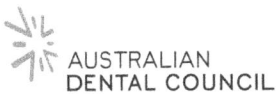

APPLICATION FOR PRACTICAL EXAMINATION–DENTIST
FORM PED V2

REFERENCE NO. [z   ]
For ADC use only

Please complete the application form in English. Please complete in **CAPITAL LETTERS** using a blue or **black** pen.

Please post the application form, including the necessary supporting documentation, to the Australian Dental Council (ADC) once completed. As we need to assess the form and the certified supporting documentation, we cannot accept scanned or emailed application forms.

Sections accompanied by ✐ indicate sections where supporting documentation is required as evidence of the information you have supplied.

Please ensure the declaration in section F is signed before submitting your application. Applications which are not signed, will not be processed.

Processing time for your application: **Please allow a turnaround of approximately four weeks from date of receipt.**

SECTION A. PHOTOGRAPHIC IDENTIFICATION

Please supply two **certified**, colour passport sized photographs of yourself for the purposes of identification.

The photographs must be less than nine months old and include the **certification date**.

Please staple photograph here ✐

SECTION B. APPLICANT DETAILS

ADC reference no.	z
Surname or family name	
Given name (s)	
Middle name (s)	
Previous name (s)	
Date of birth (DD/MM/YYYY)	☐☐ / ☐☐ / ☐☐☐☐

Please provide the correct address for the candidate named in the section above.

Number and street

Suburb/Town/City Postcode

Country

Home phone number + ☐☐ ☐☐☐ Mobile number + ☐☐ ☐☐☐
(Including country code) (Including country code)

Candidate email address

SECTION C. AUTHORITY TO ACT

You may nominate a person, or an agent, to receive all correspondence regarding the practical examination on your behalf. If you choose to do so, you will need to complete an *Authority to act* form.

Do you wish to nominate someone to act on your behalf?

Please mark ☒ one option only.
- ☐ Yes. I have complete and attached an *Authority to act* from and understand all correspondence regarding the practical examination will be forwarded to my chosen nominee.
- ☐ No, I do not wish to have someone act on my behalf.

SECTION D. APPLICATION DATES

Examination dates and relevant application periods for practical examination sessions and will be provided on the ADC website (www.adc.org.au). Applications will be accepted from candidates who:
- ☐ Meet the eligibility criteria for the examination period, and
- ☐ Do not have an existing practical examination booking, pending practical examination results, or pending appeals.

Applications will not be accepted from candidates who do not meet the above criteria or if they are received outside the application period.

SECTION E. RESIDENCY STATUS

a. Are you a permanent resident or citizen of Australia? ☐ Yes ☐ No
   Please mark ☒ one option only.

b. If you are not an Australian permanent resident or citizen, are you planning to migrate to Australia? ☐ Yes ☐ No
   Please mark ☒ one option only.

SECTION F. DECLARATION

Please read and ensure you understand the following declaration before signing.

- ❏ I have read the *Practical Examination Handbook for Dentists* and understand the requirements of the practical examination
- ❏ I agree to be available for my allocated practical examination session and understand failure to sit my allocated session is considered a withdrawal under the *Australian Dental Council withdrawal process*.
- ❏ I understand the enclosed examination fee is non-refundable in the event of a failure.
- ❏ I understand under the *Australian Dental Council withdrawal process*, a financial penalty will be incurred if I withdraw from the practical examination session allocated.
- ❏ I agree to inform the ADC of any changes to my circumstances or details via the *Notification of change of contact details* form.
- ❏ I have read the explanatory notes for this application and understand the requirements of applying for this examination.
- ❏ I understand if I do not complete all relevant sections of this application form, provide all necessary supporting documentation or pay the relevant examination fee, there may be a delay in the processing, or refusal of, this application.
- ❏ I understand the ADC reserves the right to contact me for further documentation in order to process this application.
- ❏ I am the person named in this application and all attached documents.
- ❏ The information and documentation provided in the submission of this application form is true and correct.
- ❏ I give consent to the ADC to make enquiries and/or exchange information with the relevant authorities of any Australian state or territory, or other country, regarding my qualifications and/or practice as a dentist or otherwise regarding matters relevant to this application.
- ❏ I give consent to the ADC to contact me for quality control, educational and/or research purposes.

Candidate signature

Date (DD/MM/YYYY)

SECTION G. PAYMENT

Applications are not processed until the practical examination fee of **AUD$4,500** is paid in full. A receipt will be issued upon clearance of payment.

Payment by bank cheque or Australian Money Order	Payment by credit card
Payment type ☐ Bank cheque ☐ Australian Money Order (AMO) Payment by bank cheque or AMO **must** be made in Australian dollars only. **Please note we are unable to accept cheques from the State Bank of India/Bank of India, or those with adhesive tape on the cheque face.**	Credit card type ☐ Visa ☐ Master Card Card Number ☐☐ ☐☐ ☐☐ ☐☐ Name on card Card expiry date (MM/YYYY) ☐☐ / ☐☐☐☐ Cardholder signature

EXPLANATORY NOTES AND CHECKLIST

Introduction

All personal information included in this application will be handled in accordance with the *Australian Privacy Act*. Details may be verified with, or provided to, other agencies where necessary, or required by law.

Please take the time to carefully review your application and ensure all certified documentation is provided before submitting it to the ADC.

A *complete* application includes the required, correctly certified documentation. If time permits, you will be notified in writing if any additional information is needed to process your application. Incomplete applications will result in processing delays or refusal of your application.

You will be notified in writing of the outcome of your application and the next steps in the process. In order to prevent delays, and ensure you are updated on the states of your application, an up-to-date email address must be provided.

Certification

The ADC asks you provide certified copies of any documentation required as part of your application. Failure to provide correctly certified copies can result in a processing delay or refusal of your application.

To prevent application processing delays, please ensure all accompanying documentation is certified in line with the Certification guidelines available at adc.org.au

Please do not send original documents to the ADC as part of your application. The ADC will not return any original documents submitted as part of the application process.

Translation of Documents

Any documentation provided to the ADC, which is written in a language other than English, must be accompanied by an English translation.

The ADC reserves the right to request applicants provide certified translations completed by a National Accreditation Authority for Translators and Interpreters (NAATI), formally known as Level 3, accredited translator.

All translated documentation must include the translator's details, such as their name and address, in English. Furthermore, if the document certification statement has been completed in a language other than English, this must also be translated.

Identity/Change of Name

You must state your full legally registered name **exactly** as it appears in your passport.

If your name is different to the one displayed in your passport, official documentation showing the link to your previous name (e.g. a marriage certificate) must be supplied. The ADC does not accept affidavits/statutory declarations for this purpose.

Applicant's Personal Contact Details

Section B of this application must be completed to ensure you receive all communication relevant to the practical exam.

Re-issuing of documentation/correspondence will incur an administrative fee.

Agents

The ADC will deal directly with you throughout the practical examination process. Under Australian privacy legislation, the ADC is prohibited from discussing your application with third parties unless specifically authorised to do so.

If you want someone else, such as a family member or other agent, to communicate with the ADC on your behalf, you will need to complete an Authority to Act form. The Authority to Act form can be accessed via the ADC website adc.org.au

Once this form has been processed, all correspondence will be sent to your nominated third party.

Allocation

We expect to offer a seat in an examination held during the period of February to April 2019.

Application Dates

Applications for practical examination sessions announced on our website are open to candidates who:
- meet the eligibility criteria for the examination period, and
- do not have an existing practical examination booking, pending practical examination results, or pending appeals.

Once an application period has closed, successful candidates will be allocated an examination date and notified within 4 weeks of the application period closing date.

In fairness to all candidates, we cannot consider applications received outside the assigned application period or from candidates not meeting the eligibility criteria.

Payment

If you are paying by Visa or Master Card, please ensure there are sufficient funds in your account to cover the fee transaction. The ADC will only attempt to process the fee payment from your nominated credit card once.

Examination Sessions

Practical examinations will be undertaken at the ADC Examination Centre at Level 6, 469 La Trobe Street, Melbourne.

Each practical examination will be held over two days. Examinations will be held twice a week, most weeks of the year.

All visa and travel arrangements must be arranged by you. It is your responsibility to ensure you are available to travel at the time of your practical examination.

If necessary, you should seek the advice of the Department of Home Affairs in your state or territory. Visit homeaffairs.gov.au for more information. The ADC will confirm your examination place in writing. It is recommended all travel and accommodation requirements are made once written confirmation is received.

English Language Test–OET and IELTS Results

You are not required to provide evidence of English language proficiency to sit the **ADC Practical** Examination.

Please be advised, on completion of the ADC process, evidence of English language skills may be required for registration purposes by AHPRA (ahpra.gov.au) or for migration purposes by the Department of Home Affairs (homeaffairs.gov.au).

We advise you consult these organisations for further information regarding English requirements.

Withdrawal from the examination

If you withdraw from an examination, you must advise ADC in writing via the *Notification of Withdrawal from an ADC Examination* form available via adc.org.au

The ADC does not accept withdrawal statements via email or telephone. For further details, please refer to the Practical Examination Handbook. Applications and examination fees are non-transferable.

Please note:

Failure to undertake the examination because of an inability to obtain necessary visas or to arrange travel, etc. will be considered a withdrawal and the withdrawal process will apply.

CHECKLIST

Please check to ensure the following information is completed in your application.

Section A	☐	Two certified colour passport sized photographs.
Section B	☐	All details completed using CAPITAL letters.
	☐	Certified copy of change of name evidence, where applicable.
	☐	Certified copy of relevant passport pages, including signature page.
Section C	☐	*Authority to act* form, if applicable.
Section D	☐	All details acknowledged.
Section E	☐	The ADC asks you indicate your current Australian residency status, or intention to apply for Australian residence. This has no bearing on your application and is for ADC internal use only.
Section F	☐	Read, understood, and signed the declaration.
	☐	If in doubt, please contact the ADC on (03) 9657 1777.
Section G	☐	All payment details disclosed, or cheque provided. **See adc.org.au for more information**.

Post applications and certified documents to: PO Box 13278, Law Courts Vic 8010, Australia

If you plan on sending your documents via courier, please post to Level 6, 469 Latrobe Street, Melbourne Vic 3000.

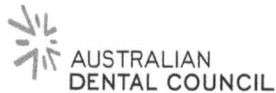
AUSTRALIAN
DENTAL COUNCIL

APPLICATION FOR WRITTEN EXAMINATION
FORM WEA V2

REFERENCE NO. [z]
For ADC use only

Please complete the application form in English. Please complete in **CAPITAL LETTERS** using a **blue** or **black** pen.

Please post the application form, including the necessary supporting documentation, to the Australian Dental Council (ADC) once completed. We cannot accept scanned or emailed application forms.

Sections accompanied by 📎 indicate sections where supporting documentation is required as evidence of the information you have supplied.

Please ensure the declaration in section F is signed before submitting your application. Applications which are not signed will not be processed.

Processing time: **Please allow a turnaround of approximately four weeks from date of application receipt.**

SECTION A. PHOTOGRAPHIC IDENTIFICATION

Please supply two **certified**, colour passport sized photographs of yourself for the purposes of identification.

The photographs must be less than nine months old, include the **certification date** and **details of the certifying officer**

Certification guidelines are available on the ADC website
https://www.adc.org.au/Resource-And-Publications/Assessment-Publications

Please staple photograph here 📎

SECTION B. APPLICANT DETAILS

Please provide certified copy of passport/evidence of any name change ADC 📎

ADC reference no.	z
Surname or family name	
Given name(s)	
Middle name(s)	
Previous name(s)	
Date of birth (DD/MM/YYYY)	☐☐ / ☐☐ / ☐☐☐☐

Please provide the correct address for the candidate named in the section above.

Number and street	
Suburb/Town/City	Postcode
Country	
Home phone number (Including country code)	+ ☐☐ ☐
Mobile number (Including country code)	+ ☐☐ ☐
Candidate email address	

SECTION C. EMERGENCY CONTACT DETAILS

Name (s)	
Relationship to you (e.g. Husband / Wife)	
Home phone number (Including country code)	+ ☐☐ ☐
Mobile number	+ ☐☐ ☐
Email Address	

SECTION D. EXAMINATION CATEGORY

Please indicate ☒ the examination category below.
- ☐ **General dentistry written examination**
- ☐ **Dental hygiene written examination**
- ☐ **Dental therapy written examination**
- ☐ **Dental hygiene and dental therapy combined written examination**
- ☐ **Dental prosthetist written examination**

SECTION E. AUTHORITY TO ACT

You may nominate a person, or an agent, to receive all correspondence regarding the written examination on your behalf. If you choose to do so, you will need to complete an *Authority to act* form.

Do you wish to nominate someone to act on your behalf?

Please mark ☒ one option only.
- ☐ Yes. I have completed and attached an *Authority to act* form and understand all correspondence regarding the written examination will be forwarded to my chosen nominee.
- ☐ No, I do not wish to have someone act on my behalf.

SECTION F. DECLARATION

Please read and ensure you understand the following declaration before signing.

- ❑ I have read the written examination handbook relevant to my profession and understand the requirements of the examination.
- ❑ I accept that the examination fee is non-refundable in the event of failure. I also understand that if I withdraw or fail to sit the examination, a penalty will be incurred according to the withdrawal process detailed in the handbook.
- ❑ I undertake to inform the ADC of any changes to my circumstances or details.
- ❑ I have read the explanatory notes for this application form, and understand all the requirements of applying for this examination.
- ❑ I acknowledge that the ADC may verify documents provided in support of this application as evidence of my identity.
- ❑ I understand that failure to complete all relevant sections of this application form, including all supporting documentation, may result in delaying the processing of this application or refusal of this application.
- ❑ I understand that the ADC reserves the right to require further documentation in order to progress this application.
- ❑ I am the person named in this application and all attached documents.
- ❑ The information and documentation provided in the submission of this application form is true and correct.
- ❑ I give consent to the ADC to make enquiries and/or exchange information with the relevant authorities of any Australian state or territory, or other country, regarding my qualifications and/or practice as a dental practitioner or matters relevant to this application.
- ❑ I give consent to the ADC to contact me for quality control, educational and/or research purposes.

Candidate signature _____

Date of birth (DD/MM/YYYY) ☐☐ / ☐☐ / ☐☐☐☐

SECTION G. PAYMENT

Applications are not processed until the written examination fee is paid in full. A receipt will be issued upon clearance of payment. Refer to the fee schedule available at www.adc.org.au for a list of current fees.

Payment by bank cheque or Australian Money Order	Payment by credit card
	Credit card type
Payment type	❑ Visa
❑ Bank cheque	❑ Master Card
❑ Australian Money Order (AMO)	Card Number
Payment by bank cheque or AMO **must** be made in Australian dollars only.	
	Name on card
Please note we are unable to accept cheques from the State Bank of India/Bank of India, or those with adhesive tape on the cheque face.	Card expiry date (MM/YYYY)
	☐☐ / ☐☐
	Cardholder signature

EXPLANATORY NOTES AND CHECKLIST

Introduction

All personal information included in this application will be handled in accordance with the *Australian Privacy Act*. Details may be verified with, or provided to, other agencies where necessary, or required by law.

Please take the time to carefully review your application and ensure all certified documentation is provided before submitting it to the ADC.

A ***complete*** application includes the required, correctly certified documentation. If time permits, you will be notified in writing if any additional information is needed to process your application. Incomplete applications will result in processing delays or refusal of your application.

You will be notified in writing of the outcome of your application and the next steps in the process. In order to prevent delays, and ensure you are updated on the status of your application, an up-to-date email address must be provided.

Certification

The ADC asks you to provide certified copies of any documentation required as part of your application. Failure to provide correctly certified copies can result in a processing delay or refusal of your application.

To prevent application processing delays, please ensure all accompanying documentation is certified in line with the Certification guidelines available at adc.org.au

Please do not send original documents to the ADC as part of your application. The ADC will not return any original documents submitted as part of the application process.

Translation of Documents

Any documentation provided to the ADC, which is written in a language other than English, must be accompanied by an English translation.

The ADC reserves the right to request applicants provide certified translations completed by a National Accreditation Authority for Translators and Interpreters (NAATI), formally known as Level 3, accredited translators.

All translated documentation must include the translator's details, such as their name and address, in English. Furthermore, if the document certification statement has been completed in a language other than English, this must also be translated.

Identity/Change of Name

You must state your full legally registered name **exactly** as it appears in your passport.

If your name is different to the one displayed in your passport, official documentation showing the link to your previous name (e.g. a marriage certificate) must be supplied. The ADC does not accept affidavits/statutory declarations for this purpose.

Applicant's Personal Contact Details

Section B of this application must be completed to ensure you receive all communication relevant to the written examination.

Re-issuing of documentation/correspondence will incur an administrative fee.

Agents

The ADC will deal directly with you throughout the written examination process. Under Australian privacy legislation, the ADC is prohibited from discussing your application with third parties unless specifically authorised to do so.

If you want someone else, such as a family member or other agent, to communicate with the ADC on your behalf, you will need to complete an *Authority to Act* form. The *Authority to Act* form can be accessed via the ADC website adc.org.au

Once this form has been processed, all correspondence will be sent to your nominated third party.

Application Dates

If you are eligible to sit a written examination, you can submit a written examination application during the published application period. The application period is outlined below.

Examination: 18 & 19 March 2019
Application period: 12 - 30 November 2018

Examination Session

Candidates cannot postpone an examination. If, for any reason, you are unable to attend your nominated session, you will need to withdraw from the examination and reapply. Please refer to the withdrawal information in the written examination handbook relevant to your profession.

Examination Venue

For **general dentistry** candidates, the written examination is delivered by the Pearson VUE in multiple locations in Australia and Overseas.

Whilst every effort is made to accommodate a candidate's venue preference, in some circumstances the requested venue may not be available and an alternative will be offered.

For **dental hygiene, dental therapy and dental prosthetist** candidates, the written examination is delivered in Melbourne, Australia only.

Please note:
All visa and travel arrangements are the responsibility of the candidate. Candidates should ensure that they are able to travel to the venue at the required time.

Payment

If you are paying by Visa or MasterCard, please ensure there are sufficient funds in your account to cover the fee transaction. The ADC will only attempt to process the fee payment from your nominated credit card once.

English languge test—OET and IELTS Results

You are **not required** to provide evidence of English language proficiency to sit the ADC written examination.

The examination is only conducted in English.

Withdrawal from Examination

If you withdraw from an examination, you must advise the ADC in writing *via a Notification of withdrawal* from an ADC examination form available via adc.org.au

The ADC does not accept withdrawal statements via email or telephone. For further details, please refer to the written examination handbook relevant to your profession.

Applications and examination fees are non-transferable.

Please note:
Failure to undertake the examination because of an inability to obtain necessary visas or to arrange travel, etc. will be considered a withdrawal and the withdrawal process will apply.

CHECKLIST

Please check to ensure the following information is completed in your application.

Section A	❏	Two certified colour passport sized photographs.
Section B	❏	All details completed using CAPITAL letters.
	❏	Certified copy of change of name evidence, where applicable.
	❏	Certified copy of relevant passport pages, including signature page.
Section C	❏	Name and contact details of an emergency contact person (no supporting documents required).
Section D	❏	Category selected
Section E	❏	*Authority to act form*, if applicable.
Section F	❏	Read, understood, and signed the declaration. If in doubt, please contact the ADC on (03) 9657 1777.
Section G	❏	All payment details supplied, or cheque provided.

See adc.org.au for more information.

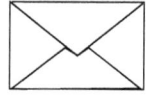

Post applications and certified documents to: PO Box 13278, Law Courts Vic 8010, Australia

If you are sending your documents via courier, please use the ADC physical address: Level 6, 469 La Trobe Street, Melbourne, 3000.

EU GSPR Authorised Reprsentative
Logos Europe, 9 rue Nicolas Poussin
1700, La Rochelle, France
Phone: +33 (0) 6 67 93 73 78
E-mail: contact@logoseurope.eu

www.ingramcontent.com/pod-product-compliance
Ingram Content Group UK Ltd.
Pitfield, Milton Keynes, MK11 3LW, UK
UKHW050455150426
5217IPUK00025B/1697